# Advances in Wound Care and Wound Management

*Editors*

TUBA SENGUL
MELANIA HOWELL
HOLLY KIRKLAND-KYHN

# NURSING CLINICS OF NORTH AMERICA

www.nursing.theclinics.com

*Consulting Editor*
BENJAMIN SMALLHEER

March 2025 • Volume 60 • Number 1

**ELSEVIER**

1600 John F. Kennedy Boulevard • Suite 1800 • Philadelphia, Pennsylvania, 19103-2899

http://www.theclinics.com

**NURSING CLINICS OF NORTH AMERICA Volume 60, Number 1**
**March 2025 ISSN 0029-6465, ISBN-13: 978-0-443-29598-0**

Editor: Kerry Holland
Developmental Editor: Malvika Shah

*Nursing Clinics of North America* (ISSN 0029-6465) is published quarterly by Elsevier Inc., 360 Park Avenue South, New York, NY 10010-1710. Months of issue are March, June, September, and December. Periodicals postage paid at New York, NY and additional mailing offices. Subscription price per year is, $168.00 (US individuals), $275.00 (international individuals), $231.00 (Canadian individuals), $100.00 (US and Canadian students), and $135.00 (international students). For institutional access pricing please contact Customer Service via the contact information below. To receive student/resident rate, orders must be accompanied by name of affiliated institution, date of term, and the signature of program/residency coordinator on institution letterhead. Orders will be billed at individual rate until proof of status is received. Foreign air speed delivery is included in all *Clinics* subscription prices. All prices are subject to change without notice. Orders, claims, and journal inquiries: Please visit our Support Hub page https://service.elsevier.com for assistance.

*Nursing Clinics of North America* is covered in *EMBASE/Excerpta Medica, MEDLINE/PubMed (Index Medicus), Social Sciences Citation Index, Current Contents, ASCA, Cumulative Index to Nursing, RNdex Top 100,* and Allied Health Literature and International Nursing Index (INI).

# Contributors

## CONSULTING EDITOR

**BENJAMIN SMALLHEER, PhD, RN, ACNP-BC, FNP-BC, CCRN, CNE, FAANP**
Assistant Dean, Master of Science in Nursing Program, Associate Professor, Duke
University School of Nursing, Durham, North Carolina, USA

## EDITORS

**TUBA SENGUL, RN, PhD, CWON**
Associate Professor, Department of Nursing, Koç University School of Nursing, Topkapı,
Istanbul, Turkey

**MELANIA HOWELL, DNP, RN, AGCNS-BC, CWOCN, DAPWCA**
Co-director, Wound, Ostomy, & Continence Nursing Education Program, Winona State
University, Winona, Minnesota, USA

**HOLLY KIRKLAND-KYHN, PhD, FNP-c, GNP-c, CWCN, FAANP**
Assistant Clinical Professor of Nursing, Betty Irene Moore School of Nursing, Associate
Director of IN-Led Mobile Clinic, UC Davis Health, University of California Davis,
Sacramento, California, USA

## AUTHORS

**AHMED M. AFIFI, MD**
Research Associate, Division of Vascular, Endovascular, and Wound Surgery, University
of Toledo, Toledo, Ohio, USA

**FRANK AVILES Jr, PT, CWS, FACCWS, CLT-LANA, ALM, AWCC**
Director of Lymphatic and Wound Healing Services, Hyperbaric Physicians of Georgia,
Cumming, Georgia, USA

**KAREN L. BAUER, DNP, APRN-FNP, CWS, FAAWC**
Clinical Assistant Professor, Director of Vascular and Wound Services, Division of
Vascular, Endovascular and Wound Surgery, University of Toledo, Toledo, Ohio, USA

**ELIZABETH FAUST, MSN, MBA, ANP-BC, CSWC, CWOCN-AP**
Wound and Ostomy Nurse Practitioner, Owner, Lizzie Wounds, LLC, Douglassville,
Pennsylvania, USA

**BETH GALL, MSN, RN, PHN, WOCN, FNP-BC**
Assistant Clinical Professor and NP Clinical Supervisor, Betty Irene Moore School of
Nursing, University of California Davis, Davis, California, USA

**LISA GRAY, DNP, FNP-BC, RN**
Clinical Assistant Professor, Betty Irene Moore School of Nursing, UC Davis Health,
University of California Davis, Sacramento, California, USA

**EMILY GREENSTEIN, APRN, CNP, CWON-AP, FACCWS**
Nurse Practitioner, Vibra Health Fargo, Horace, North Dakota, USA

**ASIYE GUL, RN, PhD**
Professor, Department of Nursing, Faculty of Health Science, Istanbul Kültür University, Istanbul, Turkey

**MELANIA HOWELL, DNP, RN, AGCNS-BC, CWOCN, DAPWCA**
Co-director, Wound, Ostomy, & Continence Nursing Education Program, Winona State University, Winona, Minnesota, USA

**IRENE JANKOWSKI, RN, MSN, ANP, CWOCN/Ret/Emeritus**
Managing Partner, Care Improvement Strategies, LLC, East Elmhurst, New York, USA

**AYIŞE KARADAG, RN, PhD, ET/WOC**
Professor of Nursing, Koç University School of Nursing, Istanbul, Turkey

**HOLLY KIRKLAND-KYHN, PhD, FNP-c, GNP-c, CWCN, FAANP**
Assistant Clinical Professor of Nursing, Betty Irene Moore School of Nursing, Associate Director of IN-Led Mobile Clinic, UC Davis Health, University of California Davis, Sacramento, California, USA

**SALOMÉ M. LOERA, DNP, ACCNS-AG, PCCN, CCRN-CMC, SCRN**
Clinical Assistant Professor of Nursing, Conway School of Nursing, The Catholic University of America, Washington, DC, USA; Clinical Nurse Specialist, Inova Health System, Falls Church, Virginia, USA

**ZYRENE MARSH, DNP, FNP-BC, RN**
Assistant Professor, Betty Irene Moore School of Nursing, UC Davis Health, University of California Davis, Sacramento, California, USA

**SANAZ MARTIN, MS, FNP-c**
Vascular Surgery Clinic Nurse Practitioner, UC Davis Health System, Sacramento, California, USA

**DIANE RITA MAYDICK YOUNGBERG, EdD, ACNS-BC, CWOCN**
Managing Partner, Care Improvement Strategies, LLC, East Elmhurst, New York, USA

**MUNIER NAZZAL, MD, MBA, MEd, FRCS, FACS**
Professor, Department of Surgery and Medical Education, Chief, Division of Vascular, Endovascular, and Wound Surgery, University of Toledo, Toledo, Ohio, USA

**RON BILLANO ORDONA, DNP, FNP-BC, GS-C, WCC**
Volunteer Clinical Faculty, Betty Irene Moore School of Nursing, University of California, Davis, Sacramento, California, USA; Clinical Director, Senior Care Clinic House Calls, Health Services Director, Care Home by RNs, Houston, Texas, USA

**LISA PETERSON, MSN, RN, CNOR**
Clinical Nurse 3, Children's Surgery Center, UC Davis Health– ATTN, Sacramento, California, USA

**TUBA SENGUL, RN, PhD, CWON**
Associate Professor, Department of Nursing, Koç University School of Nursing, Topkapı, Istanbul, Turkey

**CHARLEEN SINGH, PhD, MBA, MSN/ED, FNP-BC, CWOCN, WOCNF, CNE, RN**
Associate Professor, Betty Irene Moore School of Nursing, Program Director, DNP-FNP Program, UC Davis Health, University of California Davis, Sacramento, California, USA

# Contents

## Clinical Advances in Wound Care

Chronic wounds are complex conditions categorized into pressure injuries, diabetic foot ulcers, venous leg ulcers, and arterial ulcers. In managing these wounds, the selection of appropriate wound care products is of critical importance. Commonly used dressings include hydrocolloid, hydrogel, alginate, foam, and silver-containing dressings. Effective wound management requires addressing systemic causes, selecting suitable wound care products, and fostering collaboration within a multidisciplinary team. Looking ahead, nanotechnology and biotechnological innovations promise to revolutionize chronic wound care.

This article provides a comprehensive overview of the pathophysiology, treatment methods, outpatient rehabilitation, and future directions related to burn injuries. It details the classification of burns, treatment strategies, wound care management, and rehabilitation processes. Modern approaches, such as AI-supported models and telemedicine, are highlighted in burn treatment. The article aims to present evidence-based best practices in burn care to healthcare professionals, offering insights into future research areas. Emphasis is placed on how recent innovations and technological advancements in burn management can improve patient outcomes.

There is a significant care burden on wound care patients in the acute care space. During hospitalization, additional risk factors can cause wounds to develop, particularly in the emergency room, operating room, and intensive care units. This article will highlight common wound types, their potential complications in the acute care setting, and implications for practice.

migration, international travel, tourism, and work visits to the tropical regions have contributed to the increase. Climate change and global warming may be causing tropical diseases and vectors to spread to areas previously spared. The last decade has shown a resurgence in tropical diseases in the United States. Many of these diseases will have symptoms affecting the skin.

This study investigates the unique challenges of wound care among the unhoused population, focusing on assessment, treatment, and documentation strategies in low-resource settings. The research underscores the prevalence of trauma, chronic illnesses, and environmental exposures that complicate wound management. The paper illustrates the diverse and complex nature of wounds encountered in this population through detailed case studies, providing practical insights for health care providers. The findings highlight the necessity of resource management and innovative approaches to address the health care needs of this vulnerable group.

## Innovative Approaches and Collaborative Strategies in Wound Care

This article presents clinically focused, evidence-based summary of common wounds and alterations in tissue/skin associated with oncologic treatment, with a focus on risk factors, identification, prevention, and management of acute radiation dermatitis and chemotherapy-induced extravasation.

Surgical site infections (SSIs) pose a significant challenge in surgical care, leading to increased patient morbidity, mortality, and health care costs. This article examines the risk factors for SSIs, particularly within the operating room environment, and highlights effective prevention strategies. Key pathogens, such as *Staphylococcus aureus*, are identified, and the role of infection control practices, including hand hygiene, surgical techniques, and environmental controls, is discussed. A multi-faceted approach to prevention, involving both patient-related and procedural factors, is essential for reducing SSI rates and improving patient outcomes.

The transition of care (TOC) from acute to community-based settings presents significant challenges, especially for patients with chronic wounds. Effective communication and standardized discharge planning are critical to prevent readmissions and adverse events. This article explores the complexities of TOC, the role of skilled nursing and community-based long term care facilities, and the importance of interdisciplinary team approaches in wound care. It highlights the need for improved training, caregiver support, and the integration of advanced wound care practices to enhance the quality of life in community settings.

Melania Howell, Tuba Sengul, and Holly Kirkland-Kyhn

Wound care patients often have a variety of chronic medical conditions that result in poor outcomes, such as delayed healing and nontraumatic limb loss. Many of these suboptimal patient outcomes result from healthcare disparities linked to social determinants of health (SDOH). Race and ethnicity influence SDOH by impacting patients' access to consistent quality healthcare. Understanding and addressing why and how ethnic and cultural factors influence SDOH is crucial for making substantial changes.

Diane Rita Maydick Youngberg and Irene Jankowski

The increasing complexity of health care and the growing demand for safe, high-quality health care have underscored the crucial need for interdisciplinary teams in health care. As people are living longer, a myriad of complex health care needs arise, necessitating specialized care from various health care professionals. Interdisciplinary teams include a group of health care professionals with various areas of expertise who work together to achieve mutual goals on behalf of a patient and their other significant individuals. Consequently, the role of interdisciplinary teams in health care continues to strengthen, providing more effective responses to the evolving needs of both individuals and health care systems.

Ayise Karadag, Tuba Sengul, and Holly Kirkland-Kyhn

The Wound, Ostomy, and Continence (WOC) nurses undertake critical duties after an earthquake. These tasks include emergency triage and treatment, prevention and management of infection, prevention of organ loss, psychological support to the injured, and close cooperation and support with other health care professionals. Although WOC nurses have received advanced training in wound management in the basic training and certified training programs they receive, wound management in earthquake conditions is not a part of their training. To prevent complications and improve patient outcomes, WOC nurses need to receive training on wound management under earthquake conditions and gain experience with simulations.

Tuba Sengul, Ayise Karadag, and Holly Kirkland-Kyhn

Chronic wounds are a significant global health issue, yet they are not adequately addressed in nursing education. This lack of focus results in nursing students graduating with insufficient knowledge in chronic wound care, leading to inadequate clinical practice. Consequently, nurses often struggle to manage wounds effectively, which negatively impacts patient care quality. To address this, it is crucial to enhance the nursing curriculum by incorporating more comprehensive content on chronic wound management. This will help ensure that nurses are better equipped with the necessary clinical competencies, ultimately improving patient outcomes.

Chronic wounds are a common condition that affects a patient's quality of life and drives the cost of health care delivery high. Vigilant wound assessment and close monitoring using adequate and reliable methods and technology are vital to wound care management. Wound assessment, including visual evaluation of tissue and surrounding skin, and measurements are essential in developing an appropriate care plan. Usually, this visual evaluation is accomplished by photographic images, measuring guides, and depth probing. Artificial intelligence may offer ways to increase assessment accuracy, enhance treatment plans, optimize patient–clinician face time, and increase clinicians' access to improve wound care outcomes.

# NURSING CLINICS

---

**SERIES OF RELATED INTEREST**

*Advances in Family Practice Nursing*
*www.advancesinfamilypracticenursing.com*

---

**THE CLINICS ARE AVAILABLE ONLINE!**
Access your subscription at:
www.theclinics.com

# Foreword

# A Comprehensive Approach to Modern Wound Management

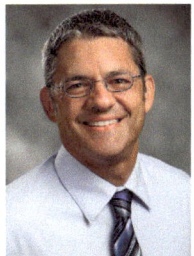

Benjamin Smallheer, PhD, RN, ACNP-BC, FNP-BC, CCRN, CNE, FAANP
*Consulting Editor*

In today's rapidly evolving healthcare landscape, advancements are occurring at an unprecedented pace. According to a National Institutes of Health study, healthcare knowledge is estimated to double every 73 days. This rapid expansion of knowledge leads to continuous improvements in comprehensive care, contributing to increased longevity. As people live longer, managing chronic illnesses over extended periods becomes more pressing. Part of living longer with multiple chronic conditions involves working not just the conditions themselves but also their sequelae: acute and chronic wounds.

Caring for acute and chronic wounds is challenged by numerous variables, such as the wound's origin, patient age, living environment, cultural and ethnic considerations, and comorbid factors that either contribute to the development of the wound or hinder its resolution. We are having to manage wounds among unhoused individuals refugee communities, and because of previously unanticipated tropical diseases. Wounds resulting from arterial, venous, and lymphatic complexities present challenges to the individual and the health care team. The increased use of immunosuppressive therapy to manage a wide variety of conditions is leading to either wound infections or wounds that do not progress along the anticipated healing trajectory. The complexity of wound care and wound management necessitates ongoing development. Therefore, it is critical to teach and disseminate them to the broader nursing community.

In this issue, we have brought together a comprehensive selection of topics addressing clinical advances in wound care, innovative approaches, and collaborative strategies. Recognizing that several "73-day" periods have passed since the authorship and publication of these articles, we hope this issue on "Advances in Wound

Nurs Clin N Am 60 (2025) xiii–xiv
https://doi.org/10.1016/j.cnur.2024.09.003
0029-6465/25/© 2024 Published by Elsevier Inc.

Care and Wound Management" will serve as a pivotal resource, capturing a comprehensive moment to propel this critical work forward.

Benjamin Smallheer, PhD, RN, ACNP-BC, FNP-BC, CCRN, CNE, FAANP
Duke University School of Nursing
307 Trent Drive
DUMC Box 3322
Durham, NC 27710, USA

*E-mail address:*
benjamin.smallheer@duke.edu

# Preface

# Advances in Wound Care and Wound Management

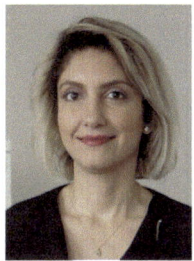 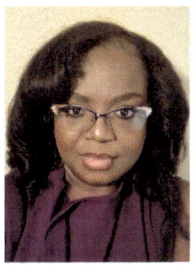 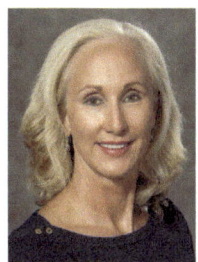

Tuba Sengul, RN, PhD, CWON

Melania Howell, DNP, RN, AGCNS-BC, CWOCN, DAPWCA

Holly Kirkland-Kyhn, PhD, FNP-c, GNP-c, CWCN, FAANP

*Editors*

Wound care and management are essential components of health care. These areas continually advance by integrating new technologies, innovative educational methods, and strategies for managing complex wounds in diverse patient populations. This special issue, "Advances in Wound Care and Wound Management," focuses on the latest developments in managing wounds across various populations, addressing rare and chronic wounds and the importance of wound care education. Within this issue, readers will find in-depth discussions on managing challenging cases, such as rare and chronic wounds, the role of education in improving wound care practices, and the innovations that are transforming this field. The articles presented offer valuable insights for clinicians and researchers working In these specialized areas to enhance patient outcomes through better wound management practices. This collection reflects ongoing efforts to meet the growing demands of global health care systems, particularly in wound care. The insights and strategies discussed in these articles serve as a valuable resource for our readers, helping them navigate the complexities of wound care in their practice.

Nurs Clin N Am 60 (2025) xv–xvi
https://doi.org/10.1016/j.cnur.2024.08.011
0029-6465/25/© 2024 Published by Elsevier Inc.

nursing.theclinics.com

## DISCLOSURES

All guest editors contributing to this article declare that there are no commercial or financial conflicts of interest, and no funding sources were involved in the project.

Tuba Sengul, RN, PhD, CWON
Koç University School of Nursing
Davutpaşa street No: 4, 34010
Topkapı, İstanbul, Türkiye

Melania Howell, DNP, RN, AGCNS-BC, CWOCN, DAPWCA
Wound, Ostomy, & Continence Nursing Education Program
Winona State University
Winona, MN 55987, USA

Holly Kirkland-Kyhn, PhD, FNP-c, GNP-c, CWCN, FAANP
Betty Irene Moore School of Nursing
UC Davis
Sacramento, CA 95817, USA

*E-mail addresses:*
tsengul@ku.edu.tr (T. Sengul)
mhowell4@alumni.jh.edu (M. Howell)
kirklandwalsh@ucdavis.edu (H. Kirkland-Kyhn)

# Clinical Advances in Wound Care

# Chronic Wounds and Dressings
## An Overview of Management and Effectiveness

Tuba Sengul, RN, PhD, CWON[a],*,
Holly Kirkland-Kyhn, FNP-c, GNP-c, CWCN, FAANP[b],
Ayişe Karadag, RN, PhD, ET/WOC[a]

## KEYWORDS

- Chronic wounds • Wound healing • Wound dressings
- Nanotechnology, Multidisciplinary care

## KEY POINTS

- In wound management, addressing systemic causes, accurately classifying the wound, and selecting the appropriate dressing are crucial for effective care.
- Hydrocolloid, hydrogel, alginate, foam, and silver-containing dressings are the most commonly used.
- Successful wound management relies on collaboration among healthcare professionals using a multidisciplinary approach.
- In the future, nanotechnology and biotechnology will offer new solutions for treating chronic wounds.

## INTRODUCTION

Chronic wounds are defined as wounds that do not progress through the normal healing process despite active treatment and do not heal within 6 weeks.[1] They pose a significant burden on both patients and health care systems.[1,2] Due to their high prevalence, impact on quality of life, and financial burden on health care systems, they represent significant public health concerns.[3] These wounds are sometimes referred to as "hard-to-heal" or "difficult-to-heal" wounds/ulcers, and the duration before they become chronic can vary between 4 weeks and 3 months.[4] Chronic wounds are categorized into 4 main types: pressure ulcers, diabetic ulcers, venous ulcers, and arterial insufficiency ulcers.[4] Elderly individuals are at the highest risk for chronic wounds owing to the slowing of wound healing and the prevalence of

[a] Koç University School of Nursing, Davutpaşa St. No: 4, Topkapı 34010, Istanbul, Turkey;
[b] Betty Irene Moore School of Nursing, UC Davis CA, Sacramento, CA, USA
* Corresponding author.
E-mail address: tsengul@ku.edu.tr

Nurs Clin N Am 60 (2025) 1–13
https://doi.org/10.1016/j.cnur.2024.08.008     nursing.theclinics.com

conditions such as cardiovascular diseases and diabetes.[5] In addition to imposing an economic burden on the health care system, chronic wounds also pose a significant financial burden on society by reducing productivity.[3,6–8] Various factors can contribute to the failure of a wound to heal, leading to severe complications, such as infection, amputation, and death.[1,4] Locally, factors such as neuropathic, arterial, venous, or lymphatic causes, pressure, trauma, nonhealing burns, infections, and autoimmune diseases can contribute to the chronicity of wounds.[1,4] The optimal approach to chronic wound management is first to address systemic causes and then focus on local factors.[4] Therefore, healthcare professionals must thoroughly understand the underlying causes of wounds' chronicity.[1]

### Function of Skin

The skin is unique in interacting with the external environment. It performs critical homeostatic functions, from regulating thermotaxis to sensing external stimuli.[9,10] The skin is the primary defense barrier, preventing dehydration and protecting internal structures from mechanical, chemical, thermal, and photic damage.[9,10] This defense extends to an immune barrier that protects against pathogenic infections and supports commensal microorganisms through the host-microbiota axis.[9,10]

## WOUND HEALING PROCESS

The wound healing process is divided into four phases: hemostasis, inflammation, proliferation, and remodeling.[9,10]

### Hemostasis

Immediately after injury, damaged blood vessels constrict to prevent blood loss and form a clot.[9–11] Platelets become active upon contact with collagen in the vessel walls, adhering to each other to create the clot.[9–12] This clot halts bleeding and covers the wound, protecting against bacteria and containing growth factors.[9–12] Platelets release chemical signals to attract immune cells to the injury site and produce antimicrobial substances against microbes.[9–12] Once sufficient clotting has occurred, the clotting process is regulated to prevent excessive clot formation.[9–12]

### Inflammation

When an injury occurs, the natural inflammation process begins.[9–12] Necrotic cells and bacterial components activate immune cells, triggering the inflammatory response.[9] Mast cells, Langerhans cells, T cells, and macrophages participate in this process.[9–12] Neutrophils rapidly migrate to the wound site following injury and phagocytize pathogens.[9–12] As neutrophils decrease after a few days, macrophages enter the wound and initiate tissue repair.[9] Macrophages clean up necrotic cells and pathogens and regulate inflammation.[9–12] Pro-inflammatory macrophages combat infection, while anti-inflammatory macrophages promote tissue repair. Regulatory T cells with anti-inflammatory properties reduce inflammation and accelerate healing.[9–12]

### Proliferation

The proliferative phase of healing is characterized by a period in which various cells play active roles in wound closure, matrix accumulation, and the formation of new blood vessels.[9–12] Mechanical stress, hydrogen peroxide, pathogens, growth factors, and cytokines activate keratinocytes.[9–12] This activation causes keratinocytes to become more invasive and mobile, a process known as re-epithelialization.[9–12] Keratinocytes cover the wound surface by secreting matrix metalloproteinases (MMPs) and generating new extracellular matrix (ECM) proteins.[9–12] Fibroblasts replace the fibrin-rich matrix with mature ECM proteins and granulation tissue.[9–12] Signals from platelets, endothelial cells, and macrophages guide fibroblasts to produce ECM proteins and differentiate into myofibroblasts.[9–12] Angiogenesis, triggered by hypoxia, forms new blood vessels.[9,10] Endothelial cells proliferate, migrate, and form new vessels.[9,10] Vascular endothelial growth factor prevents apoptosis of endothelial cells and supports angiogenesis.[9–12] Macrophages further support new vessel formation by secreting proteases and chemotactic factors.[9–12]

### Remodeling

ECM remodeling begins after injury and forms a mature wound rich in type I collagen.[9,10] Initially, the fibrin clot accumulates, and fibroblasts replace it with hyaluronan, fibronectin, and proteoglycans.[9,10] Subsequently, fibroblasts produce mature collagen fibrils.[9] During the healing process, type III collagen is replaced by type I collagen, increasing the wound's strength.[9] Changes in the ECM require a delicate balance between collagen degradation and synthesis, maintained through the temporal regulation of MMPs.[9,10] Increased expression of transforming growth factor-beta and mechanical tension stimulate the differentiation of myofibroblasts.[9,10] Myofibroblasts promote wound contraction, accelerating healing.[9,10] The wound-healing response concludes when macrophages, endothelial cells, and fibroblasts undergo apoptosis or are removed from the injury site, and a scar is developed.[9,10]

## TYPES OF CHRONIC WOUNDS

Chronic wounds are persistent and complex wounds that do not heal within the expected timeframe, typically owing to underlying conditions or complications.[10,13] This section discusses 4 common types of chronic wounds: pressure injuries, diabetic foot ulcers, venous leg ulcers, and arterial ulcers. Each type is explored in terms of its definition, stages, risk factors, and the scales used for risk assessment and healing evaluation.

### Pressure Injuries

#### Definition and stages
Pressure injuries, also known as pressure ulcers or bedsores, result from prolonged pressure or shear on the skin and underlying tissues, often over bony prominences.[14] They are classified into stages.

- *Stage 1:* Nonblanchable erythema of intact skin.
- *Stage 2:* Partial-thickness skin loss with exposed dermis.
- *Stage 3:* Full-thickness skin loss with possible exposure to fat.
- *Stage 4:* Full-thickness skin and tissue loss with exposed bone, muscle, or tendon.
- *Unstageable:* Full-thickness skin and tissue loss obscured by slough or eschar.
- *Deep Tissue Injury:* Persistent, nonblanchable deep red, maroon, or purple discoloration.[14]

#### Risk factors
The primary risk factors for pressure injuries include immobility, poor nutrition, moisture from incontinence, reduced sensory perception, shearing, and poor blood flow (Gefen and colleagues, 2020) or poor perfusion.[15] Immobility prevents regular blood flow, leading to ischemia and cell death; poor nutrition may impair skin integrity, while moisture can cause skin maceration.[16–19]

### Wound Assessment and Healing

Wound assessment and healing are expected to be measured with every wound assessment and treatment. In the past, healing scales were available, but with digital photography, healing can be assessed and documented for sharing with staff, patients, and families to document treatment outcomes over time.[16–19]

### Lower extremity ulcers
### Diabetic foot ulcers

**Definition and stages** Diabetic foot ulcers (DFUs) are severe complications of diabetes mellitus, affecting approximately 15% of diabetic patients.[20] They result from peripheral neuropathy, arterial disease, and minor trauma.

**Risk factors** The risk factors for DFUs include poor glycemic control, peripheral neuropathy, peripheral vascular disease, foot deformities, previous ulcers or amputations, and duration of diabetes.[21] Peripheral neuropathy leads to a loss of protective sensation, making patients unaware of minor injuries that can progress to ulcers.[20] Poor circulation further impedes healing, and hyperglycemia impairs immune function, increasing the risk of infection.[21]

### Assessment and Healing Scales

- *Wagner Classification:* Grades ulcers from 0 to 5 based on depth and tissue involvement.[22]
- *University of Texas Classification:* Stages ulcers by depth, infection, and ischemia.[23]
- *Diabetic Foot Ulcer Scale (DFUS):* Assesses the impact of DFUs on the quality of life.[24]

### Venous leg ulcers

**Definition and stages.** Venous leg ulcers (VLUs) result from venous insufficiency, where veins fail to return blood efficiently, causing pressure and tissue breakdown.[25] They are the most common leg ulcers, accounting for 70% to 90%.[25]

**Risk factors.** Risk factors for VLUs include a history of deep vein thrombosis, chronic venous insufficiency, obesity, prolonged standing, and age.[25] Venous hypertension causes fluid leakage, inflammation, and skin breakdown.[25]

### Assessment and Healing Scales

- *Venous Clinical Severity Score (VCSS):* Evaluates the severity of venous disease and response to treatment.[26]
- *CEAP Classification (Clinical, Etiology, Anatomy, Pathophysiology):* Categories based on clinical signs, etiology, anatomy, and pathophysiology.[27]
- *Leg Ulcer Measurement Tool (LUMT):* Monitors healing by assessing wound size and appearance.[28]

### Arterial ulcers

**Definition and stages.** Arterial ulcers, also known as ischemic ulcers, result from insufficient blood flow due to arterial occlusion or severe peripheral arterial disease, often on the lower legs, toes, and pressure points.[29]

**Risk factors.** Arterial ulcers include peripheral arterial disease, diabetes, hypertension, smoking, hyperlipidemia, and age. Reduced blood flow impairs healing and increases necrosis risk.[29]

## Assessment and Healing Scales

- *Ankle-Brachial Index (ABI):* Measures blood pressure ratio in lower legs to arms.[30]
- *Rutherford Classification:* Categorizes disease severity from asymptomatic to severe ischemia with ulceration.[31]
- *Wi-Fi Classification:* Assesses wounds, ischemia, and infection severity to guide treatment.[32]

## WOUND DRESSINGS

Wound care products provide a physical barrier to promote wound healing and protect against infection. These products are selected according to the type and condition of the wound base and surrounding tissues and are available in different forms.[10,20]

### Gauze/Bandage

Gauze or woven bandages are dry wound dressings used in wound care for many years. Cotton gauze is frequently preferred in wound care owing to its moisture-absorbing properties, biocompatibility, and skin-friendly structure.[33] However, traditional cotton gauze does not actively promote wound healing unless used to keep the wound bed moist while providing an antibacterial product.[33] Therefore, various methods have been developed to improve the properties of cotton gauze and make it more effective.[33] Modified gauze provides ease of use for nurses. It is simple to apply.[33] Cotton gauze fabrics are old-style classic wound dressings used worldwide owing to their low cost, easy production, market availability, permeability, and high absorption.[33]

### Transparent Films

Although transparent film dressings were initially used to secure intravenous catheters, they were later adopted for use in the treatment of certain wounds.[34] Transparent film dressings play an important role in wound care and creating a sterile environment in the catheter area.[34] Semipermeable film dressings are thin, flexible, transparent polyurethane sheets with an adhesive backing. They allow water vapor and gas to pass through but do not allow bacteria and water to pass through.[10,34] They have a small absorption capacity but will enable the wound bed to be seen and adapt to body contours.[10] Semipermeable film dressings can generally be used on superficial wounds with little drainage, abrasions, partial-thickness wounds, sutured wounds, and graft donor sites.[10,34] They can also be used on granular wounds and areas subject to friction.[10,34] A protectant should be applied to the surrounding skin to prevent maceration.[10,34] Film dressings should not be used on infected wounds, wounds with moderate to heavy drainage, or patients with sensitive skin.[10,34]

### Hydrocolloids

Hydrocolloid dressings contain hydrophobic polymers containing gelatin, pectin, and carboxymethylcellulose. They usually consist of a gel or foam on a self-adhesive polyurethane film carrier.[10,34–36] These dressings suit mild to moderately exuding wounds and provide a moist healing environment. The colloid composition traps exudate and forms a gel at the wound site, reducing pain and accelerating healing.[10,34–36] Hydrocolloid dressings are widely used in wounds such as pressure sores and venous ulcers.[10,34–36] Thanks to the colloid layer, it retains moisture in the wound area and prevents bacterial infections, thanks to the bacteria-proof feature of its outer layer.[10,34–36] Bacteria and debris are also trapped and removed with dressing changes in gentle, painless mechanical debridement.[10,34–36] Hydrocolloid dressings also have some disadvantages as they may cause a foul odor and require daily dressing changes, and allergic contact dermatitis has been reported.[10,34–36] Additionally, they are unsuitable for wounds producing moderate to high amounts of exudate.[10,34–36]

### Hydrofibers

Hydrofiber dressings are moisture-retaining dressings composed of soft, nonwoven sodium carboxymethylcellulose fibers that form a gel when in contact with wound fluid and have a high exudate-absorptive capacity.[10,34–36] The gel retains wound exudates through vertical absorption while supporting a moist wound-bed healing environment. Fibrin collects between the dressing and the wound surface and acts as an adhesive, securing the dressing in place so that tissue does not grow into the dressing.[10,34–36] This provides ease of application and removal for caregivers and patients and reduces pain during dressing changes.[10,34–36] These dressings are ideal for wounds that produce heavy exudate and minimize the risk of infection. They can be used in venous ulcers, diabetic foot ulcers, and surgical wounds.[10,34–36]

### Foams

They consist of 2 layers: a hydrophilic silicone or polyurethane-based foam that rests on the wound surface and a hydrophobic, gas-permeable backing to prevent leakage and bacterial contamination. Some foams require a secondary adhesive dressing.[10,34–36] These dressings absorb exudate from the wound, provide a moist healing environment, reduce the risk of infection, and protect the wound surface.[10,34–36] Foam dressings have antibacterial, anti-inflammatory, and re-epithelialization-promoting properties.[10,34–36] Foam dressings may not be suitable for minimally exuding wounds as they may cause drying.[10,34–36] They are widely used in pressure ulcers, venous ulcers, and diabetic foot wounds.[10,34–36]

### Alginates

Alginate dressings consist of natural complex polysaccharides obtained from various algae species. These dressings form gels when bound to wound exudate owing to their structure consisting of calcium and sodium salts.[10,34–36] Water-insoluble alginates form an amorphous gel that packs and covers the wound by exchanging calcium ions with sodium ions in the sodium-rich wound fluid environment.[10,34–36] Alginates come in a variety of forms, including ribbons, beads, and pads, and their absorbent capacity varies depending on the type of polysaccharide used.[10,34–36] Alginate dressings are ideal for moderately to heavily exuding wounds such as diabetic foot ulcers, venous ulcers, and pressure sores owing to their high exudate absorbency.[10,34–36] They can also be used as wound fillers to treat deep and hollow wounds.[10,34–36] However, disadvantages of alginates include the need for a secondary dressing that must be removed to monitor the wound, can be very drying in a minimally exuding wound, and has an unpleasant odor.[10,34–36] Therefore, alginates are not recommended for dry wounds or wounds that produce minimal exudate.[37]

### Antibacterial Dressings

Some topical antimicrobials may be associated with potential benefits in select patient populations. The characteristics of some commonly used agents are briefly reviewed in the following subsections.

### Iodine-based dressings

Iodine-containing antiseptics have been widely used for many years because of their effective antimicrobial properties. Povidone-iodine (PVP-I) was patented in the United

States in 1952 and introduced for medical use.[38] PVP-I is a water-soluble compound consisting of polyvinylpyrrolidone (povidone) and elemental iodine combined with hydrogen bonds.[38] Although povidone has no antimicrobial activity, it provides a controlled release of free iodine.[38] The amount of free iodine in PVP-I solutions varies depending on the concentration of the solution. The most commonly used form is a 10% aqueous solution, which can also be found in concentrations of 7.5%, 5%, 3%, and 2.5%.[38] Iodine is effective against various pathogens, including antibiotic-resistant bacteria, fungi, mycobacteria, viruses, spores, and protozoa. PVP-I dressings are more economical than cadexomer iodine and silver-containing dressings and have a lower risk of developing bacterial resistance.[38]

### Silver-based dressings

Silver has been widely used in wound care for many years to help manage local infection.[10] Historically, silver has been presented as metallic (silver foil), solution (eg, silver nitrate), or cream (eg, silver sulfadiazine).[10] Ionic silver (Ag+), the oxidized active form of silver, has received renewed interest and research for its use as a prophylactic antimicrobial agent in wound dressings owing to its broad-spectrum antibacterial range, including aerobic, anaerobic, gram-negative, and gram-positive bacteria, as well as yeast and fungi.[10] Several mechanisms can explain the antimicrobial action of silver: silver interferes with the respiratory chain in the cytochromes of mycobacteria; silver ions also interfere with components of the microbial electron transport system, binding to DNA and inhibiting DNA replication.[10] Little recent evidence of emerging microbial resistance to silver has been reported.[37]

### Honey

Honey has broad spectrum antimicrobial activity because of its high osmolarity and high hydrogen peroxide concentration. Medical-grade honey products are available as gels, pastes, and adhesives, impregnated with alginate and colloid dressings.[39] Based on systematic reviews evaluating the efficacy of honey in healing a variety of wounds, there are insufficient data to support its routine use for all wound types; certain wound types, such as burns, may provide benefit, while others, such as chronic venous ulcers, may not.[35,39]

### Hydrogel Dressings

Hydrogels are 80% to 99% water or glycerin-based and are available in sheets, gels, or impregnated gauze. They have a three-dimensional structure of hydrophilic substances.[10,34,35] These dressings, made of water-based gels, are suitable for wounds with low to moderate exudate production. They are insoluble in water and can absorb water from 10 to thousands of times their weight. Hydrogels keep the wound moist and play a positive role in cleaning necrotic tissue thanks to this excellent moisturizing ability.[10,34,35] Hydrogels can absorb minimal fluid and provide moisture to dry wounds. They allow the passage of gas and water. Most hydrogels are nearly nonadherent and, therefore, require a second dressing.[10,34,35] They reduce pain and accelerate healing by providing a moist healing environment. In addition, because hydrogels are usually transparent, it is possible to observe the wound under the dressing. Hydrogels are suitable for wounds with minimal or moderate drainage and can reduce pain.[10,34,35] However, they should not be used in infected wounds or with heavy drainage because they slowly absorb fluid. To date, various hydrogel dressings have been developed with injection, self-healing, antibacterial, antioxidant, and drug-eluting properties.[10,34,35] Due to these properties, hydrogels are widely used in wounds such as pressure sores, surgical wounds, burns, and radiation dermatitis.[10,34,35]

## Wound Contact Layers

Wound contact layers (WCLs) are commonly used primary dressings in the management of both acute and difficult-to-heal wounds.[10] These layers are placed in close contact with the wound and surrounding tissues and promote wound healing by protecting the newly formed granulation and epithelial tissue. WCLs consist of thin, nonadherent gauze dressings impregnated with various compounds that promote low adhesion.[10] Contact dressings, such as paraffin-impregnated gauze, can dry out if kept in place for long periods and can adhere to the wound bed, causing trauma and pain on removal. Newer dressing design aims to reduce these problems through features such as tissue proximity, the addition of moisturizing agents or layers made of silicone.[10] WCLs provide a barrier between the newly formed tissue and the external environment and facilitate gas and fluid exchange, helping to remove wound exudate and absorb it into the overlying absorbent dressing. Examples of contemporary WCL that overcome the challenges of previous designs incorporate silicone. Silicone-based WCLs are formulated as sheets or incorporated into other dressings, such as foams. In this way, the effect of tissue trauma that may occur because of the removal of the adherent wound dressing is reduced, and better wound healing is achieved.[10]

## Different Dressings

- *Paraffin or Vaseline-Impregnated Gauze:* Protects by isolating the wound from the external environment. Such dressings support the wound to remain moist and prevent the wound edges from drying out.[10] Paraffin gauze dressings are used primarily for superficial wounds such as surgical incisions, burns, and skin tears.[10] In addition, these dressings make it easier to apply another dressing over the wound.[10]
- *Barrier Creams and Dressings:* Play an important role in protecting the skin. They protect the skin from moisture and irritants, preventing irritation and wound formation.[10] They are mainly used in bed sores and incontinence dermatitis.[10] These products strengthen the skin's barrier function and minimize damage to the skin.[10]
- *Collagen Dressings:* Promote tissue regeneration and accelerate the wound healing process. Collagen bio-adapts to the wound bed and promotes healing by increasing cellular activity.[10] Such dressings are used in various chronic and acute wounds, such as diabetic foot wounds, pressure sores, and surgical wounds. Collagen dressings support the production of natural collagen, which is particularly deficient in the wound-healing process.[10]
- *Growth Factor Dressings:* Promote cell proliferation and tissue repair. These dressings accelerate healing, allowing wounds to close faster.[10] Growth factors modulate various biological processes in wound healing, increasing cell motility and proliferation.[10] These dressings are often preferred in difficult wound-healing situations such as burns, surgical, and diabetic wounds.[10]
- *Hyaluronic Acid Dressings:* Dressings containing hyaluronic acid provide a moist healing environment and support tissue regeneration.[10] Hyaluronic acid is a component with a high water retention capacity and helps the wound surface remain moist.[10]
- *Enzymatic Debridement Products:* Enzymatic debridement products selectively target collagen, protein, fibrin, and elastin by acting on necrotic tissue.[10] These products promote healthy tissue formation by cleansing the wound bed.[10]

## EFFECTIVENESS AND CLINICAL APPLICATIONS

In the management of chronic wounds, clinical guidelines provide health care professionals with best practices and standard treatment protocols.[40] These guidelines are based on extensive scientific research and clinical experience.[40] It is essential to regularly assess the type, size, depth, exudate amount, and signs of wound infection.[14] Regular assessments help monitor the effectiveness of the treatment plan, and these evaluations should be documented using standard documentation methods.[14] Cleaning the wound surface with sterile saline or appropriate antiseptic solutions reduces the risk of infection and speeds up the healing process.[41] Debridement of necrotic tissue through surgical, autolytic, enzymatic, or mechanical methods promotes wound healing.[41] The choice of wound dressing should be based on the type of wound and the amount of exudate, and dressings that provide a moist healing environment should be used.[42] Infected wounds should be managed with antibiotic therapy and antimicrobial wound dressings, and infection signs should be carefully monitored.[43] As an important component of person-centered care, patients and caregivers should be encouraged to actively participate in wound care and be educated about wound management.[44] Patients' and caregivers' roles in wound management should be emphasized, and adherence to care instructions should be ensured.[44] Chronic wound management requires the collaboration of various health care professionals, including nurses, doctors, physiotherapists, and dietitians.[44] Multidisciplinary teams should work together to optimize the patient's overall health status and wound-healing process.[45] Team-based wound care is critical in optimizing patient healing and increasing overall satisfaction.[45] Telehealth services are recommended when necessary.[46]

## FUTURE DIRECTIONS

With the advancement of nanobiotechnology, nano-sized biomaterials have begun to play a significant role in treating chronic wounds.[47] These technologies are used in scaffold construction, infection prevention, and substance delivery.[47] Nanotechnologies like electrospinning produce biomimetic structures that mimic natural skin and assist in the healing of resistant wounds.[47] Some nano-scaffolds support chronic wound healing by promoting cell adhesion and migration.[48] Metal nanoparticles, such as silver nanoparticles (AgNPs), have been used in antimicrobial therapy, but the accumulation of these metals can lead to DNA and cell damage.[49] Therefore, nanomaterials that can prevent infection without causing toxicity should be developed.[49] During chronic wound healing, biomaterials that can adapt to the continuously changing skin environment are being developed.[47] These materials can be used in dynamic monitoring systems for wound care because of their properties, such as photothermal effect, chemo-dynamic effect, fluorescence, and thermo-sensitivity.[48]

Biologic dermis grafts effectively treat deep wounds using autologous allogeneic and artificial dermis grafts.[10] Dermis grafts obtained through tumor engineering, utilizing fibroblast and adipose tissue-derived stromal vascular fraction cells, differ from traditional methods and accelerate the healing process.[10] Fibrin glue is a cell delivery vehicle that provides significant microvascular anastomosis advantages.[10] This glue supports wound closure while reducing the risk of infection when enriched with antibiotics.[10] Growth factor therapy, along with advanced techniques like nanotechnology, real-time monitoring, and bioactive hydrogels, offers important innovations in accelerating wound healing and promoting tissue regeneration with components such as platelet-derived growth factor (PDGF), essential fibroblast growth factor (bFGF), and epidermal growth factor (EGF).[10,47–49] Cell therapies support wound healing using various cells, including fibroblasts, keratinocytes, and adipose tissue-derived stromal vascular fraction cells.[10,47–49] Complementary treatments such as nutritional support, electrical stimulation, ultrasound, and oxygen therapy contribute to the healing process and improve patients' quality of life.[10,47–49] Recently, many nanomaterials and techniques have been used to repair chronic wounds.[10,47] These technologies offer innovative solutions, such as smart dressings with real-time monitoring and response capabilities.[48] Future goals include the development of more sophisticated nanobiotechnology-based wound management systems.[10,47–49] Additionally, innovations such as 3D-printed micro-fat grafts and new staged excision techniques are groundbreaking advances in reconstructive surgery.[48]

## SUMMARY

In conclusion, managing and treating chronic wounds is a complex process that requires integrating elements such as risk assessment, knowledge of healing phases, and multidisciplinary teamwork. Risk assessment, correct management of healing phases, and understanding how to evaluate wounds ensure successful results in treating chronic wounds. Different wound dressings' effectiveness and clinical applications significantly contribute to the healing process when each dressing is applied to the correct wound. New biotechnological wound dressings and nanotechnology offer significant advances, especially for resistant wounds. In the future, innovations such as real-time monitoring and AI-powered personalized wound care will revolutionize chronic wound management. These innovations will improve patients' quality of life and enable more effective outcomes in chronic wound care.

## CLINICS CARE POINTS

- Appropriate wound classification and Regular assessment of wound characteristics (size, depth, exudate, and infection signs) should guide dressing selection and treatment adjustments.[14,41-43]
- Using Evidence-based tools can improve the accuracy of wound healing monitoring.[14,41-43,50]
- While risk assessment and healing determination tools provide critical information, clinicians should not rely solely on the scores from these scales.[14,50]
- Nurses and other caregivers must combine clinical judgment with assessment tools to formulate an appropriate risk level for each patient.[14,50]
- Use moisture-retentive dressings to promote an optimal healing environment for chronic wounds.[14,41-43]
- Hydrocolloids, foams, and alginate dressings have accelerated healing by maintaining moisture balance.[14,50]
- Dressings should be selected based on wound type and exudate levels.[50]
- High-exudate wounds benefit from foam or alginate dressings, while low-exudate wounds may require hydrocolloids or thin-film dressings.[14,50]

## DISCLOSURE

The authors have nothing to disclose.

## REFERENCES

1. Atkin L. Chronic wounds: the challenges of appropriate management. Br J Community Nurs 2019;24(Suppl 9):S26–32.

2. Sen CK, Gordillo GM, Roy S, et al. Human skin wounds: a major and snowballing threat to public health and the economy. Wound Repair Regen 2009;17(6): 763–71.
3. Järbrink K, Ni G, Sönnergren H, et al. The humanistic and economic burden of chronic wounds: a protocol for a systematic review. Syst Rev 2017;6(1):15.
4. Werdin F, Tennenhaus M, Schaller HE, et al. Evidence-based management strategies for treatment of chronic wounds. Eplasty 2009;9:e19.
5. Gould L, Abadir P, Brem H, et al. Chronic wound repair and healing in older adults: current status and future research. J Am Geriatr Soc 2015;63(3):427–38.
6. Gosain A, DiPietro LA. Aging and wound healing. World J Surg 2004;28(3):321–6.
7. Olsson M, Järbrink K, Divakar U, et al. The humanistic and economic burden of chronic wounds: a systematic review. Wound Repair Regen 2019;27:114–25.
8. Augustin M, Brocatti LK, Rustenbach SJ, et al. Cost-of-illness of leg ulcers in the community. Int Wound J 2014;11(3):283–92.
9. Wilkinson HN, Hardman MJ. Wound healing: cellular mechanisms and pathological outcomes. Open Biol 2020;10(9):200223. https://doi.org/10.1098/rsob.200223.
10. Han S-K. Innovations and advances in wound healing. 3rd edition. Springer; 2021.
11. Zaidi A, Green L. Physiology of haemostasis. Anaesth Intensive Care Med 2019; 20:152–8.
12. Scully D, Sfyri P, Wilkinson HN, et al. Optimising platelet secretomes to deliver robust tissue-specific regeneration. J Tissue Eng Regen Med 2020;14:82–98.
13. Frykberg RG, Banks J. Challenges in the treatment of chronic wounds. Adv Wound Care 2015;4(9):560–82.
14. National Pressure Ulcer Advisory Panel (NPUAP), European Pressure Ulcer Advisory Panel (EPUAP), and Pan Pacific Pressure Injury Alliance (PPPIA). Prevention and Treatment of Pressure Ulcers/Injuries: Clinical Practice Guideline. Emily Haesler (Ed.). Osborne Park, Western Australia: Cambridge Media; 2019. Available at: https://www.npuap.org/resources/clinical-practice-guidelines. (Accessed 4 August 2024).
15. Kirkland-Kyhn H, Teleten O, Wilson M. A retrospective, descriptive, comparative study to identify patient variables that contribute to the development of deep tissue injury among patients in intensive care units. Ostomy/Wound Manag 2017; 63(2):42 7.
16. Sengül T, Karadag A. Determination of nurses' level of knowledge on the prevention of pressure ulcers: the case of Turkey. J Tissue Viability 2020;29(4):337–41.
17. Sengül T, Gul A, Yılmaz D, et al. Translation and validation of the ELPO for Turkish population: risk assessment scale for the development of pressure injuries due to surgical positioning. J Tissue Viability 2022;31(2):358–64.
18. Gul A, Sengül T, Özge Yavuz H. Assessment of the risk of pressure ulcer during the perioperative period: adaptation of the Munro scale to Turkish. J Tissue Viability 2021;30(4):559–65.
19. Sengül T, Gul A. Pressure injury in the perioperative period during COVID-19 pandemic: incidence and patient-related risk factors in a hospital in Turkey. J Tissue Viability 2022;31(4):714–7.
20. Armstrong DG, Boulton AJM, Bus SA. Diabetic foot ulcers and their recurrence. N Engl J Med 2017;376(24):2367–75.
21. Boulton AJM, Armstrong DG, Kirsner RS, et al. Diagnosis and management of diabetic foot complications. Diabetes Care 2020;43(9):2098–103.
22. Mathes SJ, Nahai F. Classification of the vascular anatomy of muscles: experimental and clinical correlation. Plast Reconstr Surg 1981;67(2):177–87.

23. Lavery LA, Armstrong DG, Wunderlich RP, et al. Diabetic foot syndrome: evaluating the prevalence and incidence of foot pathology in Mexican Americans and non-Hispanic whites from a diabetes disease management cohort. Diabetes Care 2003;26(5):1435–8.
24. Ramsey SD, Newton K, Blough D, et al. Incidence, outcomes, and cost of foot ulcers in patients with diabetes. Diabetes Care 1999;22(3):382–7.
25. O'Donnell TF, Passman MA, Marston WA, et al. Management of venous leg ulcers: clinical practice guidelines of the Society for Vascular Surgery® and the American Venous Forum. J Vasc Surg 2014;60(2 Suppl):3S–59S.
26. Kakkos SK, Kakisis I, Tsolakis IA, et al. Endarterectomy achieves lower stroke and death rates compared with stenting in patients with asymptomatic carotid stenosis. J Vasc Surg 2017;66(2):607–17.
27. Eklöf B, Rutherford RB, Bergan JJ, et al. American Venous Forum International Ad Hoc Committee for Revision of the CEAP Classification. Revision of the CEAP classification for chronic venous disorders: consensus statement. J Vasc Surg 2004;40(6):1248–52.
28. Houghton PE, Kincaid CB, Lovell M, et al. Effect of electrical stimulation on chronic leg ulcer size and appearance. Phys Ther 2003;83(1):17–28.
29. Mayrovitz HN, Wong S, Mancuso C. Venous, arterial, and neuropathic leg ulcers with emphasis on the geriatric population. Cureus 2023;15(4):e38123.
30. Al-Qaisi M, Nott DM, King DH, et al. Ankle brachial pressure index (ABPI): an update for practitioners. Vasc Health Risk Manag 2009;5:833–41.
31. Rutherford RB. The CEAP classification system and assessing outcome. Vasc Surg 1997;31(3):291–5.
32. Mills JL Sr, Conte MS, Armstrong DG, et al. The society for vascular surgery lower extremity threatened limb classification system: risk stratification based on wound, ischemia, and foot infection (WIfI). J Vasc Surg 2014;59(1):220–34.
33. Liang Y, He J, Guo B. Functional hydrogels as wound dressing to enhance wound healing. ACS Nano 2021;15(8):12687–722.
34. Atay S, Yilmaz Kurt F. Effectiveness of transparent film dressing for peripheral intravenous catheter. J Vasc Access 2021;22(1):135–40.
35. Armstrong DG, Meyr AJ. Update on basic wound therapy - wound dressing. In: Eidt JF, Mills JL Sr, Bruera E, et al. eds. UpToDate. 2022. Available at: https://www.uptodate.com. (Accessed 4 August 2024).
36. Rani Raju N, Silina E, Stupin V, et al. Multifunctional and smart wound dressings—a review on recent research advancements in skin regenerative medicine. Pharmaceutics 2022;14(8):1574.
37. Barnea Y, Weiss J, Gur E. A review of the applications of the hydrofiber dressing with silver (Aquacel Ag®) in wound care. Therapeut Clin Risk Manag 2009;6:21–7.
38. Zhang M, Yang M, Woo MW, et al. High-mechanical strength carboxymethyl chitosan-based hydrogel film for antibacterial wound dressing. Carbohydr Polym 2021;256:117590. https://doi.org/10.1016/j.carbpol.2021.117590.
39. Holloway S. Skin integrity and wound management education in the pre-registration nursing curricula. Wounds U K 2022;18(1):10–1.
40. Barrientos S, Brem H, Stojadinovic O, et al. Clinical application of growth factors and cytokines in wound healing. Wound Repair Regen 2014;22(5):569–78.
41. Wounds UK. Best practice statement: The use of topical antiseptic/antimicrobial agents in wound management. Aberdeen: Wounds UK; 2010.

42. National Institute for Health and Care Excellence (NICE). Pressure ulcers: prevention and management. Clinical guideline [CG179]. 2019. Available at: https://www.nice.org.uk/guidance/cg179, (Accessed 9 August 2024).
43. European Wound Management Association (EWMA). Antimicrobials and non-healing wounds: evidence, controversies and suggestions. 2021.
44. Kirkland-Kyhn H, Generao SA, Teleten O, et al. Teaching wound care to family caregivers. Am J Nurs 2018;118(3):63–7.
45. Moore Z, Butcher G, Corbett LQ, et al. Exploring the concept of a team approach to wound care: managing wounds as a team. J Wound Care 2014;23(Suppl 5b): S1–38.
46. Karadag A, Sengül T. Challenges faced by doctors and nurses in wound care management during the COVID-19 pandemic in Turkey and their views on tele-health. J Tissue Viability 2021;30(4):484–8.
47. Jiang T, Li Q, Qiu J, et al. Nanobiotechnology: applications in chronic wound healing. Int J Nanomed 2022;17:3125–45.
48. Youssef K, Ullah A, Rezai P, et al. Recent advances in biosensors for real time monitoring of pH, temperature, and oxygen in chronic wounds. Mater Today Bio 2023;22:100764.
49. Kong L, Wu Z, Zhao H, et al. Bioactive injectable hydrogels containing desferrioxamine and bioglass for diabetic wound healing. ACS Appl Mater Interfaces 2018; 10(36):30103–14.
50. Staebel K. Wound care: Five evidence-based practices: The best practices for the best outcomes. Am J Nurs 2023;18(2):25–8.

# Postacute Overview of Burn Injuries

## Pathophysiology, Management, and Future Directions

Tuba Sengul, RN, PhD, CWON[a],*,
Holly Kirkland-Kyhn, PhD, FNP-c, GNP-c, CWCN[b], Asiye Gul, RN, PhD[c]

**KEYWORDS**

- Burns • Wound healing • Wound dressing • Burn rehabilitation • Outpatient
- Artificial intelligence

**KEY POINTS**

- *Classification and Management of Burns*: Classifying burn injuries by depth and extent is critical in determining treatment strategies.
- *Wound Care and Dressings:* Various types of wound dressings can accelerate the healing of burn wounds and reduce infection risk.
- *Telemedicine and Artificial Intelligence:* Telemedicine and artificial intelligence-supported models in burn care facilitate remote assessment and optimize treatment plans.
- *Rehabilitation and Scar Management*: Post-burn rehabilitation and scar management are essential for enhancing patients' quality-of-life.

## INTRODUCTION

Burn injuries occur when the skin comes into contact with a heat source.[1] Burns are the fourth most common type of injury worldwide, following traffic accidents, falls, and physical violence.[2] In the United States (US), approximately 500,000 burns occur annually that require emergency treatment, leading to 40,000 hospitalizations.[3] The incidence of burns has decreased due to increased awareness and education on burn prevention.[3,4] However, due to a lack of centralized reporting, it is challenging to estimate the global incidence of burn-related deaths from all causes, but there are approximately 180,000 fire-related deaths annually, with 95% of them occurring in low- and middle-income countries.[3–5] Burn injuries are among the most costly

[a] Koç University School of Nursing, Davutpaşa Street No: 4, Topkapı 34010, Istanbul, Turkey;
[b] Betty Irene Moore School of Nursing, UC Davis, Sacramento, CA, USA; [c] Nursing Department, Faculty of Health Science, Istanbul Kültür University, Istanbul, Turkey
* Corresponding author.
*E-mail address:* tsengul@ku.edu.tr

Nurs Clin N Am 60 (2025) 15–25
https://doi.org/10.1016/j.cnur.2024.08.009     **nursing.theclinics.com**

traumatic injuries due to the extended hospital stays and rehabilitation periods, as well as the expensive nature of wound and scar treatment.[4] It is emphasized that most burns are preventable, making prevention strategies crucial.[3–6]

### Common Causes and Epidemiology

Factors that can cause burn injuries include flames (fire), hot liquids (scalds), contact with hot or cold objects, electricity, friction, radiation, and chemicals.[1] The most common etiologies of thermal injury are flame and scald burns, which account for 76% of injuries, followed by flash burns and contact burns.[7] The risk and severity of injuries caused by chemical burns vary greatly depending on the substance involved, its concentration, and the duration of exposure.[3] Tissue damage caused by strong acid spills is typically less deep than that caused by strong bases. Acids denature proteins and desiccate tissues, making the tissue less permeable to the acid.[5] Electrical injuries, especially in cases of high voltage, can cause significant internal injuries beneath normal-looking skin.[3–7] Two-thirds of all burns occur at home, often affecting children under the age of 10, adult males, and an increasing number of elderly individuals. Flammable liquids often burn young adults, while hot liquids scald toddlers in about 60% of cases.[6]

### Classification of Burns

The skin provides a strong barrier against energy transfer to deeper tissues; therefore, most injuries are confined to this layer.[5,6] The extent of the injury ranges from the skin surface to deeper structures, depending on the temperature of the burning agent and the duration of exposure to the heat source.[1–6] According to the American Burn Association (ABA), burns are classified based on the depth of injury, size, and severity.[7]

### Depth of the Burn

Burn depth is classified according to the degree of injury to the epidermis, dermis, subcutaneous fat, and underlying structures.[8] The burn depth determines how the wound will heal and whether a graft will be necessary.[7] One method defines the injury as first, second, third, and fourth-degree burns. The ABA recommends using the terms partial-thickness burns and full-thickness burns to classify burns (**Fig. 1**).[9]

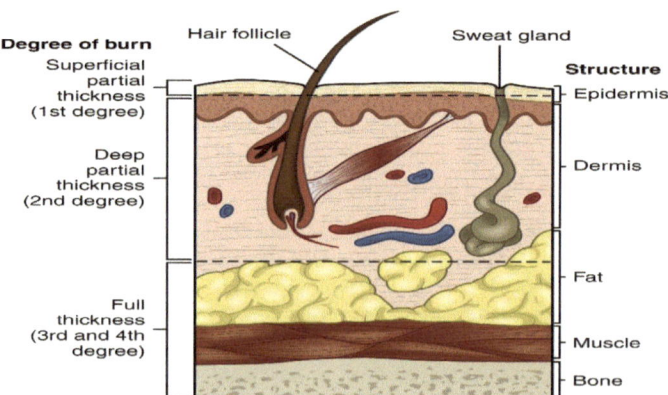

**Fig. 1.** Depth of the burn. (*From* Bidigare C. Burns. "Lewis's Medical-Surgical Nursing", Twelfth Edition editor "Harding, Mariann M., 2023:494-514.)

*Superficial Burns (First Degree):* These burns are limited to the epidermis.[6,7] They are hyperemic and sensitive, with erythema and pain subsiding within 2 to 3 d.[5,6] Sunburn is the most common example.[5]

*Partial Thickness Burns (Second Degree):* These burns are divided into superficial and deep partial-thickness burns.[6]

*Superficial Partial Thickness Burns:* These burns extend to the epidermis and papillary dermis, appearing erythematous, painful, blanching upon touch, and often blistered.[6] Healing is rapid (10–14 d) with a low-risk of scarring.[1]

*Deep Partial Thickness Burns:* These burns extend to the epidermis and reticular dermis. They appear paler and mottled, do not blanch upon touch, but are painful.[6] Epithelial regeneration takes longer (3–6 w), with a high likelihood of hypertrophic scarring.[1] Differentiating between deep partial-thickness burns, best treated with early excision and grafting, and superficial partial-thickness burns, which heal spontaneously, is always challenging through physical examination alone.[5]

*Full Thickness Burns (Third or Fourth Degree):* These burns extend through the epidermis and dermis to the subcutaneous fat and may damage underlying tissues such as muscle, tendon, and bone.[6,7] They are characterized by being painless and covered with a hard, leathery eschar that can be black, white, or cherry red.[6] These burns are typically insensate due to the destruction of nerve endings, but the surrounding areas can be extremely painful.[5] Optimal treatment for full-thickness burns involves early excision and grafting.[1–5] Estimating the depth of a skin burn based on clinical examination is challenging. The final depth of the injury often becomes apparent 48 to 72 h after the injury.[5]

*Size of the Burn:* The burn size is traditionally assessed manually using the "rule of nines."[6] In adults, each upper extremity and the head and neck are assumed to constitute 9% of the total body surface area (TBSA), each lower extremity and the anterior and posterior trunk constitute 18%, and the perineum and genitalia constitute 1% of the TBSA.[6] The Lund and Browder chart is widely accepted as it accounts for different body proportions in infants and children.[5,6] First-degree burns are not considered in the calculation of burn TBSA.[5] Another helpful metric is that the patient's palm represents approximately 1% of the body surface area in patients of any age.[10] This method is helpful when assessing scald burns and other burns with different distributions.[6]

### Severity of the Burn and Hospitalization

Burn injuries are classified as minor, moderate, or major. The severity of a burn injury and the associated ultimate morbidity and mortality are influenced by a combination of factors, including the patient's medical history, the extent and depth of the burn, the affected body region, the presence of concurrent trauma during the burn, and the patient's age.[11] A minor burn typically involves less than 10% of the TBSA and consists primarily of superficial burns. A burn is considered severe if it covers more than 10% TBSA in elderly patients, more than 20% TBSA in adults, and more than 30% TBSA in children.[8–11] Inhalation injury is a significant source of morbidity in burn patients.[3]

### TREATMENT METHODS
### First Aid and Emergency Treatment

The emergency care of a patient with a burn injury depends on the cause of the injury (thermal, chemical, or electrical), the location of the injury, and the availability of resources.[8] The first step is to stop the burning process and move the patient to a safe area.[3–8] If the individual's clothing is on fire, it is recommended to smother the flames by covering the burning clothing; otherwise, water or another fire extinguisher should be used.[8–11] Burning clothes should be removed immediately.[11]

- For a chemical burn, thorough irrigation with water is recommended, as the use of neutralizing agents is contraindicated due to the heat they generate.[8] Dry or powdered chemicals should be removed by brushing off or using other mechanical cleaning methods while still dry.[3]
- The burned area should be washed with cold tap water (neither ice nor iced water) at a temperature of 15°C to 25°C (59°F–77°F) using high-flow, low-pressure water for 20 min.[3–5] This is not recommended for extensive burns due to the theoretic risk of hypothermia and shock.[7] However, cold baths for the face should be applied. It is also noted that cooling is beneficial up to 3 h after the injury, and it should be done even if there is a delay in access to cooling methods.[12]
- After cooling the injured area, it should be covered with a thin cloth or sterile sheets to reduce the risk of contamination and maintain body temperature.[3–8] Covering the wounds is the first step in reducing pain by preventing contact with exposed nerve endings.[6]
- Standard airway, breathing, and circulation resuscitation should be applied. Tetanus prophylaxis should be administered to those not vaccinated in the past 2 y.[5]
- In burns from flames, inhalation injury should always be suspected, and 100% oxygen should be administered via a face mask. All rings, watches, jewelry, and belts should be removed as they retain heat and can create a tourniquet-like effect.[3–6]
- The primary goal of initial treatment is to rapidly restore intravascular fluid volume and maintain tissue perfusion to minimize tissue ischemia. Current information indicates oral rehydration solutions can provide adequate fluid for burns up to 40% TBSA.[5]

### Surgical Treatments

#### Debridement
The primary goals of surgical treatment for burn wounds are to remove damaged or non-viable tissue and replace it with viable tissue.[5] Eschar is the non-viable tissue that forms after a burn injury. Eschar provides an excellent environment for bacterial growth, and loose eschar must be adequately debrided.[8,13,14] The surgical removal of necrotic tissue down to a viable (bleeding) surface is typically performed within the first 4 d after injury while in hospital.[12]

#### Skin grafting
After excising burned tissue, wound closure is ideally achieved using the patient's skin.[6] An autograft, typically taken from the abdomen or thighs, is the gold standard for burn treatment if sufficient donor sites are available.[13,14] Revascularization begins around 48 h post-grafting, with re-epithelialization usually occurring within 10 d to 2 w, depending on dermal depth.[14,15] While skin grafts suffice for most wounds, flaps may be preferable for exposed bones and tendons.[6–15] Xenografts, like porcine skin, offer temporary coverage, while homografts can be sourced from living or deceased donors.[13]

#### Cultured epidermal autografts and dermal substitutes
Cultured epidermal autografts, derived from the patient's keratinocytes, provide a permanent solution for those with limited intact skin.[6–9] For extensive burns where

autografts are unavailable, dermal substitutes made from synthetic materials can temporarily cover wounds until the patient's skin is ready[9–13] and are only used in hospitals.

## BURN WOUND CARE MANAGEMENT AND DRESSING

Burn care is a complex and challenging process, particularly for healthcare professionals, as it involves managing physical and psychologic sequelae.[16–18] The role of nurses in burn treatment is critical.[16,17] Nurses caring for burn patients are responsible for tasks such as wound care, monitoring vital signs, pain management, and infection control. Nurses must have up-to-date knowledge to enhance patients' quality-of-life and improve clinical outcomes.[16] Proper management of burn wounds is crucial for reducing infection risk and promoting rapid healing.[16–18] By following wound care protocols, nurses can increase patient comfort and expedite healing.[16]

Burn dressings should possess biocompatibility, biodegradability, porosity, and appropriate mechanical properties to support healing.[17,19,20] These dressings should adhere well to the wound surface, be easily removed, and provide a barrier that reduces the risk of infection.[17,19–21] Additionally, they should be transparent, have an adequate water vapor transmission rate, and be cost-effective.[19,20] Hydrogel dressings offer significant advantages over traditional dressings and are used to cover the wound, prevent infection, maintain moisture, and reduce pain.[17–19] Dressings are available in various forms, including film, foam, composite, spray, and gel.[17–19]

*Hydrocolloid Dressings:* Hydrocolloid dressings contain hydrophobic particles that form a gel when they come into contact with the wound.[17,19,20] These dressings create a moist wound environment that accelerates healing and reduces the risk of infection.[17,19,20] Hydrocolloid dressings are commonly used for mild to moderate burns and provide convenience in wound care.[17,19,20]

*Medical grade Honey:* Phytochemical, pharmacologic, and ethno-pharmacologic uses of honey have proven highly beneficial in wound care.[22–24] Despite its many benefits and drawbacks, systematic research is needed to provide comprehensive scientific evidence of honey's efficacy in tissue engineering and to address any doubts.[22–24] Future research should focus on a better understanding of dosage and side effects in human studies.[22–24] Clinically, honey has gained significant importance in regenerative medicine due to its constructive properties that support the rapid healing of a wide range of injuries.[17,22–24] The distinctive characteristics of honey are attributed to its active components, such as sugars, enzymes, and vitamins.[17,22–24] Additionally, honey's active biomolecules aid in improving autolytic debridement and tissue granulation.[22–24]

*Alginate Dressings:* Alginate dressings are natural polysaccharides derived from seaweed.[19,20] These dressings have high absorbent properties, helping to control the amount of exudate and providing a moist healing environment.[19,20] Alginate dressings effectively manage deep and highly exudative burns.[19,20] The specific application of burn dressings varies depending on the type, wound depth, and the patient's overall health condition. While hydrocolloid dressings are preferred for superficial and moderate burns, alginate dressings are used for deep and heavily exudative burns. Foam dressings are ideal for mechanical protection in burns with large surface areas and deep wounds.[19]

*Hydrogel dressings:* Hydrogels are essential in treating burn wounds, offering a soft and flexible material that can be easily applied to the wound surface.[17,19,23] These dressings can absorb and release water reversibly, maintaining moisture at the wound site and accelerating the healing process.[19–25] The unique properties of hydrogels make them well-suited to the physiologic needs of burn wounds, speeding up healing, reducing pain, and minimizing the risk of infection.[17,19,25] Types such as antibacterial hydrogels and stem cell-loaded hydrogels can be designed to meet various clinical needs, including infection prevention and tissue regeneration support.[19–26]

*Foam Dressings:* Foam dressings promote healing by maintaining a moist environment and reducing the risk of infection.[17–19] These dressings have high absorbent capacity, effectively managing exudate, and providing mechanical protection to the wound.[17–19] Foam dressings are preferred for burns with large surface areas and deep wounds.[17–19]

*Silver-Containing Dressings:* Infections are a leading cause of mortality in burn patients.[27] Topical silver agents are commonly used to inhibit the growth of microorganisms on the wound surface.[27] Various silver-containing dressings are effective in infection control due to their antibacterial activities and have fewer side effects compared to traditional silver sulfadiazine cream.[17–19,28,29] Silver-containing dressings used in burn patients can shorten the wound healing time and effectively reduce inflammatory reactions compared to conventional treatments.[17–19,28,29] However, more research and analysis are needed to ensure the safety of these treatment methods.[29]

*Biological and Synthetic Dressings:* Biologic dressings, such as human amnion and processed amnion chorionic villus products, reduce the challenges of obtaining fresh amnion, and the risk of spreading infectious diseases.[19,30] Various brands of synthetic dressings can be widely used to cover the wound surface during re-epithelialization.[31]

## BURN AND REHABILITATION

Major burns significantly restrict patients' ability to maintain daily living activities.[32,33] After discharge, patients continue to struggle with both physical and psychologic issues, such as skin problems, pain, itching, distress, low self-esteem, anxiety, depression, and post-traumatic stress disorder.[33,34] In these patients, a significant decrease is observed in the physical, psychologic, and social dimensions of quality-of-life after the burn injury.[33–35] This process involves an intensive period requiring physical therapy and wound management.[33]

### Burns in the Outpatient Clinic

Rehabilitation after burn treatment is critical in improving patients' health, self-care, and quality-of-life.[33–36] The transition process for burn patients from hospital to home is highly complex and challenging due to the involvement of primary care, patients, and caregivers.[33–37] Patients may feel anxiety and concern when returning home due to insufficient support to meet their physical, psychologic, and medical needs post-discharge.[33–39] In the home environment, the post-discharge period is crucial for the rehabilitation and follow-up of burn patients as they face various challenges, primarily financial, and emotional stress.[33–39] Cultural factors, such as the preference for traditional medicine, can negatively affect the effectiveness of interventions. On the other hand, when the follow-up of patients after discharge is short-term, positive outcomes in overcoming symptoms such as wound healing, itching, and pain may not be achieved.[39] Nearly half of burn patients are at risk of post-traumatic stress disorder 3 to 6 mo after injury. Therefore, close and long-term monitoring of a patient's health status after discharge is crucial and can be achieved through rehabilitation.[32,33]

### Scar Management

Scar management is essential to achieving better outcomes during rehabilitation.[40–43] Hypertrophic scars contain excessive collagen and do not extend beyond the original wound boundaries.[40–44] In contrast, keloid scars appear as raised, rounded bumps extending beyond the wound boundaries and do not regress over time.[40–42] Scar management in burn patients is crucial for the best functional and psychosocial outcomes. Pressure therapy, silicone gel sheets, and scar massage manage scars.[40–42] Fractional CO2 laser therapy has emerged as an effective method for improving postburn scars.[45] This treatment significantly improves the flexibility, color, and thickness of scars, notably enhancing the overall appearance of the scar.[45] Patients have reported reduced scar itching and pain following laser treatment.[45] These findings indicate that laser therapy is a strong option for managing burn scars.[45]

## FUTURE DIRECTIONS

Regenerative medicine, mainly stem cell-based therapies, is increasingly recognized for its potential to promote wound healing and reduce scar formation.[18,46,47] Mesenchymal stem cells (MSCs) can accelerate wound healing and minimize scar tissue by supporting angiogenesis and modulating immune response.[18,46,47] These cells are home to damaged tissues and secrete growth factors and cytokines that promote tissue regeneration and remodeling.[18,46,47] In the future, with the more widespread use of MSCs, more effective strategies for treating burn wounds while minimizing scar formation are expected to be developed.[18,46,47]

*Predictive Modeling:* Artificial intelligence is used in burn treatment to develop predictive modeling and decision support systems.[48,49] These systems can analyze clinical data from patients to predict the healing process and optimize treatment plans.[48,49] For example, predicting mortality rates in critically ill patients after surgical intervention has been shown to contribute to early risk assessment and decision-making processes.[48,49]

*Telemedicine:* This technology allows for accurate and rapid assessments, enabling patients to receive on-site treatment, preventing unnecessary procedures, and efficiently using healthcare resources.[50–52] Telemedicine facilitates access to treatment for patients in remote areas and supports the effective management of hospital resources.[33] It provides an almost perfect correlation with face-to-face examinations in the assessment of burn wounds, allowing for accurate evaluation of critical parameters such as TBSA and burn depth.[50,51] Patients with partial or full-thickness burns with unknown or inadequate tetanus immunization status should be vaccinated and treated with tetanus immunoglobulin (C).[17]

(*Level A:* High-level evidence from meta-analyses or systematic reviews. *Level B:* Moderate-level evidence from well-designed cohort or case-control studies; *Level C:* Expert opinions, consensus guidelines, or low-level evidence; *Level D:* Recommendations supported by insufficient evidence or expert opinion).

## SUMMARY

This study highlights significant advances in burn management, including burn grading, treatment, improved wound dressings, application for regenerative medicine, and integration of predictive modeling and telemedicine. These innovations can improve patient outcomes by enhancing wound healing, reducing infection risks, and supporting tissue regeneration. However, the complexity of burn injuries necessitates a continued focus on multidisciplinary approaches encompassing medical, surgical, psychological, and social care. Future research should refine existing technologies and explore new methods to improve the standard of burn-care, ultimately leading to better survival rates and quality-of-life for patients.

## CLINICS CARE POINTS

- Burn patients meeting ABA referral criteria should promptly be referred to a burn center (C).[17–22]
- The burn area should be cooled with running tap water for at least 20 min within the first 3 h after the burn injury (B)[17]
- Patients with partial or full-thickness burns with unknown or inadequate tetanus immunization status should be vaccinated and treated with tetanus immunoglobulin (C)[17]
- Burn patients with diabetes who develop complications such as cellulitis should be referred to a burn center for advanced treatment (C)[17]
- Patients whose burns are expected to take longer than 14 d to heal should be referred to a burn center due to the risk of hypertrophic scarring (C).[17–35]
- In children, burns on the feet, hips, posterior legs, and hands, along with an injury history that is inconsistent with the wound and the presence of unrelated injuries, may indicate abuse. Such cases should be carefully evaluated (C).[17]
- Longitudinal intervention studies have supported targeted educational initiatives, showing their effectiveness in increasing fire safety knowledge among patients and caregivers (B).[17–22]

## DISCLOSURE

The authors have nothing to disclose.

## REFERENCES

1. Zwierełło W, Piorun K, Skórka-Majewicz M, et al. Classification, pathophysiology, and treatment: a review. Int J Mol Sci 2023;24:3749.
2. Markiewicz-Gospodarek A, Kozioł M, Tobiasz M, et al. Burn wound healing: clinical complications, medical care, treatment, and dressing types: the current state of knowledge for clinical practice. Int J Environ Res Publ Health 2022;19:1338. https://doi.org/10.3390/ijerph19031338.
3. Briggs AM, Barth BE. Physical and chemical injuries: burns. In: Kellerman RD, Rakel DP, editors. Conn's Current Therapy. 2024 edition. Philadelphia, PA: Elsevier; 2024. p. 1399–405.
4. Chen L, He X, Xian J, et al. Development of a framework for managing severe burns through a 17-year retrospective analysis of burn epidemiology and outcomes. Sci Rep 2021;11(1):9374.
5. Lee RC, Teven CM, Burn. chemical, and electrical injuries. In: Song DH, Hong JP, editors. Plastic Surgery. Vol 4: Lower Extremity, Trunk, and Burns. 5th edition. Philadelphia, PA: Elsevier; 2024. p. 501–37.
6. Wolf S.E., Burns. In: Townsend C.M., Beauchamp R.D., Evers B.M., et al., eds. Sabiston Textbook of Surgery: The Biological Basis of Modern Surgical Practice. 21st edition. Elsevier; Philadelphia, PA, 2022:484-505.
7. Pappas-Taffer L., Burns. In: Ferri F.F., editor Ferri's Clinical Advisor. 2025 edition. Elsevier; Philadelphia, PA, 2025:217.e6-217.e16.
8. Jeschke MG, Gauglitz GG. Pathophysiology of burn injuries. In: Jeschke M, Kamolz LP, Sjöberg F, et al, editors. Handbook of burns volume 1. Cham: Springer; 2020. https://doi.org/10.1007/978-3-030-18940-2_18.
9. Bidigare C. Burns. In: Harding MM, editor. Lewis's medical-surgical nursing. 12th edition. 2023. p. 494–514. ISBN: 978-0-323-78961-5.

10. Lee C, Barie PS, Houng AP. Burn wound management. In: John Cameron AM, editor. Cameron trauma and emergency care. 14th edition. Elsevier; 2023. p. 1215–442. Section 17.

11. Ogle S., Patel N., Burn injuries. In: Banasik J., editor. Pathophysiology. 7th edition. Available at: https://www.clinicalkey.com/student/nursing/content/book/3-s2.0-B9780323761550000547. Elsevier; Philadelphia, PA, 2022:1115-1135.

12. McCahill B., Nursing the patient with burn injury. In: Peate I., editor. Alexander's Nursing Practice. 6th edition. Elsevier; Philadelphia, PA, 2025:683-696. Available at: https://www.clinicalkey.com/student/nursing/content/book/3-s2.0-B9780443110221000290.

13. Myers R, Wilson CM, Seigel J. Burns. In: Urden LD, Stacy KM, Lough ME, editor. Critical care nursing. 9th edition. 2022. p. 865–88. Available at: https://www.clinicalkey.com/student/nursing/content/book/3-s2.0-B9780323642958000357. ISBN: 978-0-323-64295-8. https://doi.org/10.1016/B978-0-323-64295-8.00035-7.

14. McCann C, Watson A, Barnes D. Major burns: Part 1. Epidemiology, pathophysiology and initial management. BJA Educ 2022;22(3):94–103.

15. Radzikowska-Büchner E, Łopuszynska I, Flieger W, et al. An overview of recent developments in the management of burn injuries. Int J Mol Sci 2023;24:16357.

16. Costa PCP, Barbosa CS, Ribeiro CO, et al. Nursing care directed to burned patients: a scoping review. Rev Bras Enferm 2023;76(3).

17. Lanham JS, Nelson NK, Hendren B, et al. Outpatient burn care: prevention and treatment. Am Fam Physician 2020;101(8):463–70.

18. Ibrahim Z, El-Hiti GA, Alotaibi MH, et al. Burn wound healing: clinical complications, medical care, treatment, and dressing types: the current state of knowledge for clinical practice. Int J Environ Res Publ Health 2022;19(2):1338.

19. Shu W, Wang Y, Zhang X, et al. Functional hydrogel dressings for treatment of burn wounds. Front Bioeng Biotechnol 2021;9:788461.

20. Minsart M, Van Vlierberghe S, Dubruel P, et al. Commercial wound dressings for the treatment of exuding wounds: an in-depth physico-chemical comparative study. Burns Trauma 2022;10. https://doi.org/10.1093/burnst/tkac024.

21. Hansen JK, Voss J, Ganatra H, et al. Sedation and analgesia during pediatric burn dressing change: a survey of American Burn Association centers. J Burn Care Res 2019;40(3):287–93.

22. Lindberg T, Andersson O, Palm M, et al. A systematic review and meta-analysis of dressings used for wound healing: the efficiency of honey compared to silver on burns. Contemp Nurse 2015;51(2–3):121–34.

23. Aziz Z, Hassan BAR. The effects of honey compared to silver sulfadiazine for the treatment of burns: a systematic review of randomized controlled trials. Burns 2017;43(1):50–7.

24. Krishnakumar GS, Mahendiran B, Gopalakrishnan S, et al. Honey-based treatment strategies for infected wounds and burns: a systematic review of recent pre-clinical research. Wound Med 2020;30:100.

25. George B, Bhatia N, Suchithra TV. Burgeoning hydrogel technology in burn wound care: a comprehensive meta-analysis. Eur Polym J 2021;157:110640.

26. Chakrabarti S, Islam J, Hazarika H, et al. Safety profile of silver sulfadiazine-bFGF-loaded hydrogel for partial thickness burn wounds. Cutan Ocul Toxicol 2018;37:258–66.

27. Roy S, Mukherjee P, Kundu S, et al. Microbial infections in burn patients. Acute Crit Care 2024;39(2):214–25.

28. Brown MR, Dalziel SR, Herd E, et al. A randomized controlled study of silver-based burns dressing in a pediatric emergency department. J Burn Care Res 2016;37(4).

29. Wu JJ, Zhang F, Liu J, et al. Effect of silver-containing hydrofiber dressing on burn wound healing: a meta-analysis and systematic review. J Cosmet Dermatol 2023; 22(5):1685–91.

30. Wasiak J, Cleland H, Campbell F, et al. Dressings for superficial and partial thickness burns. Cochrane Database Syst Rev 2013;2013(4).

31. Mir M, Ali MN, Barakullah A, et al. Synthetic polymeric biomaterials for wound healing: a review. Prog Biomater 2018;7:1–21.

32. Serghiou MA, Niszczak J, Parry I, et al. Clinical practice recommendations for positioning of the burn patient. Burns 2016;42(2):267–75.

33. Heydarikhayat N, Ashktorab T, Rohani C, et al. Effect of post-hospital discharge follow-up on health status in patients with burn injuries: a randomized clinical trial. Int J Community Based Nurs Midwifery 2018;6(4):293–304.

34. Liang CY, Wang HJ, Yao KP, et al. Predictors of health-care needs in discharged burn patients. Burns 2012;38:172–9.

35. Ricci H, Goncalves N, Gallani MC, et al. Assessment of the health status in Brazilian burn victims five to seven months after hospital discharge. Burns 2014;40: 616–23.

36. Hashemi F, Rahimi Dolatabad F, Yektatalab S, et al. Effect of Orem self-care program on the life quality of burn patients referred to Ghotb-al-Din-e-Shirazi Burn Center, Shiraz, Iran: a randomized controlled trial. Int J Community Based Nurs Midwifery 2014;2:40–50.

37. Hesselink G, Flink M, Olsson M, et al. Are patients discharged with care? A qualitative study of perceptions and experiences of patients, family members, and care providers. BMJ Qual Saf 2012;21:39–49.

38. Steenoven JVD, Kolkena R, Dokter J. The after care nurse in the burns outpatient clinic of the burn Centre: an overview of activities May 2006-April 2009. Burns 2009;35(suppl 1).

39. Engrav LH, Heimbach DM, Rivara F, et al. 12-year within-wound study of the effectiveness of custom pressure garment therapy. Burns 2010;36(7):975–83.

40. Tredget E, Shupp JW, Schneider JC. Scar management following burn injury. J Burn Care Res 2017;38(3):146–7.

41. Herndon DN. Total Burn Care. 5th edition. Edinburgh, Scotland: Elsevier; 2018.

42. Forbes-Duchart L, Cooper J, Nedelec B, et al. Burn therapists' opinion on the application and essential characteristics of a burn scar outcome measure. J Burn Care Res 2009;30(5):792–800.

43. Benavides L, Ferreira B, Suman OE, et al. Burn rehabilitation. In: Lee JO, editor. Essential burn care for non-burn specialists. Switzerland AG: Springer Nature; 2023. p. 434–47.

44. Sharp P, Pan B, Yakuboff K, et al. Development of a best evidence statement for the use of pressure therapy for management of hypertrophic scarring. J Burn Care Res 2016;37(4):255–64.

45. Choi KJ, Williams EA, Pham CH, et al. Fractional CO2 laser treatment for burn scar improvement: a systematic review and meta-analysis. Burns 2021;47(2): 259–69.

46. Coalson E, Bishop E, Liu H, et al. Stem cell therapy for chronic skin wounds in the era of personalized medicine: from bench to bedside. Genes Dis 2019;6(4): 342–58.

47. Kazimierczak P, Benko A, Nocun M, et al. Novel chitosan/agarose/hydroxyapatite nanocomposite scaffold for bone tissue engineering applications: comprehensive evaluation of biocompatibility and osteoinductivity with the use of osteoblasts and mesenchymal stem cells. Int J Nanomed 2019;14:6615–30.

48. Wang G, Lam KM, Deng Z, et al. Prediction of mortality in burn patients after surgery using machine learning models: a retrospective cohort study. J Personalized Med 2022;12(8):1293.
49. Abubakar A, Ugail H, Bukar AM. Assessment of human skin burns: a deep transfer learning approach. J Med Biol Eng 2020;40:321–33.
50. Moreau M, Paré G. Early clinical management of severe burn patients using telemedicine: a pilot study protocol. Pilot Feasibility Stud 2020;6:93.
51. Basaran A, Ozlu O, Das K. Telemedicine in burn patients: reliability and patient preference. Burns 2021;47(8):1871–5.
52. Monte SA, López-Masrramon B, Aguilera-Sáez J, et al. Implementation and evaluation of telemedicine in burn care: study of clinical safety and technical feasibility in a single burn center. Burns 2020;46(7):1668–73.

# Complications of Wounds in the Acute Care Setting

Elizabeth Faust, MSN, MBA, ANP-BC, CSWS, CWOCN-AP*

## KEYWORDS

- Sepsis • Complex wounds • Pressure injury • Wound care • Complications
- Surgical site complications

## KEY POINTS

- Nurses' role: Nurses are essential in recognizing and reporting skin changes, acting as the gatekeepers of skin health in health care settings.
- Hospitalization risks: Patients in acute care settings are at higher risk for developing wounds such as moisture-associated skin damage, pressure injuries, skin tears, and surgical site complications.
- Chronic versus acute wounds: Many patients are admitted to acute care due to complications from chronic wounds, which often require additional interventions for successful healing.
- Preventive measures: Regular skin assessments, patient education, and preventive measures like frequent repositioning and maintaining skin hygiene are crucial in reducing the risk of wound development.

## BACKGROUND

Within the United States (US), 6120 hospitals had 33,679,935 admissions in 2023.[1] It is estimated that there are 60 million Americans who have had a wound that resulted in 60 billion health care dollars spent. To put this in perspective, 40 billion is spent on all cancers annually.[2] Of those costs, up to $24.3 billion are associated with the acute care setting.[3] The American population is growing, as are the number of wound patients. Clinicians often do not get the specialized training or education required to treat wounds due to the multidisciplinary nature of the specialty.[4] There are 2 main categories of wounds with very different care plans and healing trajectories: acute and chronic. Acute and chronic wounds can be encountered in any health care setting. By definition, chronic wounds fail to heal promptly or, as the Centers for Medicare (CMS) defines them, have not healed after 30 days. Some wounds by the mere diagnosis fall into a chronic wound care category: pressure injuries (PIs), venous leg ulcers (VLUs), arterial ulcers, and diabetic foot ulcers (DFUs). Acute wounds are a much

Lizzie Wounds LLC, Douglassville, PA, USA
* 107 Meadowcrest Lane, Douglassville, PA 19518.
E-mail address: lizziewoundsllc@icloud.com

Nurs Clin N Am 60 (2025) 27–47
https://doi.org/10.1016/j.cnur.2024.07.012     nursing.theclinics.com
0029-6465/25/© 2024 Elsevier Inc. All rights are reserved, including those for text and data mining, AI training, and similar technologies.

larger category with a variety of different etiologies. Some examples include skin tears, medical adhesive-related skin injury (MARSI), moisture-associated skin damage (MASD), surgical incisions, and infectious wounds. Each of these acute and chronic wounds has very different etiologies and pathophysiology. Acute wounds can occur within the hospital or be present during hospitalization. Chronic wounds are often present at the time of hospitalization, though PIs can also develop within the acute care setting. We will investigate each wound type and its implications for acute care nursing.

## PRESSURE INJURY
### Etiology

PIs, previously known as bedsores, decubitus ulcers, and pressure ulcers, develop from unrelieved pressure on the skin. PIs are defined as localized damage to the skin and underlying soft tissue, primarily occurring over bony prominences or related to medical devices.[5] The incidence of PIs is 1.3 to 3 million adults in the US.[6] Patients may be admitted with a PI or develop a PI within the acute care setting. A study examining Medicare beneficiaries hospitalized between 2006 and 2007 found that 4.5% of patients developed a PI during their hospital stays.[7] Over the last 15 years, regulations have been increased against hospital-acquired PIs (HAPIs). Within the US, the CMS and Medicaid Services have used Patient Safety Indicator 90 (PSI90), a composite rate of hospital-acquired conditions (HACs), to adjust payments and score hospitals on quality since 2015. A significant decrease in HACs occurred after PSI90 was implemented, reflecting an association between PSI90 and CMS reimbursement policy. However, PI rates increased by 29.4% during this time frame, and the only HAC observed to increase was related to PSI90.[8] Patients with at least 1 PI have double the median length of stay (LOS) and treatment cost and a 5-fold increase in mortality compared with patients without PIs. Patients who are in the critical care unit are at increased risk for HAPIs for a multitude of factors: longer LOS, immobility, comorbidities, poor oxygenation, and hemodynamic instability.[9]

### Complications

A variety of complications can occur from the development of a PI. The apparent complications are pain, infection, and the need for surgical intervention. It has also been shown to increase morbidity and mortality. In a meta-analysis, patients who had PIs are estimated to have a 2 times higher risk of mortality compared to patients without PIs over a 3-year follow-up period.[10]

### Case Study/Presentation

A 27-year-old male with a past medical history significant for chronic smoking, status post motor vehicle accident 1 year prior, which led to a paraplegic state, presented to the hospital with an infected wound on the posterior trunk.

The patient's baseline was wheelchair-bound with a gel cushion and education on off-loading in the wheelchair using wheelchair pushups and shifting. The patient previously had superficial skin injuries but never had a deeper wound. The patient presented with worsening wounds with malodor. Upon initial assessment, he had bilateral ischial unstageable (eschar-covered) PIs with active signs of infection (erythema, malodor, warmth, fever, and leukocytosis). **Fig. 1**- Unstageable PIs on admission.

The patient underwent a bedside debridement of the non-viable tissue and had systemic treatment with intravenous (IV) antibiotics for infection without sepsis criteria (**Fig. 2**).

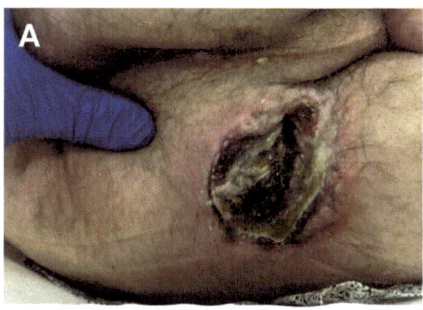
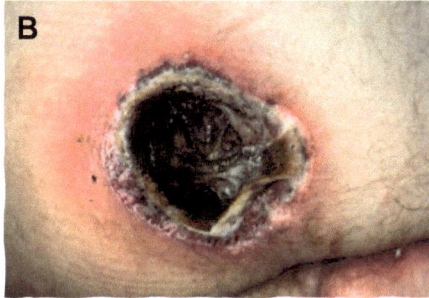

Fig. 1. (*A, B*) Unstageable ischial pressure injury on admission.

Negative Pressure Wound therapy with instillation and dwell (NPWTi-d) was applied for 1 week using a pure hypochlorous acid as the solution (**Fig. 3**).

The treatment was then changed to oral antibiotics and continuous negative pressure wound therapy (NPWT) with home health nursing to change 3 times per week. He maintained a healthy wound bed until he underwent a V to Y fascia cutaneous flap elevation inset in the reconstruction of the complex wound left and right ischial tuberosity for definitive closure (**Figs. 4** and **5**).

### Discussion

Identifying and intervening in PI risk and development is critical to patients' morbidity and mortality. Using a validated risk assessment tool and the National Pressure Injury Advisory Panel Standardized Pressure Injury Prevention Protocol Checklist 2.0[11] can decrease the burden on the patient, caregivers, and health system.

## VENOUS LEG ULCER
### Etiology

Chronic venous disease (CVD) is a common disease state in the US. This persistent and progressive disease has a vast socioeconomic, physical, and psychologic impact

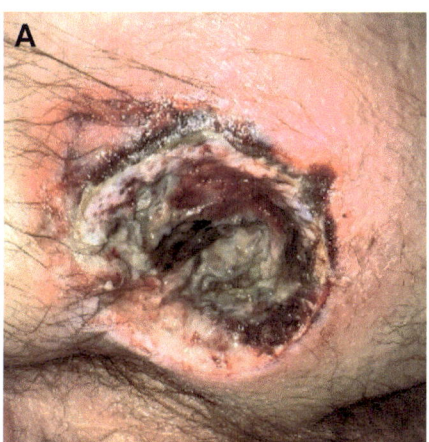
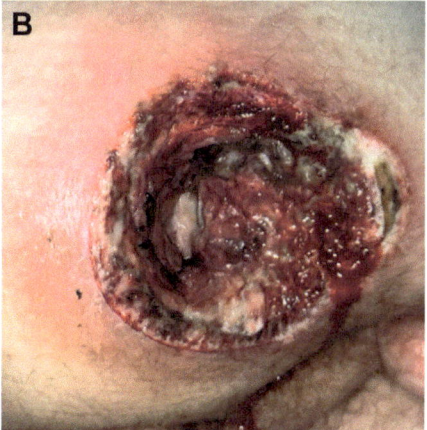

Fig. 2. (*A, B*) Ischial Pressure injury after bedside sharp debridement.

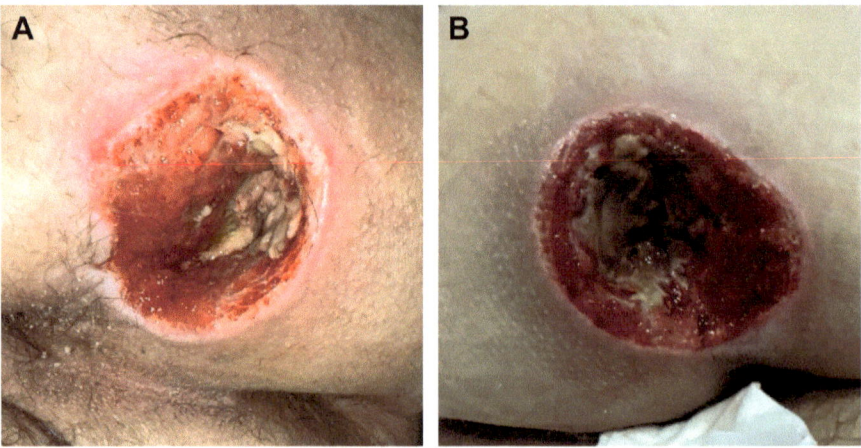

**Fig. 3.** (*A, B*) Ischial pressure injury after 1 week of NPWTi-d with pure hypochlorous acid (pHA).

on the population. CVD includes a spectrum of venous abnormalities in which blood return and/or valvular competence is compromised. A complication of CVD is the development of VLUs. VLUs are open ulcers typically occurring between the knee and ankle joint, otherwise known as the gaiter region, in the presence of CVD. VLUs are the most common cause of leg ulcers globally, accounting for 60% to 80% of leg ulcers within the US.[12] The prevalence of VLUs in all populations is 2%, but in individuals over age 65, that number jumps to 5%.[13]

Several risk factors for VLU development include older age, female sex, obesity, trauma, immobility, congenital absence of veins, deep vein thrombosis, phlebitis, and factor V Leiden mutation.[12]

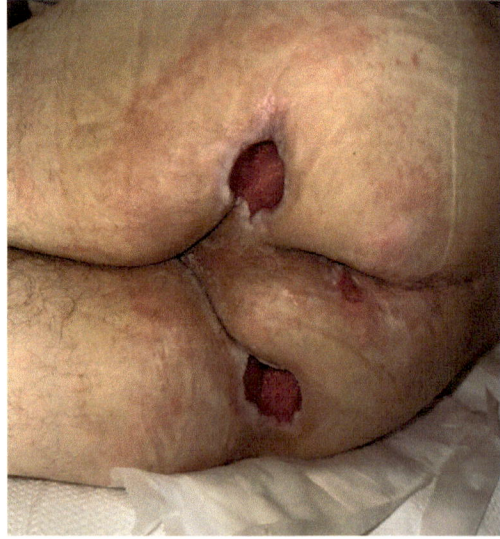

**Fig. 4.** Ischial pressure injuries after 2 months of NPWT.

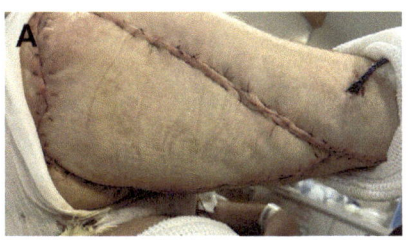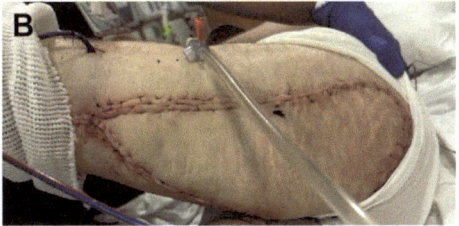

**Fig. 5.** (*A, B*) V-Y fasciocutaneous flap reconstruction for definitive closure of ischial pressure injuries.

## Complications

While 76% of VLUs heal within 16 w with the standard-of-care of advanced wound therapy and compression, the recurrence rate is 50% to 70% after 6 m. The care burden is large and significant, given the chronic and progressive nature of CVD. This translates to a lifelong financial and psychologic burden for proper management.[13] More severe complications of VLUs include cellulitis, osteomyelitis, and malignancy.[14]

## Presentation

VLUs often present as leg swelling with erythema and fluid leakage. A minor skin trauma can precipitate the ulceration, or pruritis can occur. This is reflective of the stasis dermatitis of the progressive venous disease. Patients may also exhibit a classic brawny discoloration of the skin over the gaiter region called hemosiderin staining. This is caused by the leakage in the capillaries, resulting in blood, or more specifically hemoglobin, leaking into the interstitial tissue. The iron in the blood causes this brown-tinged staining in the skin that gives the classic brawny appearance[15] (**Fig. 6**).

## Discussion

Since venous disease is progressive, early intervention is critical to preventing complications. The standard-of-care is infection management, exudate management, and compression therapy. Compression therapy can differ based on patient factors such as arterial blood flow, pain tolerance, functional capabilities, and the level of disease. Not all compression is the same, and compression used to prevent blood clots,

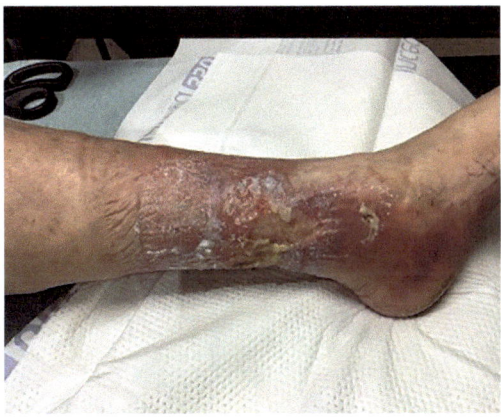

**Fig. 6.** Venous Leg ulcer with surrounding stasis dermatitis and hemosiderin staining.

such as thromboembolic deterrent hose or sequential compression devices, is not therapeutic for venous disease.[16]

## ARTERIAL ULCERS
### Etiology

Arterial wounds are caused by a lack of blood flow to an area and are often found at the distal tip of hands and feet. They account for 5% to 20% of non-healing leg ulcers. Development risk factors include advancing age, atherosclerosis, diabetes, peripheral arterial disease, and hypertension.[17] Typical characteristics are discolored tissue (gray, blue, or purple) that changes to black, well-defined edges, little to no drainage, and significant pain.

### Complications

The most common complication of arterial ulcers is amputation. Pain is also a significant complication. Treatment should be focused on restoring the blood flow, if possible. If blood flow can be restored, then principles of moist wound healing would be the standard-of-care. If blood flow cannot be restored, treatment often focuses on keeping the areas dry and bacteria-free. A Povidone/Iodine solution being painted on the area daily is a common treatment option. Over time, the area of necrosis will further demarcate and allow for the lowest level of tissue loss or auto-amputation.[18]

### Presentation

Classic presentation of distal necrosis in peripheral arterial disease (**Fig. 7**).

### Discussion

Once tissue damage from ischemia occurs, arterial ulcers are inevitable. Early detection and management of peripheral arterial disease (PAD) can prevent tissue and limb loss. It is also essential that all diabetic patients be screened for PAD to help avoid further diabetic foot complications, which will be discussed later.

## DIABETIC FOOT ULCERS
### Etiology

DFUs are a significant issue globally in persons with diabetes. The lifetime risk of developing a DFU in persons with diabetes is 19% to 34%, with the number

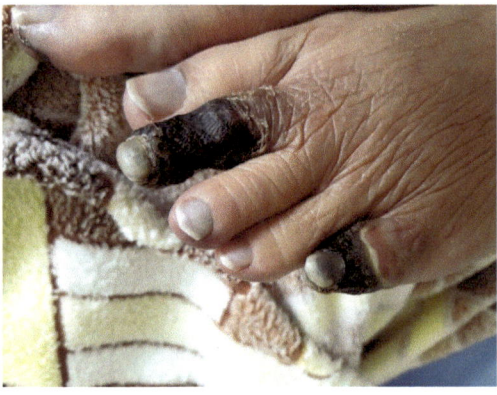

**Fig. 7.** Arterial ulcers of the 2nd and fifth digit.

increasing. Once a DFU develops, the 5-year mortality rate is 50% to 70%.[19] DFUs often develop due to high blood glucose levels, leading to the stiffening of arterials that leads to peripheral neuropathy and ischemia. These can lead to foot deformities that can increase pressures on the plantar surface of the forefoot, as well as create contractures of the toes. All diabetic patients need routine foot examinations and appropriate footwear and become established with a podiatrist as soon as possible.

### Complications

DFUs have high rates of infection. This leads to further complications of sepsis, osteomyelitis, and amputation. They additionally also have high recurrence rates of 65% within 5 years. The lifetime lower extremity amputation incidence of individuals who have had a DFU is 20%. However, that number has also been shown to be as high as 50%, depending on region, socioeconomic status, and ethnicity.[19] Infection is often a reason for admission to an acute care setting. Some infections require surgical intervention to debride necrotic or infected tissue from the foot.

### Presentation

Often, patients with DFUs have peripheral neuropathy that prevents them from feeling the pain of the ulceration. The most common locations of DFUs will be on the plantar surface of the forefoot. The area will often begin as a callus or a minor trauma. Early intervention with a trained professional is important to prevent further complications associated with DFUs. The clinical presentation of a diabetic foot ulcer is often a well-defined circular ulcer with a surrounding callus. Drainage could be minimal to moderate. Typically, the higher amounts of drainage correlate to a higher bacterial burden[20] (**Fig. 8**).

### Discussion

With the incidence of DFUs affecting approximately 18.6 million people worldwide each year, there is a large care burden associated with their treatment. Additionally, DFUs are associated with increased rates of amputation and death. Treatment should focus on surgical debridement, correcting biomechanic abnormalities, treating lower extremity ischemia and foot infection, and early referral for multidisciplinary care. Additional advanced options for the DFU include negative pressure wound therapy (NPWT), cellular, acellular, and matrix products, and hyperbaric and topical oxygen

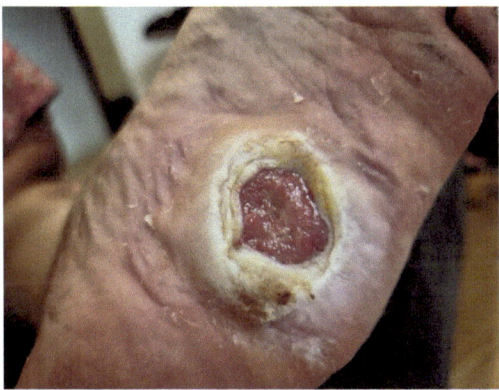

**Fig. 8.** Diabetic Foot Ulcer with surrounding maceration.

therapy. Education on the complications, the importance of adherence to the treatment plan, and glucose management should be a priority at every episode of care.[21]

## SKIN TEARS
### Etiology

Skin tears are a common occurrence in health care settings. Skin tears are acute wounds that are caused by 2 mechanic forces moving in opposite directions, causing a separation of the skin's outer layers. Skin pairs are more likely to occur in more vulnerable populations, including the elderly and the neonate population.[22] Skin tears are classified by their level of flap loss. Type 1 has no skin loss where a linear wound occurs, or the flap can be repositioned to cover the entire wound bed. Type 2 is a partial flap loss where the flap cannot be repositioned to cover the entirety of the wound bed. Type 3 is a total flap loss in which all of the skin flaps cannot be re-approximated, leaving a fully exposed wound bed.[23] Risk factors for developing a skin tear include chronic illness, impaired sensory perception, poor nutrition, history of falls, or impaired mobility—extremes of age, fragile skin, and previous skin tears.[24] Treatment of an acute skin tear should focus on cleansing the wound from debris, controlling bleeding, re-approximating the flap if possible, and then applying a non-traumatic dressing.[25]

### Complications

Not all skin tears move through the 4 phases of wound healing well. Risk factors for non-healing include edema, antiplatelet therapy, corticosteroid use and malnutrition, and dehydration.[26] Clinically, the patient may also have pain or bleeding that can complicate the healing process. It is crucial to choose a non-traumatic dressing that will not increase bleeding or pain for the patient. If a skin tear also includes deeper tissues, the patient may need further surgical interventions to allow coverage of structures.[27]

### Presentation

Type 1 skin tear has no skin loss, but a flap of epidermal tissue that covers the underlying injury (**Fig. 9**). Type 2 skin loss includes partial tissue loss (**Fig. 10**).

### Discussion

Skin tears cause a significant amount of skin injuries in the elderly population every year. These acute wounds have a high risk of becoming more complex chronic wounds. In addition to the elderly, critically ill, pediatric, and neonate populations can be at a high risk for developing skin tears. Health care providers in the acute care setting must take precautions to prevent skin tears from occurring.[24]

## MEDICAL ADHESIVE-RELATED SKIN INJURIES
### Etiology

Medical adhesive-related skin injuries, known as MARSI or tape burn, are common in fragile patient populations. MARSI occurs when the adhesive attachment to the skin is stronger than the skin-cell-to-skin-cell attachment.[28] Because of the use of medical adhesives in the acute care setting, there is a higher propensity for developing these MARSIs in the hospital setting. Common causes of MARSIs include tape applied to peripheral IV site dressings over central lines, surgical dressings, and securement devices for various tubes. The development of these skin injuries is often due to a fragile skin state, edema, or an aggressive adhesive. There are minimal data to determine the prevalence and incidence of this injury. The premature neonate population is also at particular risk for this, given their immature epithelial layer.[29]

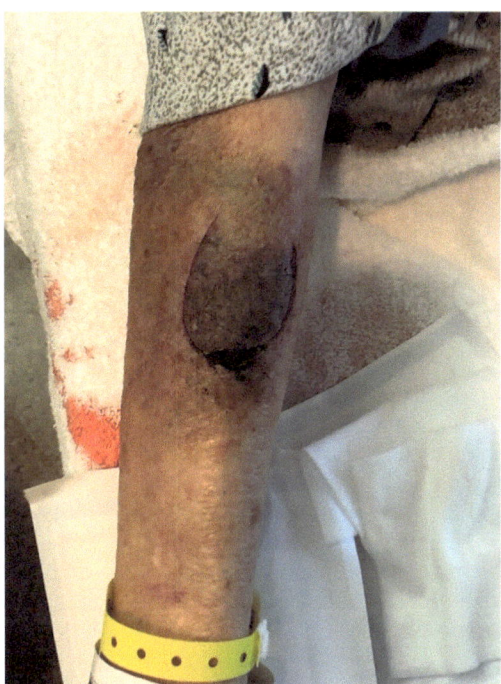

**Fig. 9.** Type 1 skin tear.

*Complications*

MARSI is a complication of using an adhesive in medical care. The skin injury the patient is left with can cause pain and bleeding and become a potential source of infection.

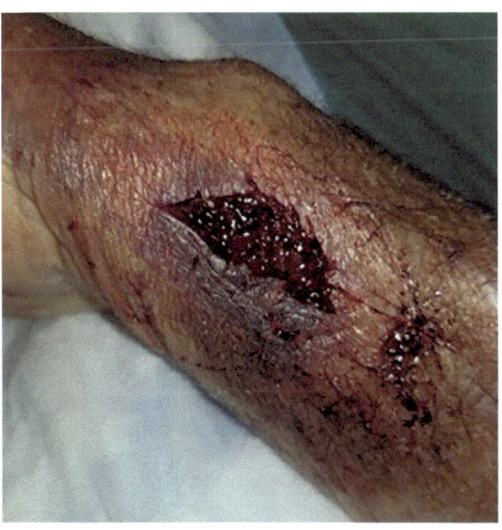

**Fig. 10.** Type 2 skin tear.

*Presentation*

The typical presentation is erythema and loss of epithelium directly under where the medical adhesive was placed (**Fig. 11**).[30]

*Discussion*

Health care clinicians should be careful when applying an adhesive to the skin, especially in fragile patient populations. Care should also be taken when removing the medical adhesive from the skin. The use of adhesive removers may help decrease the incidence of MARSI.[31]

## MOISTURE-ASSOCIATED SKIN DAMAGE
*Etiology*

MASD is also known as diaper dermatitis, incontinence-associated dermatitis (IAD), irritant dermatitis, or macerated skin. When moisture sits against the epithelial layer of the skin, it becomes overhydrated, and the acid mantle that usually protects the skin becomes weakened and disrupted. There are 4 main types of MASD: IAD, peri-wound skin damage, intertriginous dermatitis, and peristomal moisture-associated dermatitis. It was not until recently that a diagnosis code was appropriate for MASD. This resulted in varied reports of the prevalence of this skin injury. There is also a wide range of clinical manifestations, from intact epithelium with erythema to large areas of denuded skin.[32]

*Complications*

The most common complications of MASD are the pain from ulcerations or irritation and the high risk of infection. Particularly in the case of IAD, patients can be exposed to urine or feces in an area of ulceration. Infections involving fungi or yeast are also prevalent, as are bacterial infections.[33] Cleansing the area is often complicated by the pain. This leads to a negative feedback cycle where the skin and tissue become more irritated and inflamed, which then worsens the pain and can break down more areas if not adequately addressed.

*Presentation*

The presentation of MASD would be erythematous or macerated epithelium, initially followed by partial thickness ulcerations around the area of moisture exposure. In the case of IAD, these areas would be localized to the groin, the inner thighs, the perineum, the buttock, and the sacral area. For intertriginous dermatitis, the areas are within skin folds. For peri-wound MASD, the area of damage will be directly around the wound where the exudate is sitting. For peristomal MASD, the area of skin damage will be directly around the stoma where the drainage or effluent is collecting. **Fig. 12-** Diaper dermatitis in a neonate.

*Discussion*

MASD is a disease process that is often missed or undiagnosed. Treatment should be focused on decreasing causative factors and limiting exposure to moisture. Care should be taken for IAD to restrict exposure to fecal or urinary incontinence. The enzymes in feces pose a potent threat to the epithelium if left exposed. If the irritant dermatitis is related to excessive wound drainage, the dressing should be changed to a more absorptive option, or the dressing should be changed more frequently. If the MASD is related to sweat collecting in the skin folds, care should be focused on keeping the skin fold dry and clean. In peristomal dermatitis, ensuring the containment

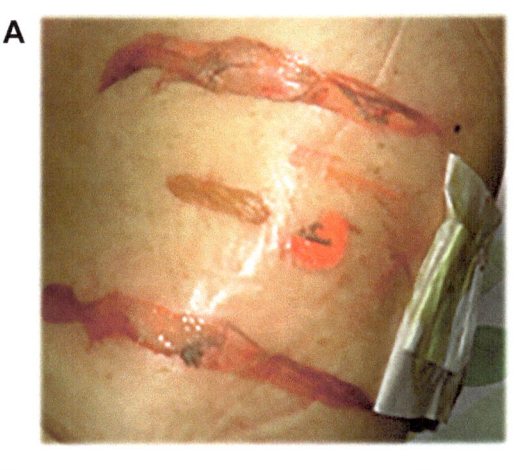

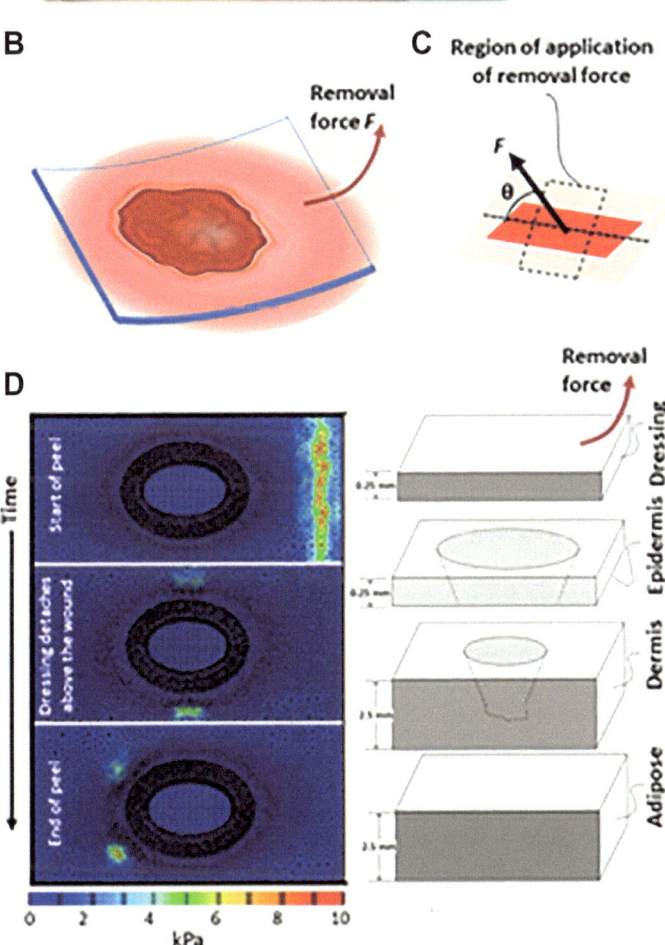

**Fig. 11.** (*A*) MARSI (*B*) simulation of dressing application (*C*) simulation of angle and forces of removal (*D*) stress to skin at removal.

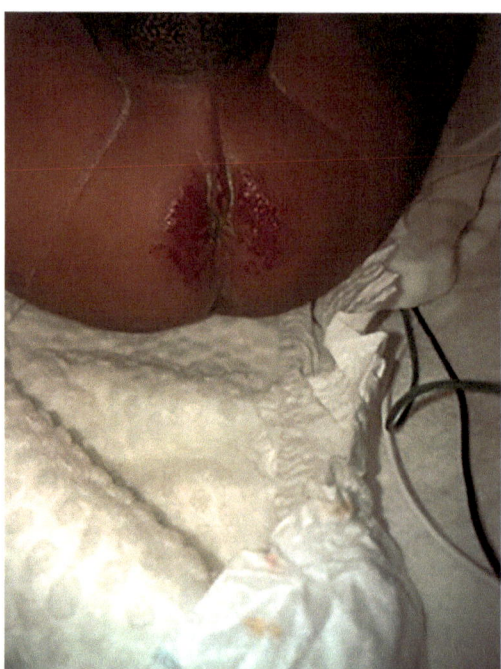

**Fig. 12.** MASD in a neonate.

device or pouch over the stoma is well-fit and preventing leaks will prevent further damage. It should be noted that friction can worsen dermatitis related to excessive moisture exposure; thus, excessive rubbing is strongly discouraged.[34]

## SURGICAL INCISIONS
### Etiology and Prevalence

In the acute care setting, patients may experience complications from their surgical procedure or have to be readmitted because of a surgical complication. These complications after surgery cause a source of significant morbidity and mortality within the US. An estimated 187 to 281 million surgical procedures are performed globally each year, with an incidence rate as high as 22% for significant complications and mortality of 0.8%.[35] It is crucial that health care professionals utilize the surgical care pathways and routinely assess and recognize these complications early.

### Complications

One of the complications is related to the surgical site or incision, such as surgical site infection, dehiscence, or a seroma or hematoma formation. The literature on surgical site complications is narrowed by type of surgery, such as orthopedic, colorectal, cardiothoracic, vascular, and Caesarian section. It is known that patients with surgical site complications have increased LOS, higher health care costs, and increased morbidity and mortality.[36]

Risk factors for surgical site complications can vary based on type. However, some common risk factors include smoking, obesity, malnutrition, previous wound complications, poor tissue quality, use of corticosteroids, emergent versus elective, and advanced age.[37] The American College of Surgeons notes there are 4 classes of surgical wound types based on the wound's level of contamination: clean, clean-contaminated, contaminated, and dirty-infected. Clean and clean-contaminated wounds should be closed in the operating room (OR).[38] The latest evidence shows that the readmission rates for each category are as follows: clean: 3.9%; clean-contaminated: 10.3%; contaminated: 12%; and dirty/infected: 11.7%.[39]

### Presentation

A 62-year-old female presented to the emergency room with abdominal pain, constipation, and fevers. She underwent a computed tomography (CT) scan that showed a bowel perforation due to diverticulitis. General surgery was consulted, and Hartmann's procedure left the midline abdominal incision open to the level of the fascia. Her post-operative course was complicated by acute kidney failure, delirium, and paranoia. For 11 days post-operatively, she received wet to moist dressings for treatment of her open incision (**Fig. 13**). Unfortunately, she was not able to eat or drink over this time due to her recent surgery, delirium, and paranoia. She was maintained on IV fluids but had little meaningful protein or caloric intake. Her incision suffered, growing. With the assistance of the certified wound, ostomy, and continence nurses, the surgical team decided to move away from wet to moist dressing changes to NPWT with instillation and dwell (NPWTi-d) (**Figs. 14** and **15**). The settings were 24 mL of pure hypochlorous acid (pHA) instilled into the foam dressing, dwell for 10 min, then turn on NPWT at −125mmHG every 2 h. This option allows the instilling of a cleansing solution into the wound cyclically, then removing the instillation, debris, and exudate in a controlled environment via a negative pressure pump. Studies show that this therapy can decrease the LOS and the number of procedures needed, and when used early, it can lead to fewer readmissions.[40]

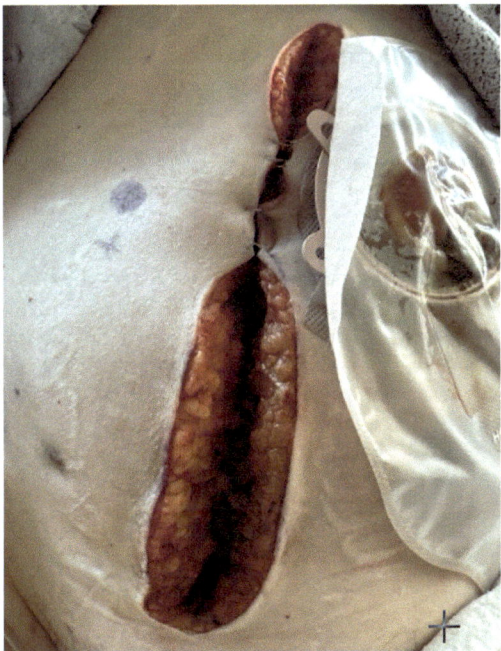

**Fig. 13.** Open incision.

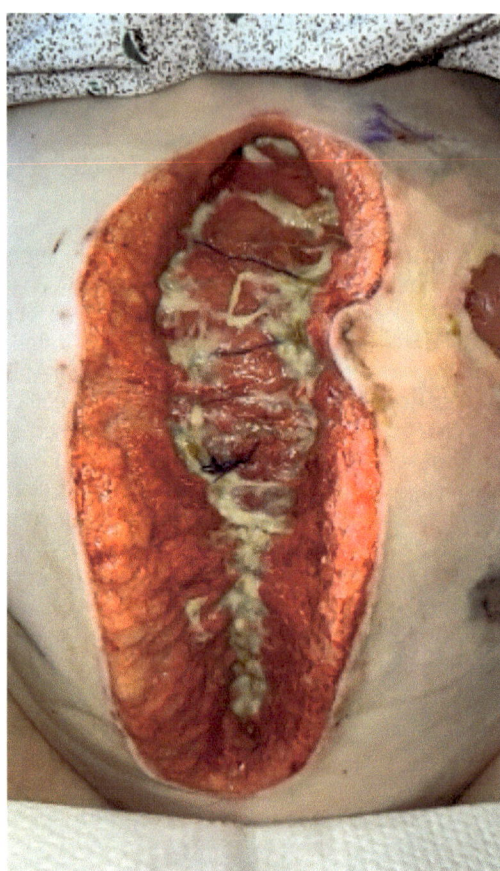

**Fig. 14.** Open incision after 11 days of wet to moist dressing changes.

The patient recovered from her acute illness but was discharged to an acute rehabilitation on NPWT, then home 43 d after her surgery (**Fig. 16**).

### Discussion

Surgical procedures, planned or unplanned, are a significant burden on today's health care system. Complications do arise in a small percentage of these, and it is important that nursing staff must be aware of early signs of surgical site complications. Common signs of infection in the surgical site include purulent drainage, spontaneous dehiscence of the wound, pain/tenderness, fever greater than 38 °C, localized edema, erythema, and presence of heat.[41]

### INFECTIOUS WOUNDS

Some wounds are unrelated to one underlying disease process or procedure but rather a bacterial or fungal invasion. When I was taught about necrotizing soft tissue infections (NSTIs) in school in 2001, they were considered extremely rare. The latest estimation is that 0.3 to 15 cases per 100,000 persons will get an NSTI.[42] Even this is considered an underestimation of the actual incidence. While relatively rare, there are high mortality rates, ranging from 25% to 35%, associated with NSTI.[43]

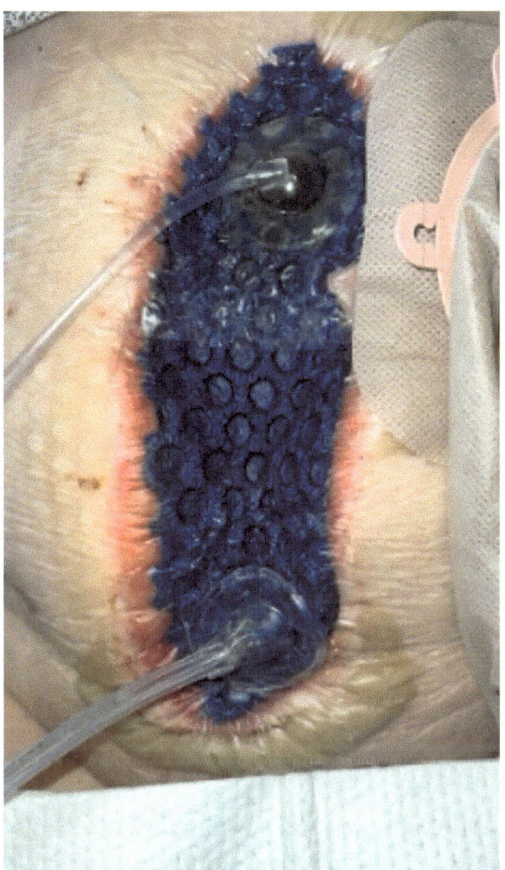

**Fig. 15.** Open incision with NPWTi-d in place.

Comorbidities that make patients at higher risk of NSTI are immunosuppression, malignancy, vascular disease, diabetes, alcoholism, and obesity. NSTI can quickly progress to sepsis and septic shock, which is why rapid diagnosis and treatment are the keys to preventing morbidity and mortality. While signs and symptoms can be vague, traditional symptoms are flu-like symptoms with a wound with extreme pain, dishwater drainage, or tissue necrosis. A thorough skin examination is crucial for early detection, particularly in diabetics who may have neuropathy that can inhibit self-reporting of pain.[43]

### Etiology

An invasion of bacteria causes NSTIs. This is classified as polymicrobial or monomicrobial. Polymicrobial necrotizing infections will produce gas within the tissues, like gas gangrene. Typical bacteria are *Pseudomonas*, *Klebsiella*, *Clostridium*, *Aeromonas*, and *Vibrio vulnificus*. For monomicrobial infections, the common bacteria are Group A Streptococcus and methicillin-resistant *Staphylococcus aureus*.[42]

### Complications

The gold standard of treatment for NSTIs is serial debridement, which removes infected and necrotic tissue in addition to management of sepsis with IV antibiotics.

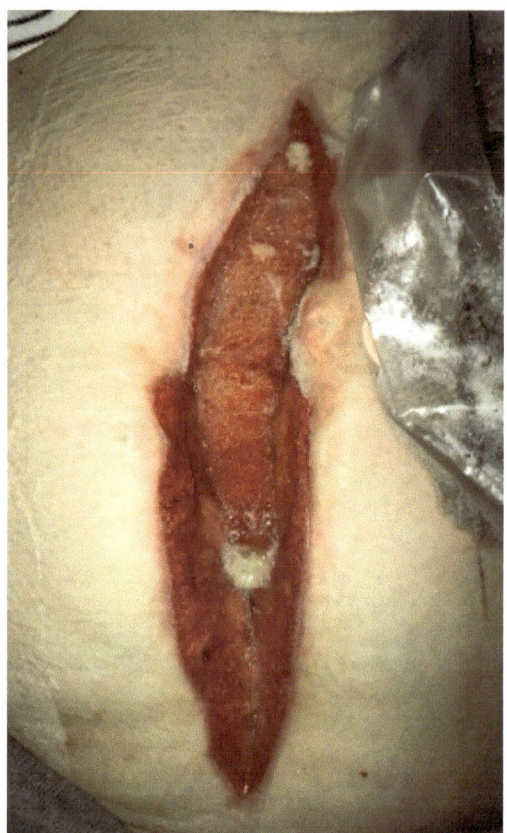

**Fig. 16.** Open incision after 1 week of NPWTi-d and 3 weeks of NPWT.

This can lead to significant soft tissue deficits. Aggressive surgical management, aggressive wound care, and staged reconstructive procedures are often required. Patients face significant debility from critical illness, extended hospitalization, and loss of soft tissue. Additionally, wound care and surgical procedures can cause considerable pain.[44]

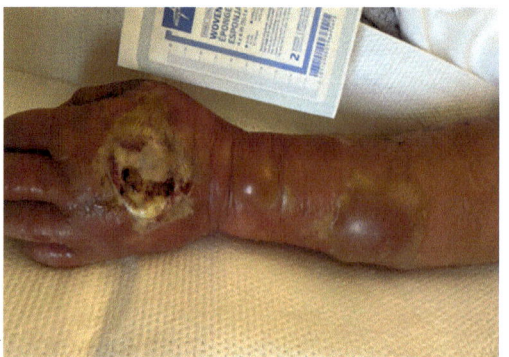

**Fig. 17.** Initial presentation of NSTI.

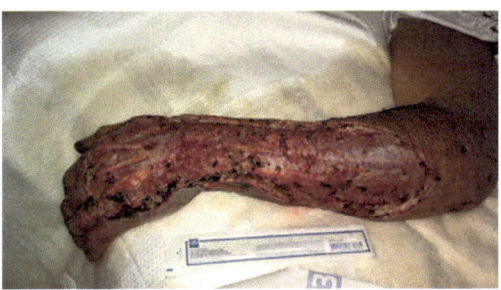

**Fig. 18.** NSTI after surgical debridement.

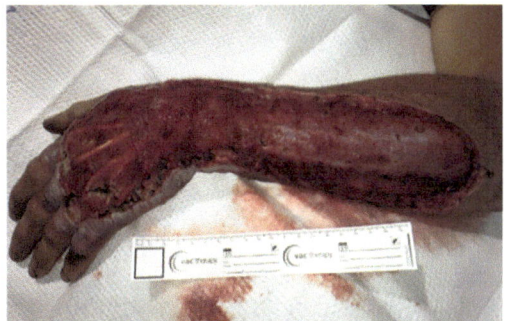

**Fig. 19.** NSTI after 4 days of NPWTI-d with pHA.

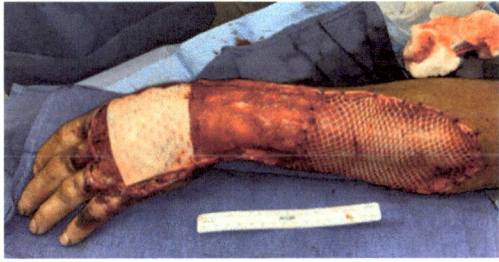

**Fig. 20.** Application of Fish Skin Xenograft to NSTI for reconstruction.

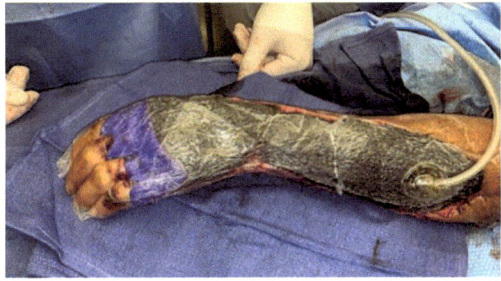

**Fig. 21.** NPWT bolster dressing over Xenograft.

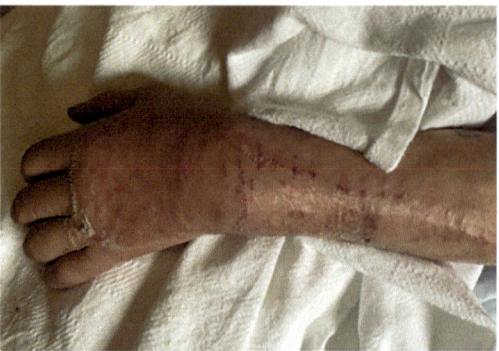

**Fig. 22.** Closed wounds from NSTI 2 months after injury.

## Case Study/Presentation

A 41-year-old male presented to the emergency room, reporting a spider bite on the left hand (**Fig. 17**). Of note, the patient has a past medical history of hypothyroidism and is homeless and living in a nearby tent encampment. After initial bloodwork and X-rays, the diagnosis of necrotizing fasciitis was made. An urgent consultation to plastic surgery was made for excisional debridement (**Fig. 18**). After this surgery, the wound was evaluated 24 h later, and the patient was transferred out of the intensive care unit, still on broad-spectrum antibiotics awaiting culture results. NPWTi-d with pHA was used to cleanse the wound and help build granulation tissue formation continually (**Fig. 19**). Ninety-two h after this therapy was started, the patient returned to the OR for a fish skin xenograft applied to the soft tissue deficit with NPWT to bolster the graft for 7 d (**Figs. 20** and **21**). After 2 more dressing changes, the patient underwent a split-thickness skin graft for definitive closure 22 d after admission. He went on to complete wound closure with minimal scarring and complete function in his hand (**Fig. 22**).

## SUMMARY

Nursing care of patients with NSTI should include aggressive wound care, sepsis symptoms management, and IV antibiotics administration. For patients admitted or in the emergency room with vague, flu-like symptoms, nurses can often recognize, and elevate a skin change that can diagnose NSTI. For patients admitted to the acute care setting, various wound types and complications can occur. Nurses are often the gatekeepers of the management of skin in the acute care space. While preventing hospital-acquired PIs is a common nursing topic, recognizing or treating skin tears, surgical site complications, and necrotizing infections are taught and discussed less frequently. Nurses must recognize that all wounds can be a source of pain, bleeding, and a portal of entry for bacteria. Open communication with the multidisciplinary team about skin and wound issues should be part of every patient's care plan. Be sure to document according to hospital policy on all wounds.

## CLINICS CARE POINTS

- Nurses are the gatekeepers of the skin and are essential to recognizing skin changes and bringing them to the attention of the healthcare team.

- Wounds can be a common cause of hospitalization.
- Patients in the acute care setting are at a higher risk for developing wounds such as moisture-associated skin damage (MASD), Pressure injuries (PI), skin tears, and surgical site complications (SSC).

## DISCLOSURE

E. Faust is a consultant for Solventum, Urgo Medical, N.A., Mediwound LTD, Molnlycke, Bruin Biometrics, Bechtel Medical, Owen & Minor, Frontier Medical Group, & Hovertech.

## REFERENCES

1. Fast facts on U.S. hospitals. AHA hospital statistics. 2024 edition 2024. Available at: https://www.aha.org/system/files/media/file/2024/01/fast-facts-on-us-hospitals-2024-20240112.pdf. [Accessed 1 May 2024].
2. Sen CK. Human wound and its burden: updated 2020 compendium of estimates. Adv Wound Care 2021;10(5):281–92.
3. Nussbaum SR, Carter MJ, Fife CE, et al. An economic evaluation of the impact, cost, and medicare policy implications of chronic nonhealing wounds. Value Health 2018;21(1):27–32.
4. Järbrink K, Ni G, Sönnergren H, et al. The humanistic and economic burden of chronic wounds: a protocol for a systematic review. Syst Rev 2017;6(1):15. Published 2017 Jan 24.
5. Mondragon N, Zito PM. Pressure Injury. In: StatPearls. Treasure Island (FL): StatPearls Publishing; 2024.
6. Chou R, Dana T, Bougatsos C, et al. Pressure ulcer risk assessment and prevention: a systematic comparative effectiveness review. Ann Intern Med 2013;159(1):28–38.
7. Lyder CH, Wang Y, Metersky M, et al. Hospital-acquired pressure ulcers: results from the national medicare patient safety monitoring system study. J Am Geriatr Soc 2012;60(9):1603–8.
8. Padula WV, Black JM, Davidson PM, et al. Adverse effects of the medicare PSI-90 hospital penalty system on revenue-neutral hospital-acquired conditions. J Patient Saf 2020;16(2):e97–102.
9. Kim P, Aribindi VK, Shui AM, et al. Risk factors for hospital-acquired pressure injury in adult critical care patients. Am J Crit Care 2022;31(1):42–50.
10. Song YP, Shen HW, Cai JY, et al. The relationship between pressure injury complication and mortality risk of older patients in follow-up: a systematic review and meta-analysis. Int Wound J 2019;16(6):1533–44.
11. NPIAP. SPIPP 2.0. NPIAP Resources. 2024. Available at: https://cdn.ymaws.com/npiap.com/resource/resmgr/s-pipp/SPIPP_2.0.FINAL.APR.2024_Wor.pdf. (Accessed 10 May 2024).
12. Vasudevan B. Venous leg ulcers: pathophysiology and classification. Indian Dermatol Online J 2014;5(3):366–70.
13. Raffetto JD, Ligi D, Maniscalco R, et al. Why venous leg ulcers have difficulty healing: overview on pathophysiology, clinical consequences, and treatment. J Clin Med 2020;10(1):29. Published 2020 Dec 24.
14. Collins L, Seraj S. Diagnosis and treatment of venous ulcers. Am Fam Physician 2010;81(8):989–96.

15. Han Y, Igawa T, Ogino K, et al. Hemosiderin deposition in lymph nodes of patients with plasma cell-type Castleman disease. J Clin Exp Hematop 2020;60(1):1–6.
16. Lim CS, Davies AH. Graduated compression stockings. CMAJ (Can Med Assoc J) 2014;186(10):E391–8.
17. Mekkes JR, Loots MA, Van Der Wal AC, et al. Causes, investigation and treatment of leg ulceration. Br J Dermatol 2003;148(3):388–401.
18. Broderick C, Pagnamenta F, Forster R. Dressings and topical agents for arterial leg ulcers. Cochrane Database Syst Rev 2020;1(1):CD001836. Published 2020 Jan 20.
19. McDermott K, Fang M, Boulton AJM, et al. Etiology, epidemiology, and disparities in the burden of diabetic foot ulcers. Diabetes Care 2023;46(1):209–21.
20. Ruke MG, Savai J. diabetic foot infection, biofilm & new management strategy. Diab Res Open Access 2019;1(1):7–22.
21. Armstrong DG, Tan T, Boulton AJM, et al. Diabetic foot ulcers: a review. JAMA 2023;330(1):62–75.
22. Holloway S, Prentice J, Samuriwo R. Preventing, assessing and treating skin tears. Nurs Stand 2023;38(10):37–45.
23. Working towards a world without skin tears. Available at: https://www.skintears.org/_files/ugd/9d080f_5c64c26040e940fcbe4279e9e5842846.pdf. [Accessed 20 May 2024].
24. International skin tear advisory panel: evidence based prediction, prevention, assessment, and management of skin tears. Available at: https://www.skintears.org/_files/ugd/9d080f_186577d4a26d417cbddde74098280af9.pdf. [Accessed 20 May 2024].
25. LeBlanc K, Campbell KE, Wood E, et al. Best practice recommendations for prevention and management of skin tears in aged skin: an overview. J Wound Ostomy Continence Nurs 2018;45(6):540–2.
26. Serra R, Ielapi N, Barbetta A, et al. Skin tears and risk factors assessment: a systematic review on evidence-based medicine. Int Wound J 2018;15(1):38–42.
27. Chou SP, Yen YH, Tseng YT, et al. Multi-disciplinary management of type 1 and 2 skin tears using a silver-based hydrofiber dressing. Medicine (Baltim) 2023;102(37):e35112.
28. McNichol L, Lund C, Rosen T, et al. Medical adhesives and patient safety: state of the science: consensus statements for the assessment, prevention, and treatment of adhesive-related skin injuries. J Wound Ostomy Continence Nurs 2013;40(4):365-E2.
29. Yang Y, Liu H, He M, et al. Multivariate analysis of medical adhesive-related skin injury at the site of peripherally inserted central catheter insertion in cancer patients: a prospective cohort study. J Vasc Access 2023. Published online August 17, 2023.
30. Gefen A, Alves P, Beeckman D, et al. Mechanical and contact characteristics of foam materials within wound dressings: theoretical and practical considerations in treatment. Int Wound J 2023;20(6):1960–78.
31. Fumarola S, Allaway R, Callaghan R, et al. Overlooked and underestimated: medical adhesive-related skin injuries. J Wound Care 2020;29(Sup3c):S1–24.
32. Woo KY, Beeckman D, Chakravarthy D. Management of moisture-associated skin damage: a scoping review. Adv Skin Wound Care 2017;30(11):494–501.
33. Dissemond J, Assenheimer B, Gerber V, et al. Moisture-associated skin damage (MASD): a best practice recommendation from Wund-D.A.CH. J Dtsch Dermatol Ges 2021;19(6):815–25.

34. Cotterell Rnld L, Boutflower R, Copson D. Managing intertriginous dermatitis (intertrigo) with a Total Barrier Protection™ strategy. Wounds U K 2020;16(4):66–71. Available at: https://search.ebscohost.com/login.aspx?direct=true&AuthType=sso&db=ccm&AN=146962860&site=eds-live&scope=site. [Accessed 12 June 2024].
35. Glaysher MA, Cresswell AB. Management of common surgical complications. Surgery 2017;35(4):190–4.
36. European Centre for Disease Prevention and Control, Surgical site infections, In: ECDC: Annual epidemiological report for 2016, 2018, ECDC; Stockholm. Available at: https://www.ecdc.europa.eu/sites/default/files/documents/AER_for_2016-SSI.pdf (Accessed 3 June 2024).
37. Willy C, Agarwal A, Andersen CA, et al. Closed incision negative pressure therapy: international multidisciplinary consensus recommendations. Int Wound J 2017;14(2):385–98.
38. User Guide for the 2012 ACS NSQIP Participant. American College of Surgeons. National surgical quality improvement program. Use data file. 2013. Available at: https://www.facs.org/media/kanfv4dl/ug12.pdf. [Accessed 4 June 2024].
39. Yin V, Cobb JP, Wightman SC, et al, Centers for Disease Control (CDC). Wound classification is prognostic of 30-day readmission following surgery. World J Surg 2023;47(10):2392–400.
40. Gabriel A, Camardo M, O'Rorke E, et al. Effects of negative-pressure wound therapy with instillation versus standard of care in multiple wound types: systematic literature review and meta-analysis. Plast Reconstr Surg 2021;147(1S-1):68S–76S.
41. Copanitsanou P. Recognising and preventing surgical site infection after orthopaedic surgery. Int J Orthop Trauma Nurs 2020;37:100751.
42. Stevens DL, Bryant AE. Necrotizing soft-tissue infections. N Engl J Med 2017;377(23):2253–65.
43. Chen LL, Fasolka B, Treacy C. Necrotizing fasciitis: a comprehensive review. Nursing 2020;50(9):34–40.
44. Stevens DL, Bisno AL, Chambers HF, et al. Practice guidelines for the diagnosis and management of skin and soft tissue infections: 2014 update by the Infectious Diseases Society of America. Clin Infect Dis 2015;60(9):1448 [published correction appears in.

# Wound Care in Children and Adolescents

Charleen Singh, PhD, MBA, MSN/ED, FNP-BC, CWOCN, WOCNF, CNE, RN[a,b,*],
Lisa Gray, DNP, FNP-BC, RN[b], Zyrene Marsh, DNP, FNP-BC, RN[b]

## KEYWORDS

- Pediatric wound care • Pediatric skin integrity • Dressing selection
- Product selection

## KEY POINTS

- Pediatric wound care utilizing a multidisciplinary team to provide patient-family-centered care and advanced dressings is recommended as the best practice to improve patient satisfaction and outcomes.
- Advanced dressings with non-traumatic silicone adhesion bordered flexible foam allow longer wear time, increase comfort, and promote moist wound healing without burdening the child or family.
- Understanding the pediatric patient and family's barriers to receiving therapeutic wound care is essential in developing the plan of care.
- Collaboration amongst wound care specialists promotes professional practice, scholarly inquiry, and support for each other's practice.

## INTRODUCTION

This article aims to provide an overview of pediatric wound care management and skin maintenance. In this ever-changing health care landscape, not only has the complexity of pediatric conditions increased, but so has the complexity of wounds.[1-3] Clinicians around the globe face similar challenges related to few pediatric-trained wound care clinicians, wound care clinicians specializing in adults tasked to treat pediatric populations, and limited access to appropriate supplies.[1-3] Wound care that is not sensitive to pediatrics can scare the child, appear harmful and confusing, disengage the child and family so that they feel something is being done to them, and perhaps be punitive.[4] Building a therapeutic relationship with the child and family is crucial to foster the healing process.[4] Building a therapeutic relationship requires listening to the child and family and incorporating growth and development concepts into the care plan.

[a] DNP-FNP Program, Betty Irene Moore School of Nursing, University of California Davis, Davis, CA, USA; [b] Betty Irene Moore School of Nursing, University of California Davis, Davis Betty Irene Moore Hall, 2570 48th Street, Sacramento, CA 95817, USA
* Corresponding author. Betty Irene Moore Hall, 2570 48th Street, Sacramento, CA 95817.
*E-mail address:* cdsingh@ucdavis.edu

Nurs Clin N Am 60 (2025) 49–56
https://doi.org/10.1016/j.cnur.2024.07.013    **nursing.theclinics.com**
0029-6465/25/© 2024 Elsevier Inc. All rights reserved, including those for text and data mining, AI training, and similar technologies.

The need for increased knowledge and awareness of pediatric wound care management persists.[1–4] As more is understood about the impacts of stress and wound healing, traumatic events in childhood, it becomes increasingly important to provide therapeutic wound care. Pediatric wound care management requires understanding childhood development and incorporating the development theory into the care plan.[4] Pediatric patients who require wound care need their social and home life incorporated into the care plan to ensure patient and family-centered care.[4] A plan of care minimizes the need for dressing changes; a more extended time between dressing changes with few steps is ideal. Like adult wound care theory, pediatric wound care includes the identification of the etiology of the wound and differentiating if the wound is the primary disease process or a secondary presentation of a disease, which requires a multisystem management approach. For example, as inflammatory bowel disease rates among children increase globally, we can anticipate an increasing incidence of pyoderma gangrenosum, which requires early identification and an appropriate treatment plan but is hard to diagnose.[5] Asthma is another complex pediatric condition with increasing global prevalence rates that often presents complex wounds related to difficult-to-manage atopic dermatitis.[6]

## THE CURRENT LANDSCAPE OF HEALTH CARE

In general, wound care needs in pediatrics range from traumatic wounds such as abrasions to complex wounds related to complex disease processes such as the graft versus host or burns. In pediatrics, a few categories of dressings can be used across the age spectrum while addressing a variety of etiologies of wounds. Using advanced dressing, clinicians can provide safe, effective, efficient, evidence-based care. The dressings listed in **Table 1** are ideal because they minimize pain and frequency of dressing changes while promoting the child's and family's independence.[4]

Following the wound care concepts, pediatric wound healing is based on moist wound healing theory. Applying the theory of wound healing in pediatrics includes differentiating between healthy wound bed tissue and non-viable tissue that would benefit from autolytic, conservative sharp wound debridement, or surgical debridement.[4] Early response to non-viable tissue is essential in facilitating wound healing. Early identification of infection that prevents the wound from moving out of the inflammatory phase with appropriate systemic and topical treatment shortens healing time (see **Table 1**). Maintaining a moist wound environment while keeping the edges open promotes wound healing by facilitating granulation and epithelization.

With advanced wound care products that are globally available, novice pediatric wound care clinicians can provide safe, effective, efficient, evidence-based care with a small formulary of products. Creating a plan of care that incorporates patient-centered pain-free dressing is possible by using a combination of bordered foam with silicone adhesion with either medical-grade honey or ionic silver for pediatric and neonatal patients.

Maintaining skin integrity for critically ill pediatric and neonatal patients requires evidence-based products that reduce or redistribute pressure over bony prominences. Reducing pressure by redistribution is achieved by placing five-layered bordered foam with silicone adhesion over bony prominences, changing the resting position of patient and devices every 2 to 4 hours, off-loading pressure using fluidized air positioner, and pressure redistributing surfaces.[7–12] (see **Table 1**) Essential to wound healing and pressure injury prevention is clean, dry skin with skin pH balanced between 4 and 6. Using products that maintain a skin pH between 4 and 6, moisturizing with a product that is both an emollient and humectant, such as dimethicone

**Table 1**
**Dressing types and use**

| Wound Type | Product Category | Use/Mechanism |
|---|---|---|
| Partial thickness/Full thickness/Intact skin over boney prominences | Bordered foam with silicone adhesion | Primary or secondary dressing; silicone non-traumatic adhesion, flexible, ideal wear time 5–7 d. Pressure injury prevention over a bony prominence or under devices. |
| Partial thickness/Full thickness | Medical grade honey | Use as a direct layer on the wound bed. Multipurpose antimicrobial stimulates healing by osmotic properties to pull fluid to the wound bed. Available as gel or calcium alginate applied during a dressing change, the wound fully absorbs calcium alginate preparation during autolytic debriding. |
| Partial thickness/Full thickness | Ionic silver is incorporated in foam alginate or hydrofiber. | Antimicrobial used for limited periods: 2 wk or less. Used as a primary dressing for shallow wounds or a primary dressing with a secondary dressing for full-thickness wounds. |
| Full-thickness wound with heavy exudate | Negative pressure dressing with contact layer | Negative pressure at a low 50–75 mm Hg setting promotes cellular proliferation and migration while maintaining a moist wound-healing environment. |
| Intact Skin Medical Adhesive Skin Injury Prevention | Elastic barrier strip cut to fit under adhesive securement | Used under adhesive that requires frequent changes or adhesive that can cause skin damage, such as NG/ET securement. |
| Moisture Maceration/Incontinence dermatitis/Candida | Prevention with barrier ointment petrolatum >70%, or dimethicone 6% Treatment with Zinc ointment. Miconazole 2% | Barrier ointment with petrolatum >70% applied as a thin layer with each diaper change prevents skin irritation/breakdown. Once the epidermis layer is damaged, treatment with zinc-based ointment is required, with an increased frequency of diaper changes. Early identification of macular-papular rashes associated with candida infection treated with miconazole 2% commercially prepared with petrolatum. |

(continued on next page)

**Table 1**
*(continued)*

| Wound Type | Product Category | Use/Mechanism |
|---|---|---|
| Moisture-associated skin breakdown around tubes, lines, drains, and skin folds | Acrylate Terpolymer, moisture-wicking fabric, moisture-transferring thin foam, bordered foam cut to fit around the tube | Protects the epidermis from oversaturation and wicks moisture away from the epidermis. The epidermis is protected from drainage related to tubes, lines, or drains. Bordered foam with silicone adhesion provides stability to the tube, preventing skin/track breakdown. |
| Pressure injury prevention support surface | Fluidized air positioner, Pressure redistribution mattress, Pediatric low-air loss mattress | Isolates and overhead warmers require pressure redistribution mattresses and fluidized air positioners to offload pressure effectively. |

6%, and wicking or protecting the skin from excessive moisture promotes skin integrity.[13,14]

## WOUND CARE LEADERSHIP AND MULTIDISCIPLINARY TEAMWORK

Pediatric clinicians should engage in wound care education, translate existing knowledge to pediatric wound care, and engage in specific pediatric research, translational science, and policy development.[15–17] Wound care leadership requires a multidisciplinary approach to meet the pediatric population's needs. To best meet the child's needs, a multidisciplinary approach is ideal.[15–17] A multidisciplinary team includes the primary provider, physical and occupational therapist, child life specialist, wound care clinician, and social services. The interdisciplinary team approach identifies barriers to care for and supports the family in overcoming barriers. Barriers to care can include transportation, family members' constraints with time off work to care for the child, or meeting clinic appointments; for families who live a distance away from pediatric centers benefit from a multidisciplinary approach for wound care by providing multiple services at one visit.

## BENEFIT OF COLLABORATION

Collaboration in pediatric wound care has many benefits. The benefits range from meeting the child and family's needs in one visit to involving the specialty service having an established relationship with the child and family.[1,15–17] The multidisciplinary approach can also include a multiplatform approach, with some practitioners being in person while others may attend the visit using video teleconference. Pediatric populations experiencing neurodevelopment or neurocognitive conditions benefit from incorporating practitioners who can guide them on how best to communicate with the child. Children who process the environment differently find the dressing change process frightening and overwhelming and benefit from clinicians who can facilitate the care. Children who require frequent or lengthy hospitalizations benefit from child life engagement to avoid the dressing change experience as punitive or harmful.

## HOW TO COLLABORATE

Collaboration begins with a culture of the child at the center of the care plan.[1,15–18] Policy and procedures guide the collaborative care approach. Collaboration is sometimes formal or informal, depending on the situation. Collaboration involves the primary team, ideally a surgical specialty representative, wound care practitioner, child life, social services, and physical or occupational therapy.[17,18] Collaboration should consider the practitioners in the community. For example, primary care providers in the community should be incorporated, and a representative from where the child spends most of his or her time, such as school or daycare. Each team member provides insight from their respective specialties to develop a holistic care plan.[2]

## PROFESSIONAL ORGANIZATIONS

Pediatric wound care specialists must be members of professional organizations that are related to pediatrics and wound care.[19] Given the limited number of pediatric wound care specialists, the professional organization provides an opportunity to connect with other pediatric wound care specialists.[18,19] For pediatric wound care specialists belonging to a professional organization, it is an opportunity for other wound care specialists to connect with pediatric wound care clinicians. Professional organizations connect clinicians and disseminate knowledge while providing an avenue for inquiry and scholarship.

## CHALLENGES

There are several challenges facing pediatrics. The first of the several includes limited access to wound care training across the globe.[20–23] Clinicians trained in wound care are limited and even more limited in pediatrics. Compounding this challenge is that more children than ever are displaced. There are an estimated 50 million children globally that are displaced, which means no infrastructure for preventative health care or treatment.[18–21] Supply limitations, including access to clean water and follow-up, especially challenge clinicians at the front lines in wound care for children. With an estimated 12 million refugee children with limited access to care, there is a foreseeable crisis related to the health of children in general.[20]

## FUTURE OF WOUND CARE

The future of wound care in pediatrics requires a greater understanding of wound healing and the impact of pediatric conditions on wound healing.[22–25] Increasing is the understanding of stress and its impact on general health and wound healing. Globally, clinicians are identifying increasing rates of wounds resistant to cephalexin or presenting with multidrug-resistant bacteria, which suggests early, and appropriate wound care treatment plans are crucial for wound healing and preventing negative sequelae. Consensus on treatment plans and policies for approaching pediatric wound care management is another area for development. Recognizing that wounds and pressure injuries require different prevention, treatment, and management approaches is a crucial element of policy development. Given the dearth of pediatric wound care literature, as well as ongoing research in pediatric wound care.

## TECHNOLOGIES

Technological advances in dressings support a therapeutic healing environment while minimizing discomfort and cost.[26] Newer negative pressure therapy dressing options are smaller and lighter with dressing interfaces that utilize silicone dressing, which decreases the discomfort associated with both the therapy and dressing changes. Newer technology incorporated into the dressing requires less frequent dressing changes, which requires few clinic visits or facilitates care at home and is supported with telehealth.[27,28] Telehealth can support children and families in several different formats, minimizing the burden of traveling to a clinic to utilize a pediatric wound care specialist.[26–28]

## SOCIAL MEDIA AND ARTIFICIAL INTELLIGENCE

Social media and artificial intelligence (AI) can help overcome the barriers to access to pediatric wound care. Social media is one platform that can connect clinicians and clinicians to families. Globally, 62.3% of the world's population utilizes social media, which presents a platform for pediatric wound care specialists to support children with wound care needs.[28] The future of AI in pediatric wound care ranges from early detection of infection in a wound bed with smart dressings to support etiology identification or clinical decisions. For social media and AI engagement in pediatric wound care management more research is required before meaningful use.

## SUMMARY

Pediatric wound care requires a multidisciplinary and interdisciplinary approach to facilitate family and child engagement related to wound healing. Treatment plans for wound care should incorporate the principles of pediatric development to support the child's growth and development during wound healing. Dressing and treatment approaches require evidence-based wound care and identifying and addressing etiology. Incorporating technology in the treatment plan, such as virtual visits, increases engagement and improves access to wound care clinicians.

## CLINICS CARE POINTS

---

- Advanced dressings such as bordered foam with Safetac technology and medical grade honey minimize the frequency of dressing changes, decrease discomfort, improve healing rates and overall satisfaction.

---

## DISCLOSURE

All authors have no financial disclosures to report and have no conflicts of interest.

## REFERENCES

1. Katkin JP, Kressly SJ, Edwards AR, et al. Task Force on Pediatric Practice Change. Guiding principles for team-based pediatric care. Houston, TX: Pediatric Telehealth Best Practices; 2022. p. 43–173.
2. Boland L, Graham ID, Légaré F, et al. Barriers and facilitators of pediatric shared decision-making: a systematic review. Implement Sci 2019;14:1–25.
3. McNamara SA, Hirt PA, Weigelt MA, et al. Traditional and advanced therapeutic modalities for wounds in the paediatric population: an evidence-based review. J Wound Care 2020;29(6):321–34.
4. Singh C. Skin and wound care for neonatal and pediatric publications. In: McNichol L, Ratliff C, Yates S, editors. Wound, ostomy and continence nurses society core curriculum: Wound management. Philadelphia, PA: Lippincott Williams & Wilkins; 2021. p. 233–55.
5. Kuenzig ME, Fung SG, Marderfeld L, et al. Twenty-first century trends in the global epidemiology of pediatric-onset inflammatory bowel disease: systematic review. Gastroenterology 2022;162(4):1147–59, diseases increasing amongst pediatrics - Google Scholar.
6. Engelkes M, Baan EJ, de Ridder MA, et al. Incidence, risk factors and re-exacerbation rate of severe asthma exacerbations in a multinational, multidatabase pediatric cohort study. Pediatr Allergy Immunol 2020;31(5):496–505.
7. Jackson JE, Kirkland-Kyhn H, Kenny L, et al. Reducing hospital-acquired pressure injuries among pediatric patients receiving ECMO: a retrospective study examining quality improvement outcomes. Wound Manag Prev 2021;67(9): 14–24.
8. Jackson JE, Kirkland-Kyhn H, Kenny L, et al. Reduction in hospital associated pressure injuries for pediatric Extracorporeal Membrane Oxygenation patients with provider education, Pediatrics, 2021, 147 (3_MeetingAbstract): 468. https://doi.org/10.1542/peds.147.3MA5.468b
9. Gefen A. The aetiology of medical device-related pressure ulcers and how to prevent them. Br J Nurs 2021;30(15):S24–30.

10. Singh CD. Use of a moisture wicking fabric for prevention of skin damage around drains and parenteral access lines. J Wound, Ostomy Cont Nurs 2016;43(5):551–3.
11. Singh CD, Anderson C, White E, et al. The impact of pediatric pressure injury prevention bundle on pediatric pressure injury rates: a secondary analysis. J Wound, Ostomy Cont Nurs 2018;45(3):209–12.
12. Singh CD, Shoqirat N. Pressure redistribution crib mattress: A quality improvement project. J Wound, Ostomy Cont Nurs 2019;46(1):62–4.
13. Chaudhary DK, Pokhrel P, Shrestha A, et al. Bacteriological Profile and Antibiotic Susceptibility Pattern of Wound Infection in Children. EC Microbiol 2017;5(3): 93–100. ECMI-05-0000137.pdf ecronicon.net.
14. Blaak J, Staib P. The relation of pH and skin cleansing. pH of the skin: issues and Challenges. Curr Probl Dermatol 2018;54:132–42.
15. Foster M, Whitehead L, Maybee P. The parents', hospitalized child's, and health care providers' perceptions and experiences of family-centered care within a pediatric critical care setting: A synthesis of quantitative research. J Fam Nurs 2016;22(1):6–73.
16. Brannon GE, Ray MR, Lark P, et al. Influence of pediatric patients' developmental or chronic health condition status as a predictor of parents' perceptions of patient-and family-centered care. Health Commun 2022;37(7):880–8.
17. Krasnosky R, Barton G, Highfield L, et al. Pediatric wound care: Establishing a consensus group to develop clinical practice guidelines. J Nurs Interprofessional Leadersh Qual Saf 2020;3(1):2.
18. Majchrzak K, Bobbink P, Probst S. Survey of physicians' and nurses' needs and expectations regarding a multidisciplinary wound clinic. J Wound Manag Res 2021;22(3):21–30.
19. McDowell B.M., Blending family-centered care and the Neuman Systems Model in caring for children experiencing traumatic stress, 2020. Available at: http://hdl. handle.net/10755/19330. Accessed May 6, 2024.
20. Hazer L, Gredebäck G. The effects of war, displacement, and trauma on child development. Humanit soc sci commun 2023;10(1):1–19.
21. Aguilar P, Heusser P. The Geneva Global Hub for Education in Emergencies: A new ally for education in emergencies. Prospects 2023;53(1):3–13.
22. Cuadrado C, Libuy M, Moreno-Serra R. What is the impact of forced displacement on health? A scoping review. Health Pol Plann 2023;38(3):394–408.
23. Väyrynen, R. (2023). Complex humanitarian emergencies: Concepts and issues. Raimo Väyrynen: a Pioneer in International Relations, scholarship and policymaking: with a foreword by olli rehn and a preface by Allan Rosas, 301-343.
24. Hao M, Sun J. Nursing intervention of children's lower limb chronic wound healing under artificial intelligence. IEEE Access 2023;11:141090–9. https://doi.org/10. 1109/ACCESS.2023.3335192.
25. Berg L, Martinez JL, Serena TE, et al. Meeting report: promoting wound healing by optimising dressing change frequency. Int Wound J 2019;10(3):44–51.
26. Alrimy T, Alhalabi W, Malibari A, et al. Desktop virtual reality offers a novel approach to minimize pain and anxiety during burn wound cleaning/debridement in infants and young children: a randomized crossover pilot study. J Clin Med 2023;12(15):4985.
27. Keegan AC, Bose S, McDermott KM, et al. Implementation of a patient-centered remote wound monitoring system for management of diabetic foot ulcers. Front Endocrinol 2023;14:1157518.
28. Aichner T, Grünfelder M, Maurer O, et al. Twenty-five years of social media: a review of social media applications and definitions from 1994 to 2019. Cyberpsychol, Behav Soc Netw 2021;24(4):215–22.

# Updates in Arterial Ulcers

Karen L. Bauer, DNP, APRN-FNP, CWS, FAAWC[a], Ahmed M. Afifi, MD[a],
Munier Nazzal, MD, MBA, MEd[b],*

## KEYWORDS

- Arterial ulcer • Peripheral artery disease • Ischemic ulcer
- Critical limb threatening ischemia • Nonhealing ulcer

## KEY POINTS

- Arterial ulceration is most often secondary to critical limb-threatening ischemia, which is the terminal stage of peripheral artery disease. Still, it is also essential to recognize a concomitant arterial component in other lower extremity ulcers.
- The main management principle is establishing in-line flow to the foot or ulcerate area using endovascular therapy or open revascularization.
- The goal of wound management in arterial ulcers before revascularization is to reduce the risk of infection and progression by keeping the area clean and dry and utilizing goal-directed medical therapy to optimize host factors.
- Wound management tactics in arterial ulcers after revascularization are similar to those in other wound types.
- Chronic limb-threatening ischemia disproportionately affects non-white populations. Thus, community awareness and public health efforts are crucial to promote early recognition of peripheral artery disease risk factors and symptoms.

## INTRODUCTION

Arterial ulcers, a complex interplay of various etiologic factors, represent a significant global health burden. Leg ulcers affect 0.12% to 1.8% of adults, with higher prevalence in those aged 65 and older **Fig. 1**.[1] Venous disease is the most common cause, but arterial disease accounts for about 22% of leg ulcer cases.[2] Arterial ulcers result from insufficient blood supply due to arterial narrowing or obstruction, with contributors like hypertension, diabetes, and hyperlipidemia.[3] Peripheral arterial disease (PAD) significantly contributes to lower extremity arterial ulcers. The prevalence of PAD increased by 72.5% from 1990 to 2019, reaching 113,443,017 cases.[4–6] PAD prevalence is higher in black patients and lower in Asian patients compared to white

[a] Division of Vascular, Endovascular and Wound Surgery, University of Toledo, Mail Stop 1095, 3000 Arlington Avenue, Toledo, OH 43614-2598, USA; [b] Division of Vascular, Endovascular, and Wound Surgery, Department of Surgery and Medical Education, University of Toledo, Mail Stop 1095, 3000 Arlington Avenue, Toledo, OH 43614-2598, USA
* Corresponding author. Department of Surgery, The University of Toledo, 3000 Arlington Avenue, Mail Stop 1095, Toledo, OH 43614.
*E-mail address:* Karen.Bauer@utoledo.edu

Nurs Clin N Am 60 (2025) 57–75
https://doi.org/10.1016/j.cnur.2024.08.003 **nursing.theclinics.com**

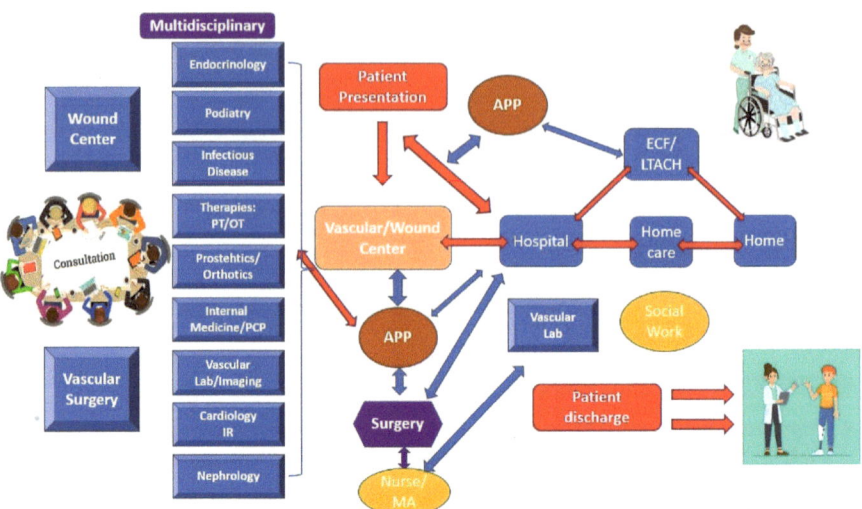

**Fig. 1.** Schematic of suggested services and interactions at chronic limb-threatening ischemia-dedicated centers. Legend: APP, Advanced Practice Provider; ECF, Extended Care Facility; IR, Interventional Radiology; LTACH, Long-Term Acute Care Hospital; MA, Medical Assistant; PT, Physical Therapy; OT, Occupational Therapy; PCP, Primary Care Provider.

patients, with diabetic black patients showing a 25.3% rate.[7] Mild-to-moderate chronic kidney disease also raises PAD risk.[6] Genetic factors account for about 21% of ankle brachial index (ABI) variability, indicating higher PAD risk for individuals with a family history.[7] Chronic limb-threatening ischemia (CLTI), the severe form of PAD with tissue loss or ischemic rest pain, has a 1-year incidence of 0.33% and a 2-year prevalence of 0.74%.[8] CLTI requires customized, multidisciplinary management, beginning with early diagnosis and treatment by primary care providers and clinicians. Thorough history taking, physical examination, and recognizing risk factors and symptoms are crucial for diagnosing PAD and CLTI, necessitating a comprehensive vascular evaluation.

## RESOURCES NEEDED WHEN MANAGING ARTERIAL ULCERS

Arterial ulcers and CLTI are complex, requiring coordinated, multi-disciplinary management to reduce limb loss. Management has evolved with new endovascular approaches and better understanding of PAD risk factors, infection, wound management, ischemia, and diabetes. Revascularization is the gold standard, but team-oriented vascular limb salvage services are increasingly popular, supported by expert consensus and research. This approach can reduce amputation rates, improve patient satisfaction, and optimize quality metrics.[9]

Involved specialties include endocrinology, infectious disease, internal or vascular medicine, interventionalists, and ancillary clinicians such as wound-trained advanced practice providers, nurses, physical therapists, and nutritionists. Recent guidelines emphasize the need for multidisciplinary care and developing limb salvage centers for arterial ulcer (CLTI) patients.[10,11] Obstacles to interdisciplinary management include timely access to vascular technologists and surgeons, skilled wound care clinicians, coordination among care settings, integration of services, limb salvage champions to oversee protocols, institutional support for resources, and sustainable educational tools.[9] Limb salvage services vary from basic community hospital services to comprehensive centers of excellence at academic hospitals. These centers are new and varied, with limited high-quality research on outcomes, mostly focusing on diabetic patients.[12,13] While multidisciplinary centers can lower amputation rates, their impact on mortality rates is unclear. Future research with clear definitions of limb-salvage services and outcomes is needed.[9]

### Clinical Presentation/Description of Ischemic Ulcers

Arterial ulcers account for about 15% of all leg ulcers.[10] They are caused by reduced blood flow, usually from PAD. Chronic limb ischemia is characterized by ischemic rest pain, nocturnal recumbent pain, or ischemic skin lesions lasting more than 2 weeks, including ulcers or gangrene, indicating end-stage PAD (10). This differs from acute limb ischemia, which presents acutely with pain, pulse deficit, poikilothermia, paralysis, pulselessness, and pallor, requiring surgical emergency. Recognizing an arterial component in other leg ulcer presentations, especially in diabetic patients, venous leg ulcers, atypical lower extremity (LE) ulcers, or LE pressure ulcers, is essential.

### Characteristics of ischemic ulcers

Purely arterial ulcers are typically found on the distal leg, especially the lateral malleolus, dorsal foot, and toes. They appear pale, dry, and "punched out" but can also present as wet or dry gangrene. Arterial ulcers are usually painful. Physical examination may reveal diminished or absent pedal pulses, dependent rubor, and surrounding pallor, cyanosis, or mottling. See **Fig. 2** for an image of an ischemic ulcer.

### Presentation in mixed etiology

A thorough history and physical examination are crucial to assessing any ulcer. Establishing a differential diagnosis and identifying primary and secondary factors in lower extremity (LE) ulcerations is crucial, as multiple etiologies may be involved.[12] Chronic venous insufficiency accounts for about 70% of leg ulcers, and up to 25% of lower leg ulcers have arteriovenous components.[14] Mixed-etiology ulcers may present with cool extremities, shiny, cracked, pale, dry, inelastic skin, sluggish capillary refill, and weak pedal pulses. These ulcers may improve slowly, worsen rapidly, or be more painful than non-arterial ulcers. Identifying and addressing risk factors, physical examination findings, and ulcer characteristics consistent with PAD or CLTI is essential.

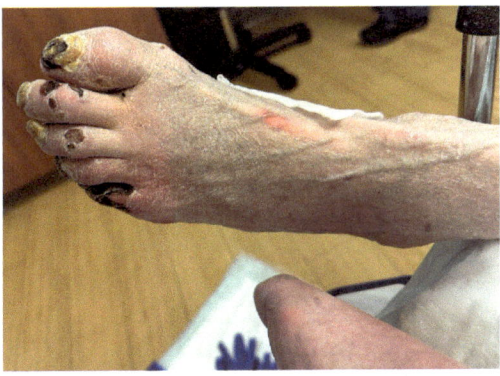

**Fig. 2.** Foot with arterial ulcers.

### Atypical and small vessel arterial ulcers

Conditions like diabetic angiopathy, embolism, Buerger's disorder, and vasospastic conditions such as Raynaud's disorder also show ischemic components and can worsen LE ulcers or present independently. Clinicians must differentiate these conditions and recognize that these patients often have good proximal blood flow with palpable larger arteries. Small vessel or vasospasm-related tissue loss usually occurs on the distal toes. It may be accompanied by pain induced by stress, cold, stimulants, friction, or activity and exacerbated by infection, inflammation, or systemic illness.[12] See **Table 1** for differential diagnosis in LE arterial ulcers.

## CLASSIFICATION SYSTEMS AND THEIR APPLICATION

Many classification systems exist to distinguish PAD severity. Pure arterial ulceration represents end-stage PAD but requires standardized grading for objective decision-making. The first classification system, developed by the European Society of Cardiovascular Surgery in 1952 and published by Fontaine and colleagues in 1954, has 4 stages and is primarily used for research.[15] The Rutherford Classification for chronic limb ischemia, devised in 1986 and revised in 1987, is frequently used for standardized PAD classification.[16] Patients with pure arterial ulceration fall into categories 5 and 6 of this classification. The system classifies patients with LE ulcers of other etiologies but

**Table 1**
**Differential diagnosis and associated factors**

| Differential Diagnosis | Cormorbid Conditions |
|---|---|
| Large-vessel disease:<br>　Acute arterial thrombosis<br>　Atherothrombotic disease (PAOD) | Vasculitis:<br>　Polyarteritis nodosa<br>　Takayasu arteritis<br>　Rheumatoid arthritis<br>　Systemic lupus erythematosus |
| Small-Vessel Disease:<br>　Thromboangitis Obliterans<br>　(Buerger's Disease)<br>　Raynaud's Phenomenon<br>　Diabetic Angiopathy | Sickle Cell<br>Polycythemia Vera |
| Embolization:<br>　Septic Emboli<br>　Cholesterol Embolization Syndrome<br>　Cardiac Embolic Source<br>　Arterio-arterial thrombo/atheroemboli<br>　Iatrogenic | Vasopressor-Induced Skin Necrosis |
| Vascular Access-Induced Steal Syndrome | Calciphylaxis (calcemic uremic arteriolopathy) |
| Warfarin-Induced Skin Necrosis | Chronic Venous Insufficiency |
| Necrotizing Fasciitis | Other Chronic Illnesses:<br>　Chronic Kidney Disease<br>　Hypertension<br>　Dyslipidemia<br>　Cardiovascular Disease<br>　Cerebrovascular Disease<br>　Smoking |

*Abbreviation*: PAOD, peripheral arterial occlusive disease.
*Data from* Bauer KL. Differentiation of Lower Extremity Skin Changes in the Intensive Care Setting. AACN Adv Crit Care. 2022;33(2):196-207. https://doi.org/10.4037/aacnacc2022737.

an arterial component for the primary etiology, such as the Clinical-Etiology-Anatomy-Pathophysiology (CEAP) classification in chronic venous disease. The WiFi classification system, developed by the Society for Vascular Surgery and published by Dr Joseph Mills and colleagues in 2014, addresses patients with concurrent diabetes and PAD/CLTI, providing a detailed analysis and estimating the risk of amputation and the benefit of revascularization.[16,17] See **Figs. 3** and **4** for the WiFi Classification System. Six angiomas in the lower extremity correlate to specific foot areas served by specific arteries, and selective revascularization based on vessel and wound location may improve outcomes, but further research is needed.[16] (**Table 2**).

## DIAGNOSIS OF ARTERIAL ULCERS
### Ankle-Brachial Index

The Ankle-Brachial Index (ABI), developed in 1969, compares systolic ankle and brachial pressures to study PAD. It is simple but less accurate in patients with calcified arteries, such as those with diabetes or chronic renal failure. A normal ABI (>1.0) without symptoms rules out significant PAD, but exercise studies are needed if symptoms arise during exertion. The toe-brachial index (TBI) is used for non-compressible arteries, as digital arteries usually avoid calcification and predict cardiovascular mortality in symptomatic lower-extremity artery disease.[18] Segmental pressures measure occlusive disease levels by comparing systolic pressures within the same limb and bilaterally. Pulse Volume Recording (PVR) measures arterial flow changes unaffected by calcification but is subject to intra-reader variations. ABI, PVR, and TBI remain

| Wound | | |
|---|---|---|
| Grade  Ulcer | | Gangrene |
| 0 | No ulcer | No gangrene |
| 1 | Small, shallow ulcer on distal leg or foot; no exposed bone, unless limited to distal phalanx | No gangrene |
| 2 | Deeper ulcer with exposed bone, joint, or tendon; generally not involving the heel; shallow heel ulcer, without calcaneal involvement | Gangrenous changes limited to digits |
| 3 | Extensive, deep ulcer involving forefoot and/or midfoot; deep, full-thickness heel ulcer ± calcaneal involvement | Extensive gangrene involving the forefoot/midfoot; full-thickness heel necrosis ± calcaneal involvement |

| Ischemia Grade | | | |
|---|---|---|---|
| | ABI | Ankle Systolic Pressure | TP |
| 0 | ≥0.80 | >100 mm Hg | ≥60 mm Hg |
| 1 | 0.6-0.79 | 70-100 mm Hg | 40-59 mm Hg |
| 2 | 0.4-0.59 | 50-70 mm Hg | 30-39 mm Hg |
| 3 | ≤0.39 | <50 mm Hg | <30 mm Hg |

| Infection Grade | |
|---|---|
| | Clinical Manifestation of Infection |
| 0 | No symptoms or signs of infection<br>Infection present, as defined by the presence of at least 2 of the following items:<br>• Local swelling or induration<br>• >Erythema 0.5-2 cm around the ulcer<br>• Local tenderness or pain<br>• Local warmth<br>• Purulent discharge (thick, opaque to white, or sanguineous secretion) |
| 1 | Local infection involving only the skin and the subcutaneous tissue<br>Exclude other causes of an inflammatory response of the skin (trauma, gout, acute Charcot, fracture, thrombosis, venous stasis) |
| 2 | Local infection with erythema >2 cm, or involving structures deeper than skin and subcutaneous tissues, and no systemic inflammatory response signs |
| 3 | No systemic inflammatory response signs<br>Local infection with the signs of SIRS, as manifested by 2 or more of the following:<br>• Temperature >38°C or <36°C<br>• Heart rate >90 beats/min<br>• Respiratory rate >20 breaths/min or $Paco_2$ <32 mm Hg<br>• White blood cell count >12 000/mm³ or <4000/mm³ or 10% immature bands |

Abbreviations: ABI, ankle–brachial index; TMA, transmetatarsal amputation; TP, toe pressure; SIRS, systemic inflammatory response syndrome.

**Fig. 3.** WiFi classification system.

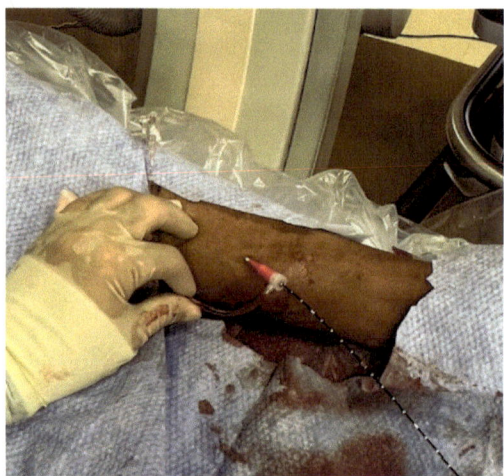

**Fig. 4.** Distal approach to anterior tibial artery.

useful for PAD diagnosis but cannot predict ulcer healing accurately. Measuring tissue oxygen around an ulcer helps predict healing, as oxygen is essential for the process.[18]

### Transcutaneous Oxygen Measurement

Transcutaneous oxygen measurement or $TcPO_2$ measures tissue oxygenation using skin electrodes near the ulcer. A saturation of more than 50 mm Hg is average, while less than 20 mm Hg suggests poor ulcer healing. $TcPO_2$ can also determine amputation levels but is influenced by external factors like temperature, probe placement, tissue edema, inflammation, and user skill. It cannot be used directly over bony prominences or the ulcer bed, and disposable probes are costly. Drawbacks include user variability, poor reproducibility, and poor correlation with healing in diabetic patients.[19]

### Hyperspectral imaging

Hyperspectral imaging captures images reflecting oxygenated tissue to produce a digital map. It records oxygen saturation in different regions of the image, correlating with PAD severity and predicting wound healing. However, its use needs more validation and widespread adoption.[20]

| Table 2<br>**Rutherford classification** | | |
|---|---|---|
| **Grade** | **Category** | **Clinical Description** |
| 0 | 0 | Asymptomatic |
|  | 1 | Mild Claudication |
| I | 2 | Moderate Claudication |
|  | 3 | Severe Claudication |
| II[a] | 4[a] | Rest Pain |
| III[a] | 5[a] | Ischemic Ulcers of Digits |
|  | 6[a] | Severe Ischemic Ulcers or Gangrene |

[a] Grades II and III, categories 4, 5, and 6 are embraced by the term chronic critical limb ischemia.
*Data from* Rutherford RB, Baker JD, Ernst C, et al. Recommended standards for reports dealing with lower extremity ischemia: revised version [published correction appears in J Vasc Surg 2001 Apr;33(4):805]. J Vasc Surg. 1997;26(3):517-538. doi:10.1016/s0741-5214(9770045-4).

### Near-Infrared Spectroscopy

Near-infrared spectroscopy measures tissue oxygen saturation by comparing oxygenated and deoxygenated hemoglobin. It is non-invasive and quick, but melanin can interfere with the reading, making it inaccurate in darker-skinned patients.[21]

### Near Infrared Fluoroscopy

This method measures perfusion in nonhealing ulcers by injecting a fluorescent dye and capturing its distribution with a special camera. Although helpful in guiding diagnosis and treatment in PAD patients, it has drawbacks like a giant, expensive camera and the need for standardization.[15] Despite many techniques for quantifying tissue perfusion, there are other gold standards. A comprehensive review of 10 techniques found they needed to be more suitable as a reference standard.[22] See **Table 3** for a summary of optical imaging modalities.

## MANAGEMENT

Management goals in CLTI include improving survival, reducing pain, closing ulcers, preventing amputation, optimizing function, and maximizing quality of life. Due to its complexity and end-stage nature, CLTI management is primarily palliative. Pharmacotherapy is used only after failed revascularization or when revascularization is not an option. Patients and caregivers must understand that arterial ulceration indicates end-stage disease.[23]

## REVASCULARIZATION IN PATIENTS WITH ISCHEMIC ULCERS

Revascularization is the cornerstone of managing arterial ulcers and can be achieved through endovascular therapy (EVT), open surgical therapy, or a hybrid approach. Advances in the endovascular field have been significant, but no technique is universally superior. Unlike patients with rest pain, arterial ulcers require restoring direct in-line flow to the foot for healing.

### Endovascular Techniques

Recent advances in endovascular therapy (EVT) have made most PAD/CLTI patients suitable for intervention. New devices improve arterial canalization, preserve patency, and minimize restenosis. However, EVT is less ideal for small vessel disease, long lesions, heavy calcification, or extreme distal disease. Disease recurrence and complications like vessel dissection can occur.

## ACCESS METHODS

- *Antegrade Approach:* Typically via the common femoral artery, preferred for its large diameter. It is often used for lower extremity interventions from the common iliac to distal calf arteries.[24]
- *Retrograde Approach:* Used when antegrade access fails. A 2019 study showed 98.6% technical success and no significant short-term complications in 97.1% of cases.[25,26] High-resolution ultrasound and arterial mapping are needed for best access points.[27]
- *Distal Access:* Via posterior tibial, anterior tibial, or pedal arteries. It can be complicated by dissection, thrombosis, and vasospasm. Combining antegrade and retrograde approaches can improve success.[27]

**Table 3**
Optical imaging modalities in arterial ulcers

| Imaging Modality | Advantages | Disadvantages |
|---|---|---|
| Hyperspectral | • Ease of use<br>• Display microvascular component | Limited depth of image |
| Thermal | • Ease of use<br>• Portable<br>• Real-time | • Limited sensitivity/specificity<br>• Limited Accuracy |
| Fluorescence | • Moderate ease of use<br>• High resolution | • needs injection of indocyanine green |
| Near-infrared spectroscopy | • Ease of Use<br>• Noninvasive<br>• Portable<br>• High Resolution | • Limited Specificity |

## ADVANCES IN ENDOVASCULAR THERAPY

- *Vessel Access:* Improved below-knee lesion access due to new wires and catheters.[28]
- *Balloons and Stents:* Specialized devices offer less traumatic recanalization and better arterial patency with fewer re-interventions. Lithoplasty energy fragments calcified arteries, improving patency when followed by drug-coated balloons are mainly used for iliac, femoral, and popliteal segments.[29] Drug-eluting stents and drug-coated balloons benefit the femoropopliteal segment, achieving patency similar to autogenous vein bypass.[30,31]

## VESSEL PREPARATION

- *Atherectomy:* Essential for removing atheromatous tissue, classified into excisional, orbital, atheroablative, and rotational types. It is often followed by drug-coated balloons or stenting. A review showed 92.3% technical success for femoropopliteal atherectomy, with complications like distal embolization (3.4%), vessel perforation (1.9%), and dissection (4%). Major amputation rates were 2.2%, with a mortality rate of 3.4%.[32] Vessel preparation in infra-popliteal artery disease showed better limb salvage with scoring balloons and mechanical atherectomy devices than plain balloon angioplasty.[33,34] (**Table 4**).

In patients without revascularization options, venous arterialization is an alternative for limb salvage, using venous circulation to heal ulcers and avoid amputation. Recently revived by endovascular techniques, a study of 105 patients showed successful deep vein arterialization in 99%, with 66.1% amputation-free survival at 6 months. Complete wound healing occurred in 25% of patients and was in progress in another 51% of patients.[35]

### Open Surgery

The complexity of PAD/CLTI management necessitates multiple intervention options. Bypassing with an autogenous vein conduit in the lower extremity offers the best results, particularly for long femoropopliteal lesions, but is invasive and unsuitable in up to 20% of cases. Two recent studies compared endovascular versus vein bypass approaches for preventing major amputation and death in chronic limb-threatening ischemia patients. The BASIL-2 trial found that endovascular techniques are the best first revascularization treatment, with better amputation-free survival (63% vein bypass vs 53%

**Table 4**
**Examples of atherectomy devices**

| Device | Type | Manufacturer |
|---|---|---|
| SilverHawk | Directional | Medtronic/Covidien |
| TurboHawk | Directional | Medtronic/Covidien |
| HawkOne | Directional | Medtronic/Covidien |
| Avinger-Pantheris | Directional | Medtronic/Covidien |
| Diamondback | Orbital | Cardiovascular Systems, Inc |
| Excimer | Laser | Spectranetics |
| Rotablator | Rotational | Boston Scientific/Scimed |
| Pathway Jetstream PV | Rotational | Boston Scientific |
| Phoenix | Rotational | Volcano Corporation |

endovascular) due to lower deaths in the endovascular group (53% vs 45%). However, reintervention was higher after endovascular procedures (19% vs 5% after vein bypass).[36] Another North American study found a lower incidence of major adverse limb events or deaths in the vein bypass group (42.6%) compared to the endovascular group (57.4%). Above-ankle amputation was higher in the endovascular group (14.9% vs 10.4%), and technical success was higher in the surgical group (98.3% vs 84.7%).[37]

### Non-Revascularization Treatments

Although revascularization is the mainstay of CLTI treatment, not all patients are candidates. Some may benefit from non-revascularization-based, non-pharmacologic therapies.[10]

### Spinal cord stimulation and lumbar sympathectomy

These procedures are believed to reduce sympathetic vasoconstriction and activate vasodilatory mechanisms to improve microcirculatory perfusion. However, no substantive data support their effectiveness, and being invasive, they are not currently recommended.[23]

## PHARMACOTHERAPY IN ARTERIAL ULCERS

More high-quality evidence regarding medical therapy in arterial ulceration must be provided due to heterogeneity in patient selection, endpoints, and intervention protocols. Adjunctive medical therapies are usually used with revascularization to improve wound healing, prevent amputation, or address atherosclerotic cardiovascular disease risk factors.[10]

### Prostanoids

Prostanoids (prostaglandin E1 and prostacyclin) inhibit platelet and leukocyte activation, promote vasodilation, and protect the endothelium. A 2018 Cochrane Review found they do not affect major amputation rates or cardiovascular mortality and provide only minor benefits in pain relief and ulcer healing, with a high risk of adverse effects.[38] Iloprost (prostacyclin) may reduce major amputation rates when combined with antibiotics in non-revascularization candidates, but studies are limited and not statistically significant. Iloprost is suggested for ulcer closure and pain management when revascularization is not possible. Shared decision-making with patients and families is essential for this therapy.

### Vasoactive Drugs

There is a lack of evidence supporting the widespread use of vasoactive drugs such as cilostazol, pentoxifylline, and naftidrofuryl in arterial ulcers. Cilostazol, the only Food and Drug Administration (FDA)-approved medication for intermittent claudication, can improve pain-free walking time in PAD patients. A 2020 meta-analysis showed potential benefits of cilostazol in amputation-free survival (HR 0.79; 95% CI 0.69–0.91), limb salvage rate (HR 0.42; 95% CI 0.27–0.66), and reduced need for repeat revascularization (RR 0.44; 95% CI 0.37–0.52), with no difference in all-cause mortality. However, its effects on wound healing have been less studied and are inconclusive.[39] Current practice guidelines report insufficient evidence that cilostazol benefits clinical outcomes in CLTI patients.[10]

### Stem Cell Therapy

Recent research has focused on stem cell therapy, primarily using bone marrow mononuclear cells delivered intramuscularly or intra-arterially. Small studies suggest potential benefits in wound healing and pain-free walking distance, but there is no conclusive evidence regarding long-term limb salvage or survival improvement.[10]

### Growth Factors

Growth factors like hepatocyte growth factor and vascular endothelial growth factor are thought to upregulate angiogenesis, potentially increasing perfusion to ischemic tissues. However, there is limited evidence, and small studies have shown no benefit in wound healing, amputation, or survival.

### Sulodexide

Sulodexide, a glycosaminoglycan composed of dermatan sulfate and fast-moving heparin, has anti-thrombotic and fibrinolytic properties, suggesting potential in arterial ulceration management. However, limited studies do not support its use in CLTI or arterial ulceration.

## GOAL-DIRECTED MEDICAL THERAPY IN PERIPHERAL ARTERY DISEASE/CHRONIC LIMB-THREATENING ISCHEMIA

Medical therapy plays a limited role in improving PAD symptoms and is not the primary treatment for arterial ulcers. CLTI is an end-stage presentation of systemic atherosclerosis and often coincides with significant atherosclerotic cardiovascular disease, leading to high mortality from myocardial infarction (MI) and stroke. While age and sex are non-modifiable risk factors, hyperlipidemia, hypertension, diabetes, smoking, and a sedentary lifestyle can be managed to reduce disease progression. Failure to address these modifiable risk factors results in poor prognosis, with a 20% to 26% mortality rate within 1 year of CLTI diagnosis.[10] The primary medical therapies for PAD include peripheral vasodilators, lipid-modifying agents, and antithrombotic agents. These should be used in a multi-modality, patient-centered framework.[40] See **Table 5** for a summary of Goal-directed medical therapy (GDMT).

### Lipid-Lowering Therapy

Systematic reviews and meta-analyses in 2020 and 2022 found that statin therapy in CLTI patients decreased amputation risk, mortality, and major adverse cardiac events (MACE) and increased overall patency rates.[41] All patients with pure arterial ulceration (CLTI) should start statin therapy, barring medical contraindications, to reduce all-cause and cardiovascular mortality.[10] PCSK9 inhibitors are a newer class of lipid-lowering agents that lower LDL levels and show promise in atherosclerotic risk modification, though they are more expensive than other cholesterol drugs.[42]

### Antithrombotic Therapy

*Antiplatelet agents:* Antiplatelet therapy benefits in PAD risk factor modification are well documented. A 2015 meta-analysis found clopidogrel monotherapy to have the best overall safety and efficacy.[43] However, studies on antiplatelet therapy have not consistently shown improvement in wound healing, limb salvage, or 1-year survival in CLTI patients.[43]

*Anticoagulation:* In CLTI, both atherosclerotic plaque and microthrombi adhesion, contribute to arterial stenosis. The Voyager trial found that low-dose (2.5 mg) rivaroxaban reduced the incidence of acute limb ischemia (ALI), major amputation, MI, ischemic stroke, and cardiovascular death better than aspirin alone in PAD patients with a history of LE revascularization.[44]

**Table 5**
Summary of Goal-directed medical therapy in peripheral artery disease /chronic limb-threatening ischemia

| Medication Class | Medication Examples | Dose | Goal | Considerations |
|---|---|---|---|---|
| Statin | Atorvastatin Rosuvastatin Simvastatin Pravastatin | Low-Intensity: LDL-C reduction < 30% Moderate- Intensity: LDL-C 30–<50% High- Intensity: LDL-C reduction. 50% | LDL-C <70 | If statin reaction occurs, dose to maximum tolerated and consider addition of non-statin lipid-lowering agent Adjust dose to needed intensity |
| PCSK9 Inhibitors | Alirocumab Evolocumab | 75 mg sq q 2 weeks or 420 mg sq q month 140 mg sq q 2 wk or 420 mg sq q month | LDL-C <70 | Guideline recommendations: second-line or third-line agents/monotherapy in statin intolerance in patients with persistent hypercholesterolemia with established ASCVD or a known familial component |
| Antiplatelet | Aspirin Clopidogrel | 75–325 mg po qd 75 mg po qd | Decrease platelet aggregation and activation to reduce risk of | Other antiplatelet medications are less used |
| Direct Oral Anticoagulants | Apixaban Rivaroxaban | 2.5 mg po bid 2.5 mg po bid | Work with antiplatelet therapy (APT) to address microthrombi in CLTI: dual-pathway inhibition | Dose adjusted for CLTI vs full therapy in VTE or A-fib Vitamin K antagonist (warfarin) not indicated in this setting) Assess bleeding risk and monitor |
| Hypertension Management | | Varies | <140/<90 | There is no evidence for one agent over another in PAD specifically |
| Diabetes Management | Metformin | 500 mg po bid or 850 mg po qd | HgbA1C <7 | Other agents can also be utilized |

*Abbreviations:* ASCVD, atherosclerotic cardiovascular disease; LDL-C, low-density lipoprotein; VTE, venous thromboembolism.

*Management of hypertension:* It is widely known that adequate management of hypertension reduces MACEs in patients with PAD.[10]

*Management of Diabetes:* Diabetes is a significant risk factor for PAD, correlating with the severity and duration of the disease. Diabetic patients with CLTI have poorer outcomes. Sodium-glucose co-transporter 2 (SGLT-2) inhibitors show potential benefits in MACE reduction, chronic kidney disease (CKD), and mortality.[10] However, a 2021 meta-analysis showed slightly increased PAD and amputation rates in diabetes mellitus (DM) patients on SGLT-2 therapy. Weight reduction and adequate hypertension management can mitigate these risks.[45] These agents should be used cautiously in DM patients with advanced PAD/CLTI. Monitoring glycosylated hemoglobin A1c is essential in LE ulceration, especially in CLTI.[10]

## LIFESTYLE MODIFICATION

Adoption of a healthy lifestyle is crucial in patients with CLTI and arterial ulceration, including smoking cessation, weight management, exercise, and a healthy diet.[10]

### Smoking Cessation

Smoking accelerates PAD progression and increases MACEs. Smoking cessation should be addressed at every patient encounter.[10]

### Weight Loss, Diet, and Exercise

While no specific studies on diet and exercise for arterial ulcers exist, high-fat, high-carbohydrate diets increase MACE risk. Diets rich in monounsaturated fats, omega-3 fatty acids, antioxidants, and plant sterols may reduce plaque burden and MACEs. Supervised exercise programs decrease MI incidence and cardiovascular mortality in PAD patients and may be beneficial post-revascularization for those who can tolerate it.[10]

### Pain Management

Arterial ulcers and lower extremity pain significantly impact quality of life. There are no specific evidence-based recommendations for pain management in CLTI, but pain should be managed tiered and side effects closely monitored. Nonmedical tactics may be adjunctive based on patient preference. Early pain management referral is recommended if adequate pain relief cannot be achieved.[10,23]

## PHARMACOGENETICS

Pharmacogenetic testing guides cardiovascular risk factor management and treatment, with CYP2C19 genotyping commonly used to guide clopidogrel management after coronary intervention.[46] Similar research exists for oral anticoagulants, statins, beta-blockers, hydralazine, and anti-arrhythmic drugs, primarily focusing on coronary artery disease (CAD) and congestive heart failure (CHF).[46]

## TOPICAL WOUND MANAGEMENT

Wound healing and pain resolution are the main goals of revascularization in CLTI. Still, up to 75% of arterial ulcers do not close following revascularization, suggesting a complex milieu of contributing factors beyond blood flow.[47] See **Table 6** for some of these factors.

### Standard Dressings

Dressings manage bacterial burden, exudate, and promote granulation tissue. For non-revascularized arterial ulcers, keep the area dry and infection-free. After

| Table 6 Factors contributing to closure of ischemic ulcers | |
| --- | --- |
| Local Factors | Moisture level: dessication/maceration Increased biofilm/bacterial burden/infection Increased ulcer depth Recurrent local trauma |
| Comorbidities | Diabetes mellitus Obesity Chronic kidney disease/end-stage renal disease Malnutrition |
| Medications | Non steroidal anti inflammatory drugs Chemotherapy Steroids |
| Lifestyle Factors | Smoking Alcohol intake |
| Revascularization Factors | Reocclusion/restensosis Non-targeted revascularization |

*From* Antonopoulos CN, Lazaris A, Venermo M, Geroulakos G. Predictors of Wound Healing Following Revascularization for Chronic Limb-Threatening Ischemia. Vasc Endovascular Surg. 2019;53(8):649-657. https://doi.org/10.1177/1538574419868863.

revascularization, manage like other ulcers. Dressing choice does not significantly impact healing.[48]

### Negative Pressure Wound Therapy

Controlled negative pressure applied to the ulcer bed removes debris and exudate within a closed system, applying tension to cells and promoting tissue generation. Low-quality evidence supports negative pressure wound therapy (NPWT) use in diabetic foot ulcers, but attention must be paid to the microcirculatory compromise in ulcers with an ischemic component. Negative pressure can be adjusted to avoid further ischemia.[47]

### Cell Therapy

Platelet-rich plasma accelerates wound healing; platelet-derived growth factor has limited results in diabetic foot ulcer (DFU) but has not been studied in arterial ulcers.[49] A 2021 meta-analysis showed that cellular products as adipose-derived stem cell (ADSCs) and bone marrow cells improve ulcer closure and reduce amputation rates (48). Stem cell transplantation shows promise but needs further study for efficacy and safety.[49]

### Hyperbaric Oxygen Therapy

Hyperbaric oxygen therapy (HBOT) is not indicated for CLTI or pure arterial ulcers and shows inconclusive results.[47] A 2017 meta-analysis found no significant difference between HBOT and standard therapy in ulcer closure or amputation risk for DFU but did show increased wound healing. HBOT may speed ulcer closure in DFU with mild ischemia after conventional therapy fails but does not significantly affect major amputation and is not recommended as an alternative to revascularization in CLTI.[10]

## CONSIDERATIONS IN MIXED ARTERIAL-VENOUS LEG ULCER

Managing the venous component is crucial for arterial-venous leg ulcer (AVLU) closure. Patients with an ankle brachial pressure index (ABPI) of 0.5 to 0.8 may benefit from modified compression therapy (20–30 mm Hg). Revascularization should be considered if no improvement is seen within 3 months. Patients with an ABPI less than 0.5 can use modified or full compression therapy post-revascularization, depending on tolerance, ulcer size reduction, and graft patency.[50] Sclerotherapy effectively manages AVLU with varicosities near the ulcer, even without revascularization.[51] An interdisciplinary approach, including vascular specialist evaluation, is essential for AVLU management.

## SUMMARY

CLTI and arterial ulcer patients face complex presentations, leading to higher risks of hospitalization, prolonged stays, readmission, and death. Despite lacking a universally accepted frailty scale, recognizing and addressing frailty is crucial in vascular surgery. The burden of CLTI on patients and health systems necessitates interdisciplinary, patient-focused, and shared decision-making to optimize quality of life. Further research is needed to guide revascularization decisions, balancing patient outcomes, wishes, and health system considerations.[52] Non-white populations experience higher rates of PAD-associated adverse events, presenting with more severe disease, atypical symptoms, and higher cardiovascular risk factors. They receive less timely care and suffer higher adverse event rates, highlighting the need for improved awareness, risk factor modification, and patient-centered care to slow CLTI progression in these communities.[53]

## CLINICS CARE POINTS

- Ischemic ulcerations are complex and multifactorial phenomena that require thorough investigation and multi-modal management.
- The standard of management of arterial ulcers is revascularization.
- Attention to wound care principles is necessary to reduce risk of infection and ulcer worsening and to promote ulcer closure.
- Multi-disciplinary nursing coordination and communication with standardized tools is necessary to promote patient success.
- In arterial ulceration, nurses are at the center of key clinical metrics and positioned well to impact patient outcomes.

## REFERENCES

1. Graham ID, Harrison MB, Nelson EA, et al. Prevalence of lower-limb ulceration: a systematic review of prevalence studies. Adv Skin Wound Care 2003;16(6):305–16.
2. Callam M, Harper D, Dale J, et al. Arterial disease in chronic leg ulceration: an underestimated hazard? Lothian and Forth Valley leg ulcer study. Br Med J 1987;294(6577):929.
3. Hafner J, Schaad I, Schneider E, et al. Leg ulcers in peripheral arterial disease (arterial leg ulcers): impaired wound healing above the threshold of chronic critical limb ischemia. J Am Acad Dermatol 2000;43(6):1001–8.
4. Vos T, Lim SS, Abbafati C, et al. Global burden of 369 diseases and injuries in 204 countries and territories, 1990–2019: a systematic analysis for the Global Burden of Disease Study 2019. Lancet 2020;396(10258):1204–22.

5. Wang H, Abbas KM, Abbasifard M, et al. Global age-sex-specific fertility, mortality, healthy life expectancy (HALE), and population estimates in 204 countries and territories, 1950–2019: a comprehensive demographic analysis for the Global Burden of Disease Study 2019. Lancet 2020;396(10258):1160–203.

6. Lin J, Chen Y, Jiang N, et al. Burden of peripheral artery disease and its attributable risk factors in 204 Countries and Territories from 1990 to 2019. Front Cardiovasc Med 2022;9:868370.

7. Vitalis A, Lip GY, Kay M, et al. Ethnic differences in the prevalence of peripheral arterial disease: a systematic review and meta-analysis. Expert Rev Cardiovasc Ther 2017;15(4):327–38.

8. Kwong M, Rajasekar G, Utter GH, et al. Updated estimates for the burden of chronic limb-threatening ischemia in the Medicare population. J Vasc Surg 2023;77(6):1760–75.

9. Nickinson ATO, Houghton JSM, Bridgwood B, et al. The utilisation of vascular limb salvage services in the assessment and management of chronic limb-threatening ischaemia and diabetic foot ulceration: a systematic review. Diabetes Metab Res Rev 2020;36(7):e3326.

10. Conte MS, Bradbury AW, Kolh P, et al. Global vascular guidelines on the management of chronic limb-threatening ischemia. J Vasc Surg 2019;69(6, Suppl): 3S–125S.e140.

11. Armstrong DG, Bharara M, White M, et al. The impact and outcomes of establishing an integrated interdisciplinary surgical team to care for the diabetic foot. Diabetes Metab Res Rev 2012;28(6):514–8.

12. Bauer KL. Differentiation of lower extremity skin changes in the intensive care setting. AACN Adv Crit Care 2022;33(2):196–207.

13. Lipsky BA, Berendt AR, Cornia PB, et al. Infectious Diseases Society of America clinical practice guideline for the diagnosis and treatment of diabetic foot infections. Clin Infect Dis 2012;54(12):e132–73.

14. Marin JA, Woo KY. Clinical characteristics of mixed arteriovenous leg ulcers: a descriptive study. J Wound, Ostomy Cont Nurs 2017;44(1):41–7.

15. Hoven P, Oams S, Manen L, et al. A systematic review of the use of near-infrared fluorescence imaging in patients with peripheral vascular disease. J Vasc Surg 2019;70:286–97.

16. Hardman RL, Jazaeri O, Yi J, et al. Overview of classification systems in peripheral artery disease. Semin Intervent Radiol 2014;31(4):378–88.

17. Mills JL Sr, Conte MS, Armstrong DG, et al. The society for vascular surgery lower extremity threatened limb classification system: risk stratification based on wound, ischemia, and foot infection (WIfI). J Vasc Surg 2014;59(1):220–34. e342.

18. Gornik H, Aronow H, et al. 2024 ACC/AHA/AACVPR/APMA/ABC/SCAI/SVM/SVN/ SVS/SIR/VESS guideline for the management of lower extremity peripheral artery disease: a report of the American College of Cardiology/American Heart association Joint Committee on clinical practice guidelines. JACC (J Am Coll Cardiol) 2024 Jun;83(24):2497–604.

19. Arsenault KA, McDonald J, Devereaux PJ, et al. The use of transcutaneous oximetry to predict complications of chronic wound healing: a systemic review and meta-analysis. Wound Repair Regen 2011;19(6):657–63.

20. Chiang N, Jain JK, Sleigh J, et al. Evaluation of hyperspectral imaging technology in patients with peripheral vascular disease. J Vasc Surg 2017;66(4):1192–201.

21. Boas DA, Franceschini MA. Haemoglobin oxygen saturation as a biomarker: the problem and a solution. Philos Trans A Math Phys Eng Sci 2011;369(1955): 4407–24.
22. Wermelink B, Ma K, Haalboom M, et al. A systematic review and critical appraisal of peri-procedural tissue perfusion techniques and their clinical value in patients with peripheral arterial disease. Eur J Vasc Endovasc Surg 2021;62:896–908.
23. Laoire ÁN, Murtagh FEM. Systematic review of pharmacological therapies for the management of ischaemic pain in patients with non-reconstructable critical limb ischaemia. BMJ Support Palliat Care 2018;8(4):400–10. https://doi.org/10.1136/bmjspcare-2017-001359.
24. Saab F, Jaff MR, Diaz-Sandoval LJ, et al. Chronic total occlusion crossing approach based on plaque cap morphology: the CTOP Classification. J Endovasc Ther 2018; 25(3):284–91.
25. Schmidt A, Bausback YM, Piorkowski M, et al. Retrograde tibioperoneal access for complex infrainguinal occlusions: short- and long-term outcomes of 554 endovascular interventions. JACC Cardiovasc Interv 2019;12(17).
26. Tsubakimoto Y, Nakama T, Kamoi D, et al. Outcomes of pedal artery angioplasty are independent of the severity of inframalleolar disease: a subanalysis of the Multicenter RENDEZVOUS Registry. J Endovasc Ther 2020;27:186–93. https://doi.org/10.1177/1526602820901838.
27. Feldman ZM, Mohapatra A. Endovascular management of complex tibial lesions. Semin Vasc Surg 2022;35(2):190–9.
28. Laird JR, Mathews SJ, Brodmann M, et al, Wing-It Trial Investigators. Performance of the Wingman catheter in peripheral artery chronic total occlusions: short-term results from the interna- tional Wing-It trial. Cathet Cardiovasc Interv 2021,97.310–6. https://doi.org/10.1002/ccd.29366.
29. Adams G, Shammas N, Mangalmurti S, et al. Intravascular lithotripsy for treatment of calcified lower extremity arterial stenosis: initial analysis of the disrupt PAD III study. J Endovasc Ther 2020;27:473–80.
30. Almasri J, Adusumalli J, Asi N, et al. A systematic review and meta-analysis of revascularization outcomes of infrainguinal chronic limb-threatening ischemia. J Vasc Surg 2018;68:624–33. https://doi.org/10.1016/j.jvs.2018.01.066.
31. Giannopoulos S, Mustapha J, Gray WA, et al. Three-year outcomes from the LIBERTY 360 study of endovascular interventions for peripheral artery disease stratified by Rutherford category. J Endovasc Ther 2021;28:262–74.
32. Gupta R, Siada S, Lai S, et al. Critical appraisal of the contemporary use of atherectomy to treat femorpopliteal atherosclerotic disease. J Vasc Surg 2022;75: 697–708.
33. Nugteren M, Welling R, Bakker O, Unlu C, Hazenbberg C. Vessel preparation in infrapopliteal arterial disease: a systematic review and meta-analysis. J Endov Ther 2022;1012.
34. Bhat TM, Afari ME, Garcia LA. Atherectomy in peripheral artery disease: a review. J Invasive Cardiol 2017;29(4):135–44.
35. Shishehbor M, Powell R, Montero-Baker M, et al. Transcatheter arterialization of deep veins in chronic limb threatening ischemia. N Engl J Med 2023;388: 1171–80.
36. Bradbury A, Moakes C, Popplewell M, et al. A vein bypass first versus best endovascular treatment first revascularization strategy for patients with chronic limb threatening ischemia who required an infra-popliteal, with or without additional more proximal infra-inguinal revascularization procedure to restore limb

perfusion (BASIL-2): an open-label, randomized, multicenter, phase 3 trial. Lancet 2023;401:1798–809.

37. Farber A, Menard M, Conte M, et al. Surgery or endovascular therapy for chronic limb threatening ischemia. N Engl J Med 2022;387:2305–16. https://doi.org/10.1056/NEJMoa2207899.

38. Vietto V, Franco JV, Saenz V, et al. Prostanoids for critical limb ischaemia. Cochrane Database Syst Rev 2018;1(1):CD006544. https://doi.org/10.1002/14651858.CD006544.pub3.

39. Desai K, Han B, Kuziez L, et al. Literature review and meta-analysis of the efficacy of cilostazol on limb salvage rates after infrainguinal endovascular and open revascularization. J Vasc Surg 2021;73(2):711–21.e3. https://doi.org/10.1016/j.jvs.2020.08.125.

40. Parvar SL, Fitridge R, Dawson J, et al. Medical and lifestyle management of peripheral arterial disease. J Vasc Surg 2018;68(5):1595–606. https://doi.org/10.1016/j.jvs.2018.07.027.

41. Sagris M, Katsaros I, Giannopoulos S, et al. Statins and statin intensity in peripheral artery disease. Vasa 2022;51(4):198–211. https://doi.org/10.1024/0301-1526/a001012.

42. Hajar R. PCSK 9 inhibitors: a short history and a new era of lipid-lowering therapy. Heart Views 2019;20(2):74–5. https://doi.org/10.4103/HEARTVIEWS.HEART VIEWS_59_19.

43. Katsanos K, Spiliopoulos S, Saha P, et al. Comparative efficacy and safety of different antiplatelet agents for prevention of major cardiovascular events and leg amputations in patients with peripheral arterial disease: a systematic review and network meta-analysis. PLoS One 2015;10:e0135692.

44. Bonaca MP, Bauersachs RM, Anand SS, et al. Rivaroxaban in peripheral artery disease after revascularization. N Engl J Med 2020;382(21):1994–2004. https://doi.org/10.1056/NEJMoa2000052.

45. Lin C, Zhu X, Cai X, et al. SGLT2 inhibitors and lower limb complications: an updated meta-analysis [published correction appears in Cardiovasc Diabetol. 2021 Jun 9;20(1):119]. Cardiovasc Diabetol 2021;20(1):91. https://doi.org/10.1186/s12933-021-01276-9.

46. Duarte JD, Cavallari LH. Pharmacogenetics to guide cardiovascular drug therapy. Nat Rev Cardiol 2021;18(9):649–65. https://doi.org/10.1038/s41569-021-00549-w.

47. Antonopoulos CN, Lazaris A, Venermo M, et al. Predictors of wound healing following revascularization for chronic limb-threatening ischemia. Vasc Endovasc Surg 2019;53(8):649–57. https://doi.org/10.1177/1538574419868863.

48. Broderick C, Pagnamenta F, Forster R. Dressings and topical agents for arterial leg ulcers. Cochrane Database Syst Rev 2020;1(1):CD001836.

49. Dong Y, Yang Q, Sun X. Comprehensive analysis of cell therapy on chronic skin wound healing: a meta-analysis. Hum Gene Ther 2021;32(15–16):787–95. https://doi.org/10.1089/hum.2020.275.

50. Lim SLX, Chung RE, Holloway S, et al. Modified compression therapy in mixed arterial-venous leg ulcers: an integrative review. Int Wound J 2021;18(6):822–42. https://doi.org/10.1111/iwj.13585.

51. Mosti G, Cavezzi A, Massimetti G, et al. Recalcitrant venous leg ulcers may heal by outpatient treatment of venous disease even in the presence of concomitant arterial occlusive disease. Eur J Vasc Endovasc Surg 2016;52(3):385–91. https://doi.org/10.1016/j.ejvs.2016.06.004.

52. Fernando ME, Blanchette V, Mishra R, et al. Frailty in people with chronic limb threatening ischemia and diabetes-related foot ulcers: a systematic review. Ann Vasc Surg 2023;89:322–37. https://doi.org/10.1016/j.avsg.2022.09.057.
53. Nedunchezhian S, Reddy TK, Wegener M, et al. A systematic review of racial/ethnic disparities in pharmacotherapy and surgical treatment outcomes in peripheral arterial disease among African American/non-Hispanic Black, non-Hispanic White and Hispanic patients. AHJ Plus 2022;18(10017).

# Wound Care in Venous Disease and Lymphedema

Frank Aviles Jr, PT, CWS, FACCWS, CLT-LANA, ALM, AWCC[a],*,
Elizabeth Faust, MSN, CRNP, CSWS, CWOCN-AP[b]

## KEYWORDS

- Lymphedema • Venous leg ulcer • Phlebolymphedema
- Chronic venous insufficiency

## KEY POINTS

- Understand the role of the venous system.
- Understand the role of the lymphatic system.
- Identify the role of therapeutic compression in treating venous-related wounds.
- Identify the role of complete decongestive therapy in treating patients with lymphatic disease.

## INTRODUCTION

The lymphatic system plays a significant role in removing fluid from the body. This article examines how an impaired venous and lymphatic system can negatively influence the wound healing trajectory, explore potential complications, and select proper treatment interventions to address the symptom or disease.

## EDEMA MANAGEMENT

The venous system transports deoxygenated blood, whereas the lymphatic system circulates lymphatic fluid. Oxygenated blood is delivered to the capillaries, where average vascular permeability transfers water, oxygen, and nutrients to cells and tissues via filtration. Concurrently, the venous system transports deoxygenated blood back to the heart, whereas lymph/waste products are eliminated via the lymphatic system. Both systems share features such as having superficial and deep components, valves, and the ability to enhance fluid movement with muscle pumps.[1] Prolonged edema leads to higher-than-normal inflammatory changes. These higher-than-normal levels of inflammation and pressure can lead to ulcerations, known as venous leg ulcers. Chronic hypoxia, permanent skin changes, frequent infections,

---

[a] Hyperbaric Physicians of Georgia, 1505 Northside Boulevard, Suite 1300, Cumming, GA 30041, USA; [b] Lizzie Wounds, 107 Meadowcrest Lane, Douglassville, PA 19518, USA
* Corresponding author. PO Box 247, Gulf Breeze, FL 32562.
*E-mail address:* Frank.Aviles@hbomdga.com

Nurs Clin N Am 60 (2025) 77–98
https://doi.org/10.1016/j.cnur.2024.07.018
0029-6465/25/© 2024 Elsevier Inc. All rights reserved, including those for text and data mining, AI training, and similar technologies.

and nonhealing wounds can occur if edema and inflammation are not adequately managed.[2]

It is important to note that both chronic venous disease and lymphedema are progressive diseases; thus, early intervention and management should be a priority. Skin ulceration can develop as patients progress through venous and lymphatic disease stages. It is essential to follow basic principles of wound healing, including wound hygiene, moist wound bed healing, and infection management. In addition to primary wound care, compression therapy is crucial for wound progression if venous and lymphatic diseases exist. The first step is to diagnose correctly. Edema can be attributed to congestive heart failure, kidney failure, pregnancy, venous insufficiency, lymphedema, May-Thurner syndrome, and medication effects, among others.[3] It is estimated that 50% of the US population older than 50 years has varicose veins. Varicose veins affect roughly 30% of the population.[4] Chronic venous insufficiency (CVI) affects 25 million adults in the United States, with nearly 6 million suffering from advanced diseases. The annual cost of venous ulcer care is estimated at $3 billion.[5] An estimated 10% to 35% of adults in the United States have CVI, with 4% of adults aged 65 years or older developing venous ulcers.[6] The formation of an ulcer carries a poor prognosis, with 40% of patients experiencing recurrence despite standard treatment.[7] Lymphedema affects an estimated 35 million patients in the United States.[8] Primary lymphedema is rare, affecting 1 in 100,000 individuals, whereas secondary lymphedema is the most common cause, affecting approximately 1 in 1000 Americans.[9] Recent studies showed that CVI is the primary cause of lower extremity lymphedema (41.8%, followed by cancer in 33.9%).[10] Szyber and colleagues reported approximately 6 million cases of lower limb lymphedema, and 60% had CVI.[11]

## PHASES OF HEALING

Acute wounds undergo a series of physiologic events that overlap and have distinct clinical features. The healing process includes four phases: clotting, inflammation, proliferation, and maturation. If an acute wound's healing process stalls, it may become chronic, reverting to the inflammatory phase. Therefore, it is crucial to accurately diagnose the cause and identify any factors that could impede the healing trajectory.[12] The assessment should include wound etiology followed by examining the wound and the surrounding skin to ascertain the current healing phase. This assessment aids in selecting suitable interventions and products to advance wound healing.[13] It is common for patients seeking care to have wounds stalled in the inflammatory phase. Characteristics of the inflammatory phase include peri-wound erythema, edema, pain, induration, and increased drainage without granulation tissue[14] (Figs. 1 and 2). In the proliferative phase, granulation tissue will be evident, with the characteristics of the inflammatory phase decreasing. Lastly, the maturation phase is the closure of skin defects with ongoing collagen maturation and may last for a year. The maximal tensile wound strength occurs after about 11 to 14 weeks. The ultimate resulting scar will never have 100% tensile strength of the skin. Instead, the tensile strength will only be about 80%[15] (Fig. 3).

## CLINICS CARE POINTS—PHASES OF HEALING

- *Patients with chronic wounds require the following throughout the healing process:*
  - Diagnosis and proper management of problem/cause (differential diagnoses such as mixed ulcers, pyoderma gangrenosum, May-Thurner syndrome, metabolic disorders, skin cancers, and others).

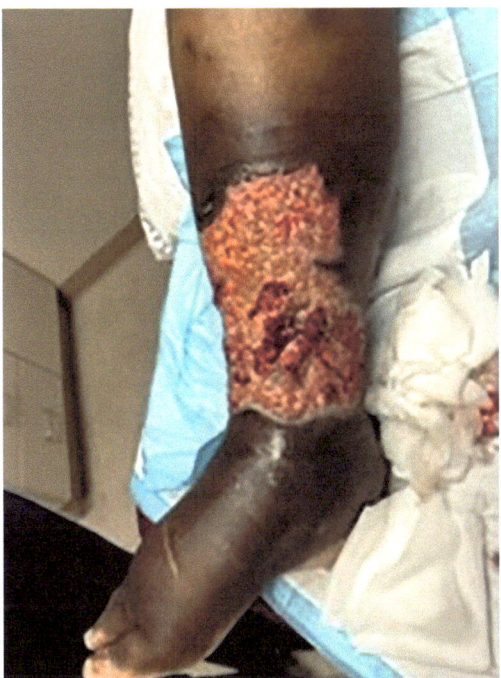

Fig. 1. A chronic nonhealing wound that is in the inflammatory phase.

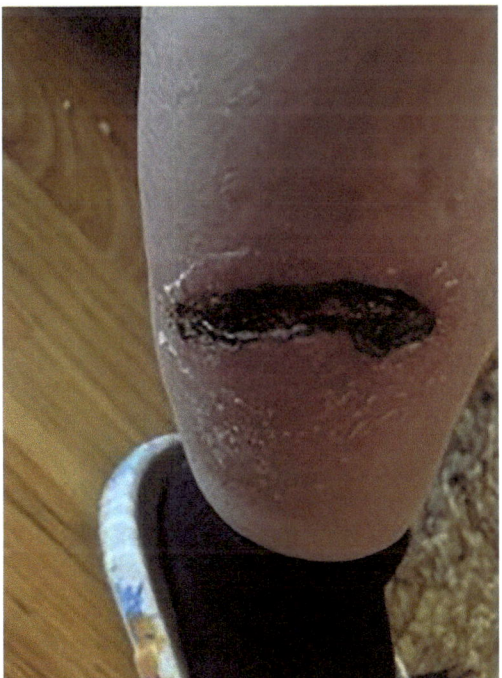

Fig. 2. Chronic wound with prolonged clinical signs of inflammation.

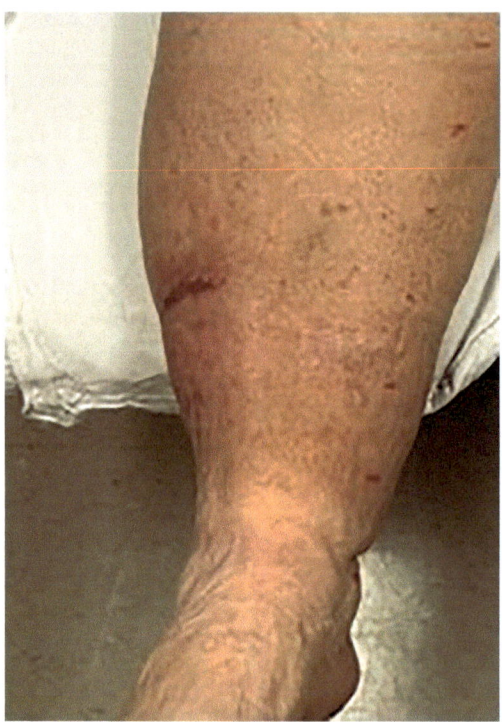

**Fig. 3.** Wound in the maturation phase. It is now closed, and the new tissue formation is gaining tensile strength.

- o Perfusion (large and small vessel arterial circulation) and average diffusion distance (edema increases diffusion distance, delaying oxygen and nutrients to the tissue).
- o Address local and systemic infection if present (the longer the wound is open, the more the likelihood of infection).
- o Adequate hydration.
- o If malnutrition is present, consult a dietitian. Address hydration, proteins, calories, and supplementation, including arginine, glutamine, and micronutrients (more than 50% of hospital admissions may be malnourished with serious consequences affecting healing potential).
- Chronic wounds require the following throughout the healing process:
  - o Delivery of oxygen to the wound bed/tissue (transcutaneous oxygen measurements < 40 mm Hg while normobaric breathing [<50 mm Hg in patients with diabetes] indicates hypoxia and below 30 mm Hg suggests severe hypoxia & poor wound healing potential).
  - o Proper wound bed temperature (studies have shown that temperatures at 33°C are critical for neutrophil, fibroblast, and epithelial cell activity decrease in vitro).
  - o Adequate pH levels (chronic wounds have a pH between 7.15 and 8.9).
  - o Address biofilm (it is estimated that 60%–100% of nonhealing chronic wounds have biofilm).
  - o Removal of wound debris, necrotic tissue, callouses, and closed edges (frequent debridement stimulates the acute repair and allows epithelial tissue to migrate from the edges).

## Understanding the Venous System

The venous and arterial systems constitute the circulatory system, forming a closed loop. The arterial system carries oxgenated blood to tissues and organs, whereas the venous system, a low-pressure network, returns deoxygenated blood to the heart. At rest, two-thirds of the blood volume resides within the venous system.[16] This system operates against gravity, unlike the arterial system's pulsatile action. Its effectiveness relies on healthy valves, unobstructed veins, and the muscle pump. Properly functioning valves prevent venous reflux, as skeletal muscle contractions propel blood toward the heart during activity. If these components are compromised, it can lead to an accumulation of deoxygenated blood, increasing pressure and potentially causing CVI. The great saphenous vein below the knee is often where valve incompetence or failure occurs,[17] leading to blood flowing backward from deep to superficial veins. The prevalence of this condition is about 7% in individuals at 50 years, increasing to approximately 20% by the age of 70 years.[18] An acute deep vein thrombosis (DVT) may also result in increased venous pressure with accumulation of interstitial fluid. The lymphatic system will work to remove this fluid, but it may become overwhelmed and eventually damaged over time. Obesity, along with an increase in intraabdominal venous pressure, can negatively affect the lower leg veins and lymphatic system.[19]

## Progression and Stages of Venous Disease

Venous disease progresses through various stages, each characterized by distinct symptoms that guide health care providers in determining the most appropriate treatment. The CEAP classification is the accepted standard for staging CVI. Venous duplex ultrasound is the gold-standard method for evaluating/confirming CVI.

CEAP stands for

- C: Clinical, indicating how the disease manifests in the body.
- E: Etiology, identifying the cause.
- A: Anatomy, specifying the location of the issue.
- P: Pathophysiology, describing the impact on blood flow.

The CEAP classification, established in 1994 and recently updated, reflects the progression of CVI. CEAP can be assessed using all four categories, but it is commonly staged using the clinical classification "C" alone.

Venous stages:
- C0: no visible signs
- C1: visible veins or blood vessels
- C2: varicose veins
- C3: edema
- C4: skin quality changes
- C5: healed ulcers
- C6: active ulcers

## SYMPTOMS OF VENOUS DISEASE

- Limb heaviness
- Pain
- Edema. Pitting edema where skin indention is noted after pressing your finger gently (**Fig. 4**)
- Varicose veins (**Fig. 5**)
- Telangiectasias

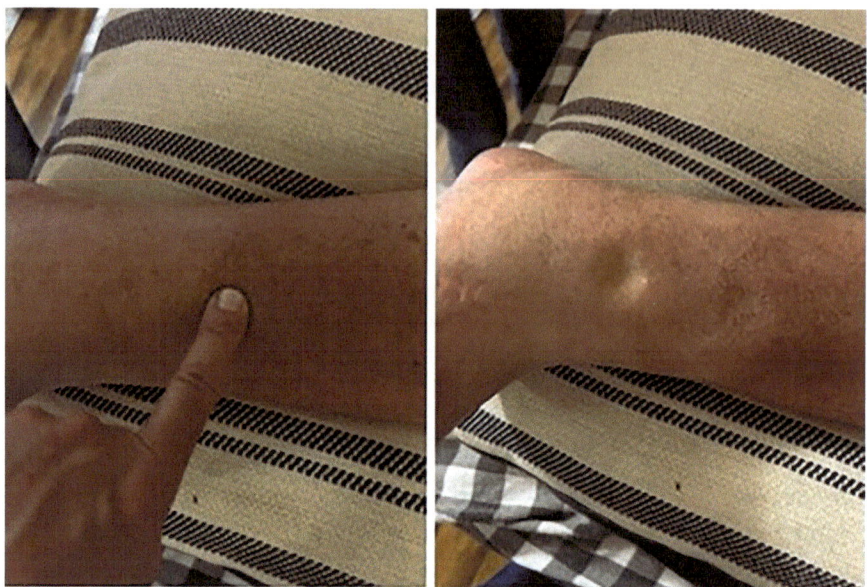

**Fig. 4.** Pitting edema noted when pressing down gently on the skin with finger, leaving an imprint.

- Lipodermatosclerosis (panniculitis that leads to skin induration or hardening, increased pigmentation, swelling, and redness) (**Fig. 6**)
- Inverted champagne bottle deformity of lower leg
- Stasis dermatitis (**Fig. 7**)

## VENOUS ULCERS

The risk factors for venous disease include age 55 years or older, family history of CVI, higher body mass index, history of pulmonary embolism or superficial/deep venous thrombosis, lower extremity skeletal or joint disease, higher number of pregnancies, parental history of ankle ulcers, physical inactivity, history of ulcers, severe lipodermatosclerosis (**Fig. 8**), and venous reflux in deep veins.[20] Approximately 76% of the cases can be determined by clinical presentation[21] or irregular wound shape (**Fig. 9**), well-defined borders, and shallow wound bed with granulation and fibrin. Common locations include medial malleolus, gaiter region, or circumferentially.[22] These wounds have edema and hemosiderin staining (brown or purple skin on the lower leg) (see **Fig. 7**).[23] Atrophy blanche (a common clinical sign that may be associated with venous hypertension and may be seen after a leg ulcer has healed) is described as a smooth white plaque surrounded by a hyperpigmented border and telangiectatic blood vessels.[24] Stasis dermatitis is an inflammatory skin condition typically experienced in patients with CVI (**Fig. 10**).

## TREATMENT INTERVENTIONS
### Lifestyle Modifications

- Maintain a healthy weight.
- Diet
- Exercise
- Avoid prolonged sitting.

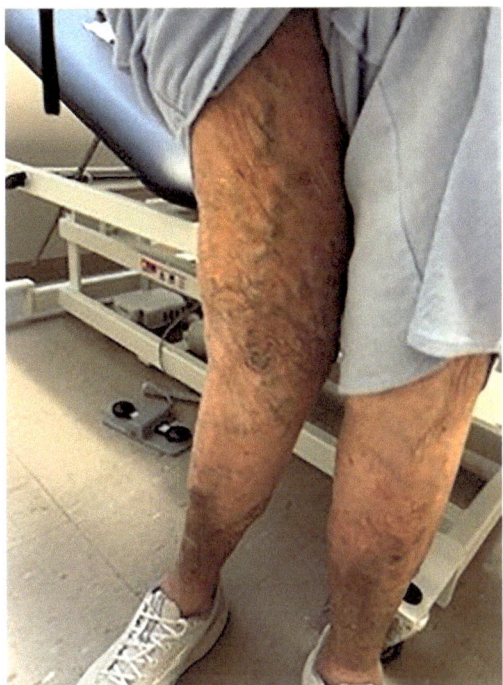

**Fig. 5.** Note the varicose veins along with the discoloration or hemosiderin deposits in the lower legs.

- Increase activity level by walking several times a week. Muscle pump activation, along with diaphragmatic breathing, can aid in returning blood to the heart
- Control high blood pressure.
- Leg elevation above heart level

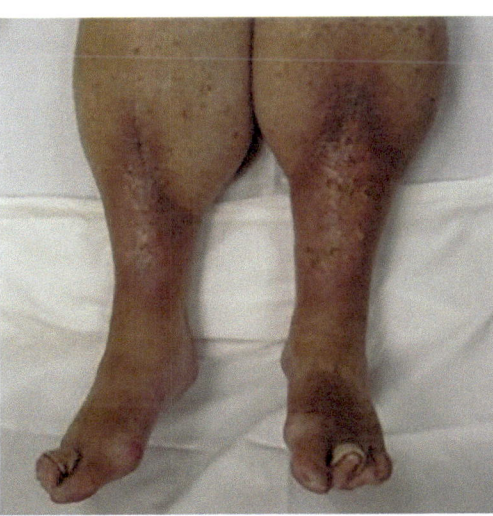

**Fig. 6.** Lipodermasclerosis. The skin hardens, and the lower legs sometimes assume this inverted champagne bottle shape. (Image credit: Karen Ashforth.)

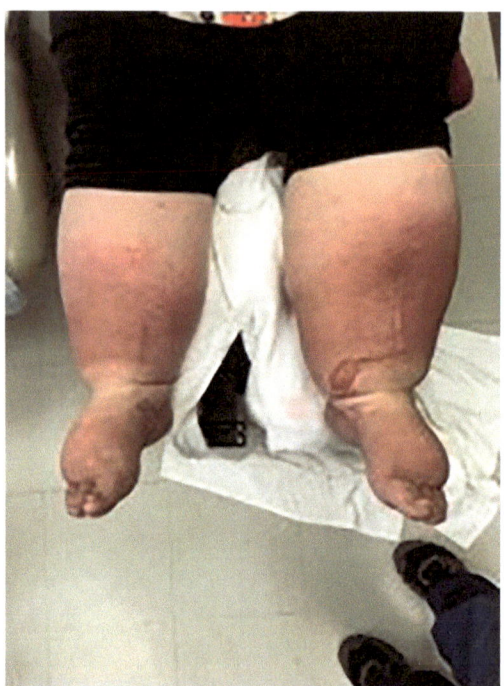

**Fig. 7.** Stasis dermatitis often confused with cellulitis.

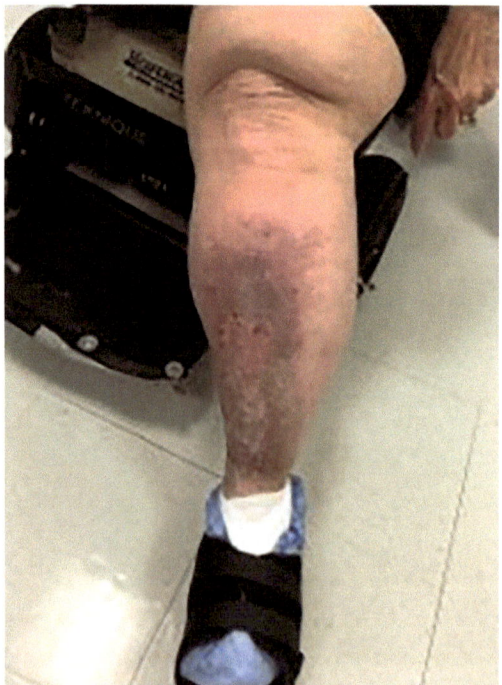

**Fig. 8.** Hemosiderin staining and lipodermatosclerosis of the lower leg.

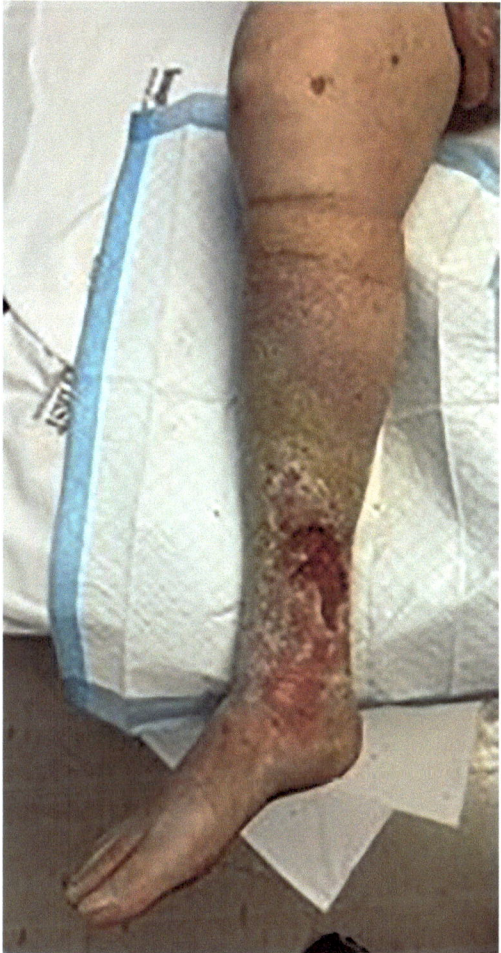

**Fig. 9.** Venous ulcer with an irregular wound border and skin changes.

### Peripheral Artery Disease Screening/Testing

Arterial screening is important as 20% of venous ulcers have arterial disease.[25]

### Wound Care

Before using compression as an adjunctive intervention, it is best practice to prepare the wound and peri-wound tissue.

### Wound Bed Preparation

#### Tissue management

This is the process of removing necrotic or devitalized tissue, bacteria, and cells that impede the healing trajectory. There are various types of debridement, such as surgical, sharp, biological, mechanical, enzymatic, and autolytic, each with pertinent indications and contraindications.[19] Wilcox and colleagues demonstrated that wounds responded favorably with frequent debridement.

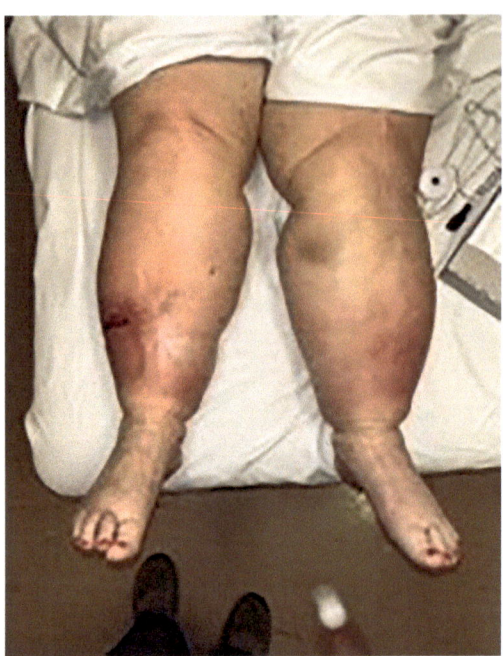

**Fig. 10.** Stasis dermatitis resolved with treatment.

### Tissue/inflammation

Bioburden can be addressed by debriding, wound cleansing, and using antimicrobials and antibiotics for systemic infections.[26]

### Moisture Balance

We provide the ideal wound moisture level to promote epithelization and the optimal effect of growth factors and proliferating cells. Utilization of specific dressing categories may be selected to match the wound characteristics. Excessive exudate can lead to wound and peri-wound maceration, skin irritations, and infections.[27]

### Epithelial (Edge) Advancement

Epithelial movement occurs from the edges of the wound as it progresses. Barriers such as rolled edges, necrotic tissue, callouses, and closed edges will prevent this migration; therefore, the clinician must address this.[28]

### Repair/Regeneration

The goal is to encourage wound closure by providing a matrix to support cell infiltration, stimulating cell activity using signal molecules or growth factors, delivering oxygen therapy, or using stem cells.[29]

### Social

Consider the patient's psychosocial and physical risk factors and comorbidity and living arrangements/conditions, as they can affect the ability for patients to heal.

### Wound Hygiene

In 2019, an international panel of wound care experts met to discuss the management of biofilm, followed by a consensus document on wound hygiene as a fundamental aspect of the care of patients with open wounds. It consists of four components: cleanse, debride, refashion edges, and dressing.

### Dressing Categories for Highly Exudative Wounds

Calcium alginates—absorb moderate to maximal amounts of exudate.

Hydro fibers—highly absorbent wicking exudate and the fibers form a gel on contact with exudate.

Foam—absorb moderate to maximal amount of exudate. There are many variations in this category from which to select.

Superabsorbents—absorb copious amounts of fluid.

Negative pressure devices—various forms are available with small to large canisters for fluid collection.

Antimicrobials—dressings that alter the wound bed bioburden available in several types or categories.

### Medications

- Oral, intravenous, or topical antibiotics for infections.
- Antiinflammatory medications—possibly for controlling pain and inflammation.
- Pentoxifylline has been used effectively along with compression for patients with venous ulcers. Milan and colleagues summarized that in seven randomized controlled trials, pentoxifylline plus compression improved healing of venous ulcers compared with placebo plus compression. Four trials showed that pentoxifylline alone improved healing compared with placebo alone.[30]
- Micronized purified flavonoid fraction (MPFF)
- MPFF studies have demonstrated an increase in the number of functional lymphatic capillaries and a decrease in their diameter and a decrease in endolymphatic pressures after 4 weeks of treatment.
- There is evidence that MPFF improves symptomatology with one dose of 1000 mg daily or 500 mg twice daily after 2 weeks of treatment.[31,32]

### Compression Therapy

Compression therapy is considered the cornerstone treatment in treating venous leg ulcers. It may be provided through medical compression bandages, garments, velcro devices, or intermittent pneumatic compression (IPC). Before applying compression, arterial insufficiency, infection, and systemic conditions such as acute congestive heart and kidney failure must be addressed.[33]

When applying compression, the goal remains to decrease edema and pain while promoting ulcer progression and preventing reoccurrence.[34] Additional goals include stabilizing skin appearance and reducing venous reflux and varicose veins. There are various forms of compression to choose from, and one must consider patient factors such as age, activity level, etc. Selection includes but is not limited to elastic bandages, nonelastic bandages, Unna boots, Duke boots, multilayers, Velcro devices, garments or stockings, and IPC pumps[35] (**Table 1**). Certified lymphedema therapists, certified compression fitters, and representatives from medical grade compression companies such as Jobst (Sweden), Sigvaris (Winterthur, Switzerland), Juzo (Julius Zorn, Inc., OH, USA), Lohmann-Rauscher (Lohmann & Rauscher GmbH & Co. KG, Rengsdorf, Germany), Medi (Medi GmbH & Co. KG, Bayreuth, Germany), and others can offer valuable information on how to fit patients properly.[36] Measuring the extremity for garments requires that the extremity already has been reduced. Contraindications include acute deep vein thrombosis, peripheral arterial disease, acute

| Table 1 Types of compression | |
|---|---|
| Compression Type: | Description |
| Long stretch (elastic) | Elastic material such as "ace bandage" providing compression at rest. High resting pressure with low working pressure |
| Short stretch (inelastic) | Stiffer material providing a high working pressure and low resting pressure. Along with the calf muscle pump, it provides effective edema reduction. Can be reused. Reapplication is beneficial as the limb decreases in circumference. |
| Multilayer | Contains various layers of padding, elastic, and/or inelastic materials. Two-layer provides approximately 20–30 mm Hg, whereas three-/four-layer provides 30–40 mm Hg. Caution: some companies have developed a two-layer 20–30 mm Hg and a two-layer 30–40 mm Hg multilayer compression. |
| Unna boot | Provides static compression when treating venous ulcer & postsurgical lower extremity wounds. It is a semirigid dressing, and ambulation/exercise is required to promote the calf muscle pump efficiency reducing edema. |
| Velcro devices | Compression device made of short-stretch material that is adjustable, providing a high working pressure. Easy application and removal. May require a foot piece along with the calf device. |
| Garments/stocking | Garments fitted after edema is reduced. Various compression levels and materials exist. Medical grade and proper fitting recommended |
| Intermittent pneumatic compression | A device that pumps air into a sleeve or garment to provide compression to the extremities, head, neck, or the torso. Can treat multiple areas to move fluid from distal to proximal. |

infection, allergy to materials, severe cardiac insufficiency, and severe neuropathy with sensory loss or microangiopathy.

Medical compression garments may be in a circular or flat knit pattern. A flat knit pattern is customized and provides adequate tissue containment.[37] Follow the manufacturer's recommendations for washing and drying garments/bandages. Do not sleep in your garments. It is best to apply it first thing in the morning and remove it before bed. If compression is required at night, alternative forms of compression are available.[38] TED hose provides approximately 8 mm Hg of compression and is used postsurgical to prevent the development of DVTs. TEDs do not benefit ambulatory patients in controlling swelling, especially patients suffering from CVI or lymphedema.[39] Garment replacement is recommended approximately every 6 months or if the garment displays signs of being damaged. There are various garment donning/doffing aids to assist patients.[40]

### Compression Levels

15 to 20 mm Hg—available from over-the-counter for mild swelling. These are not sufficient for patients with venous or lymphatic swelling.

20 to 30 mm Hg—Medical Grade Class I. Used to manage swelling, varicose veins, travel, and sports.

30 to 40 mm Hg—Medical Grade Class II. Stronger and used for moderate to severe symptoms in patients with venous ulcers and lymphedema.

40 to 50 mm Hg—Medical Grade Class III. Very strong compression and typically used for severe venous and lymphedema cases.

### Surgical—Endovascular Interventions

These procedures aim to heal the ulcer and decrease reoccurrence rates. Early endovenous ablation, when an ulcer exists to correct superficial venous reflux along with compression, demonstrated faster healing rates than compression alone or with delayed intervention if the ulcer did not heal after 6 months.[34]

### Prognosis

Poor prognostic signs for healing include ulcer duration longer than 3 months, ulcer length of 10 cm (3.9 in) or more, presence of lower limb arterial disease, advanced age, and elevated body mass index.[41] Margolis, in his 2004 study, stated that a wound less than 10 cm$^2$ and less than 12 months old at the first visit has a 29% chance of not healing by the 24th week of care, whereas a wound greater than 10 cm$^2$ and greater than 12 months old has a 78% chance of not healing.[42]

## CLINICS CARE POINTS—VENOUS

- Patients with venous ulcers and adequate arterial perfusion benefit from therapeutic compression. Match the type of compression to the patient.
- Venous disease is progressive and leads to ulcers in the latter stages. Diffusion distance on edematous legs decreases the delivery of oxygen and nutrients to the skin and ulcers. Decrease swelling = decrease diffusion distance.
- If CVI is not managed, the lymphatic system will eventually become overwhelmed. An existing venous system failure combined with lymphatic damage requires more than compression therapy, that is, complete decongestive therapy (CDT).
- Diaphragmatic breathing helps with venous and lymphatic drainage and reduces inflammation in patients with lower limb venous and lymphatic damage.

## LYMPHATIC SYSTEM
### Pathophysiology

The lymphatic system's primary function is to remove excess fluid and waste. This fluid, known as lymph, comprises water, proteins, waste products, and long-chain fatty acids.[43] The superficial lymphatic system consists of lymphatic vessels just beneath the skin, lymph nodes that filter the lymph before traveling below the fascia to the deep lymphatic system before it reenters the bloodstream.[44] Unlike the closed venous and arterial systems, the lymphatic system is open, beginning at the capillary level and ending at the venous angles/system. The initial lymph capillaries remove fluid and the larger molecules such as proteins, cell fragments, and long-chain fatty acids. The lymph fluid then travels through several vessels to regional lymph nodes for filtration. These nodes filter superficial lymph from specific areas of the body: cervical nodes filter fluid from their respective sides of the head and neck, axillary nodes filter fluid from the left/right upper extremities and anterior/posterior upper quadrants, and inguinal nodes filter fluid from the lower abdomen, lower extremities, and external genitalia. Collectors (type of vessel) are equipped with valves and smooth muscles and innervated by the autonomic nervous system. Typically, healthy lymphatic systems operate at 5% to 10% of their capacity.[45] The left venous angle processes an estimated 2 to 4 L of lymphatic fluid per day, whereas the right venous angle handles about 250 mL. This discrepancy is due to the different areas from which lymph is returned to the venous system. For instance, the left venous angle receives lymph from both inguinal, left axillary, left cervical lymph nodes, and digestive tract. In contrast, the right venous angle receives fluid from the right axillary and cervical lymph nodes.[46,47]

The lymphatic system is tasked with removing lymph, but let us focus on one type of macromolecule found in lymph fluid: proteins. Proteins create colloidal osmotic pressures that retain water in the plasma and interstitial space. A healthy superficial lymphatic system removes these hydrophilic proteins. Without functional lymphatics, survival would be compromised within approximately 24 hours.[21] The use of diuretics for managing swelling exclusively due to lymphedema is not recommended. These medications can remove water from the lymph fluid but fail to eliminate the protein, which will seek water once the medication ceases. Protein, a proinflammatory macromolecule, remains in the interstitial space, potentially causing irreversible skin and soft tissue changes and an increased risk of cellulitis.[21] It is essential to note that some patients with lymphatic conditions may also have cardiac issues that necessitate diuretic use. The patient's physician should determine the proper dosage and desirable precautions. The term phlebolymphedema is used when there is damage to the lower limbs' lymphatic and venous systems.[47] The damage to the lymphatic system is a secondary consequence of venous damage, as it is overwhelmed by its capacity to remove interstitial fluid (**Fig. 11**).

### Lymphedema Stages

The International Society of Lymphology (ISL) Consensus Document describes a staging system to identify the progression of extremity lymphedema. It consists of four stages describing noted swelling and skin condition[48] (**Figs. 12** and **13**).

- Stage 0: latent or subclinical condition. Swelling is not evident despite impaired lymph transport. This stage may exist months or years before edema is noted. Good outcomes were reported with early management during this stage, preventing the progression of the following stages.
- Stage I: reversible stage. Early visible accumulation of high protein-rich fluid, which subsides with elevation. Swelling may be pitting. Good treatment outcomes can be expected when adequately managed, that is, CDT.
- Stage II: swelling increases, and limb elevation is not adequate. Pitting is initially present, but as this stage progresses, pitting may be difficult due to tissue hardening. Improvement can occur with appropriate treatment and management.
- Stage III: lymphostatic elephantiasis with no pitting and developing of skin changes such as thickness, increased fibrotic tissue, and warty overgrowths. The tissue becomes harder. Limb size does not come into play for this stage, but instead, observable skin changes do as listed earlier in addition to hyperpigmentation, increased skin folds, and fat deposits. Treatment is beneficial, but due to the skin changes, the duration of treatment may have to be extended.[49]

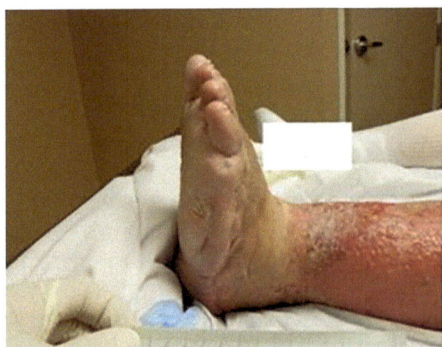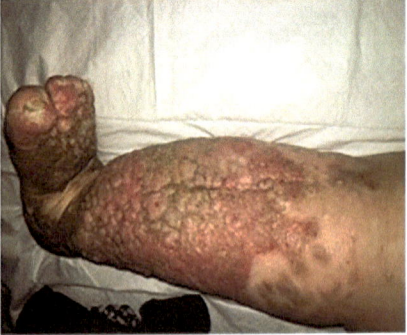

**Fig. 11.** CVI not managed leads to phlebolymphedema.

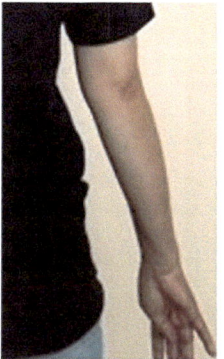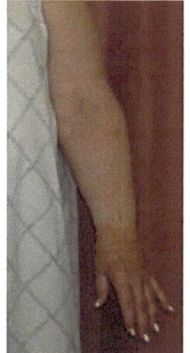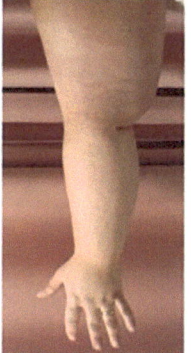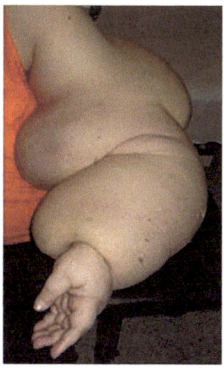

**Fig. 12.** Upper body lymphedema stages. (Image credit: Karen Ashforth.)

## CHARACTERISTICS

Diagnosis of lymphedema is based on clinical evidence, whereas imaging such as lymphoscintigraphy is only required when there is doubt about the lymphatic compromise.[50] Regardless if it is primary or secondary lymphedema, the treatment will be similarly. The severity of lymphedema is categorized as mild (<20% increase in extremity volume), moderate (20%–40%), or severe (>40%).[31]

*Primary lymphedema*: congenital and patients may be born with characteristics usually in the lower extremities, but symptoms can occur later in life, especially after puberty or injury. A family history may be evident.

*Secondary lymphedema*: damage to the lymphatic system, such as lymph node surgery, trauma, fused ankle, CVI, infection, radiation, and obesity.

### Treatment

Patients with lymphatic damage benefit from CDT, the gold standard of care. CDT is performed by a therapist usually trained as a Certified Lymphedema Therapist. There are two phases to CDT. The initial phase is where the therapist works on decongesting the body part while educating the patient on how to manage it. Then, the second phase is the self-care phase.[51]

### Manual Lymphatic Drainage

Manual lymphatic drainage (MLD) is a gentle technique to stimulate the superficial lymphatic system. When working on an extremity, we decongest from the proximal to the distal segments (**Fig. 14**).

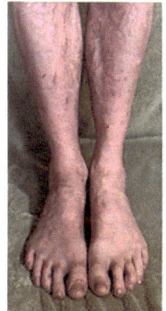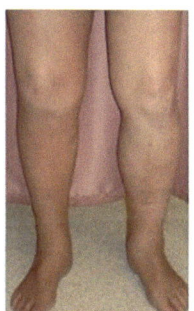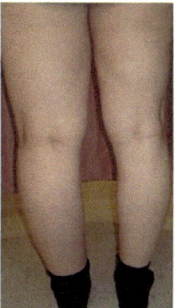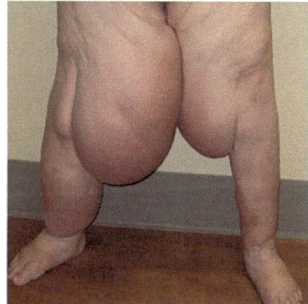

**Fig. 13.** Lower body lymphedema stages. (Image credit: Karen Ashforth.)

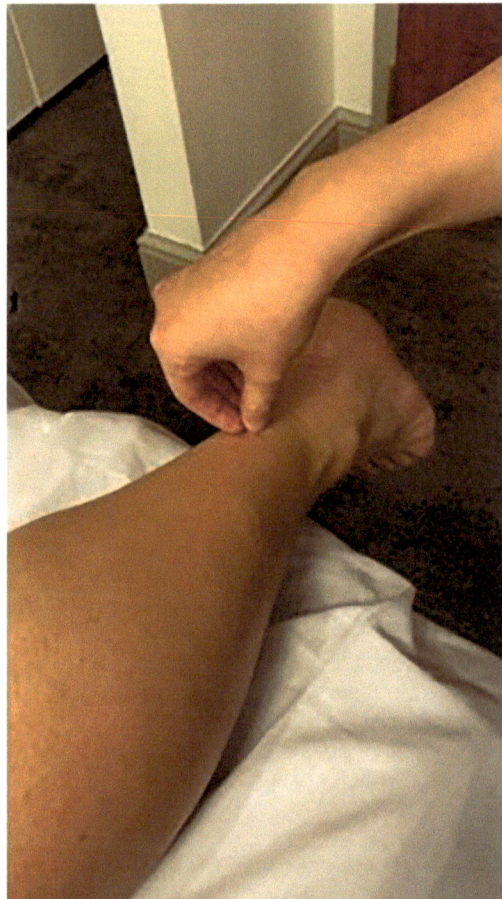

**Fig. 14.** Manual lymphatic drainage requires a superficial and gentle stroke.

## Skin Care

Patients may encounter frequent infections due to an increased diffusion distance causing increase in fluid. Clinicians use moisture-wicking products, zinc-based products, and skin wipes to protect the skin.

## Compression/Bandaging

Initially, short-stretch bandages (**Figs. 15** and **16**) are used while the extremity decongests followed by measuring for compression garments. The amount of pressure required (15–20 mm Hg is considered over-the-counter and low level of compression, 20–30 mm Hg Class I provides compression without being aggressive, 30–40 mm Hg Class II is a more substantial amount of compression, 40–50 mm Hg Class III is very strong compression) and product selection is also based on adequate arterial perfusion as well as patient considerations, Various garment styles are available (knee high, thigh high, pantyhose, open or closed toes, arm sleeve, hand, gauntlet, chest, head, and neck, etc.).

## Decongestive Exercises

The muscle pump increases the efficiency of the lymph transport. Diaphragmatic breathing exercises are also beneficial in increasing lymphatic and venous transport. Basic ambulation and leg exercises while wearing compression is adequate.

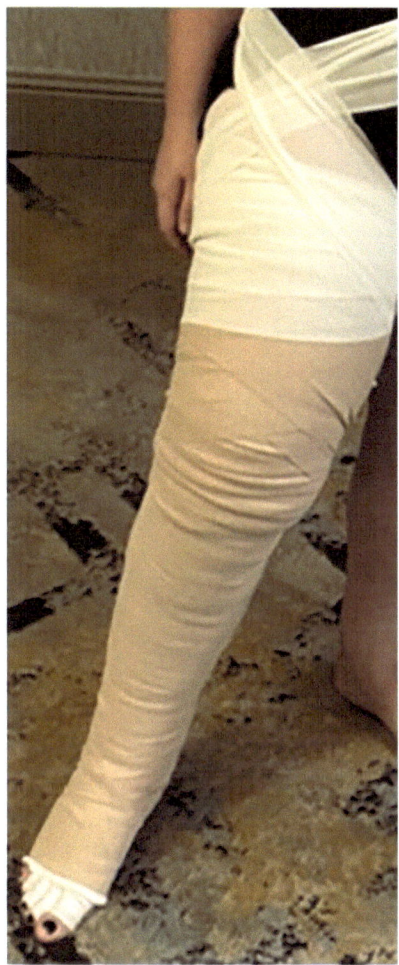

**Fig. 15.** Compression of the lower extremity using short-stretch bandaging in the early phase of CDT.

### Education

Education is provided to transition into the self-care phase of CDT treatment, such as self-MLD, self-bandaging, donning/doffing/caring for compression garments, home exercise program, and dos and don'ts.

### Kinesio Taping

Kinesio taping, developed by Dr Kenzo Kase, applies elastic adhesive tape in specific locations to help lift the skin and facilitate lymph movement[32] (**Fig. 17**).

### Intermittent Pneumatic Pumps

IPC pumps have become a useful adjunct modality for treating lymphedema but do not replace CDT. Over the years, IPC technology has improved, concluding their effectiveness in reducing limb volume and improving quality of life.[52] IPC pump with

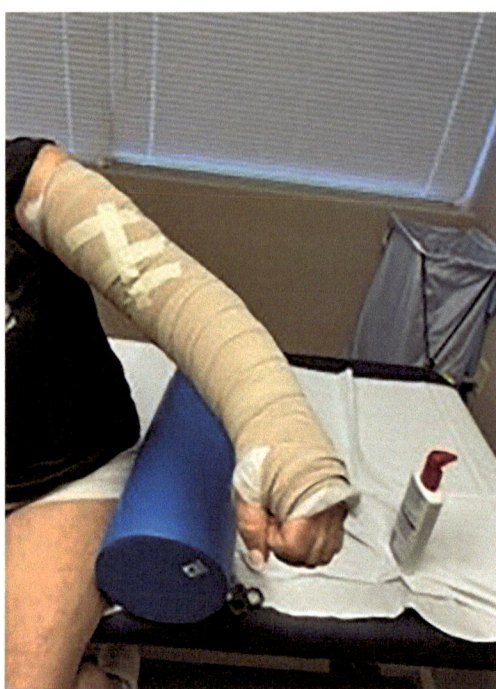

**Fig. 16.** Compression of the upper extremity using short-stretch bandaging in the early phase of CDT.

a higher number of chambers and advanced pumps providing sequential or peristaltic compression in an ascending pattern on the limb exists and is preferred over single chambers.[21,52] The amount of pressure during treatment can vary, but in one study 80 to 120 mm Hg was prescribed, resulting in a 75% mean reduction of edema,[53] whereas another study recommended pressures from 80 to 150 mm Hg for 45 to 60 minutes per day in lower limbs.[54] Taradaj and colleagues showed that patients with lower limb lymphedema being treated once a day, three times a week for four weeks concluded that when IPC was added to MLD and multi-bandaging, the most significant limb reduction with treatment pressures of 120 mm Hg (38%) was achieved compared with treatment pressures of 60 mm Hg (13%) or bandaging and MLD alone (13%).[55]

### Surgical Interventions

These techniques continue to improve, showing promising results, decreased pain, and improved quality of life. There is still no cure, and managing it is crucial.

### CLINICS CARE POINTS—LYMPHEDEMA

- The use of diuretics to decrease edema in patients with lymphatic damage is not recommended. According to Farrow (2010), this will increase the concentration of proteins in the interstitial space and the inflammatory process, leading to irreversible skin and soft tissue changes.
- Unilateral or bilateral asymmetrical extremity swelling can be a physical characteristic of lymphedema.
- CDT by a certified clinician is the gold-standard treatment.

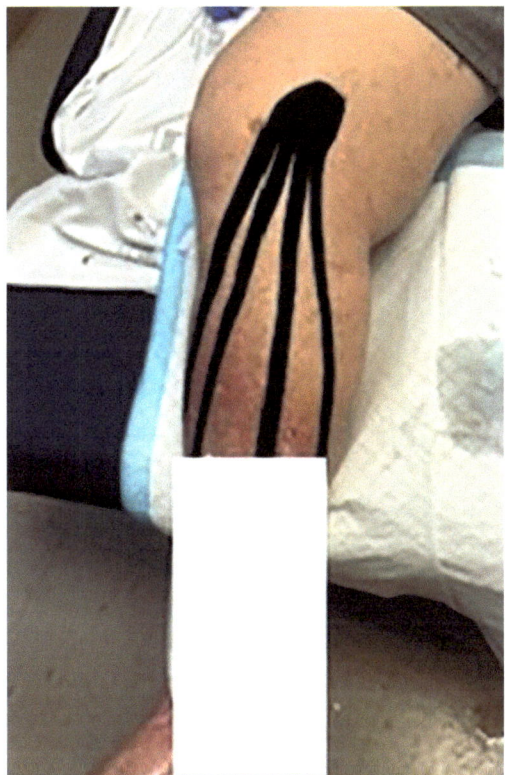

**Fig. 17.** Using Kinesio taping to direct the direction of fluid as it elevates the skin.

## SUMMARY

Venous and lymphatic diseases are chronic and progressive with no definitive cure, often leading to a decreased quality of life, particularly in advanced stages when wounds are present. Identifying the affected system and its characteristics aids clinicians in managing these conditions while adhering to the principles of wound care and understanding the importance of therapeutic compression. Patients with chronic wounds face increased complications over time, especially when the scars remain in the inflammatory phase of healing. Those with venous diseases or lymphedema are at greater risk of complications if these conditions are not appropriately managed alongside essential wound care.

## DISCLOSURE

F. Aviles—Advisor/speaker/consultant/instructor for Eva Medtec, Kent Imaging, Wound Vision, Norton School of Lymphatic Therapy, Essity, Urgo, Molnlycke Healthcare, and —AOTI Inc. E. Faust – Consultant for Mediwound, Urgo Medical, Owens & Minor, Solventum, Kerecis, Bechtel Medical, Molnlycke, Frontier Therapeutics, and Hovertech.

## REFERENCES

1. Jones O. Venous drainage of the lower limb. TeachMeAnatomy. 2023. Available at: https://teachmeanatomy.info/lower-limb/blood-vessels/venous-drainage/. Accessed July 24, 2024.

2. National Institutes of Health. Dysfunctional exosomes involved in chronic inflammation in diabetic wounds. NIH Research Matters. Available at: https://www.nih.gov/news-events/nih-research-matters/dysfunctional-exosomes-involved-chronic-inflammation-diabetic-wounds. Accessed July 26, 2024.

3. Trayes KP, Studdiford JS, Pickle S, et al. Edema: diagnosis and management. Am Fam Physician 2013;88(2):102–10.

4. Shadrina AS, Elgaeva EE, Stanaway IB, et al. Mendelian randomization analysis of plasma levels of CD209 and MICB proteins and the risk of varicose veins of lower extremities. PLoS One 2022;17(5).

5. Eberhardt RT, Raffetto JD. Chronic venous insufficiency. Circulation 2005;111:2398–409.

6. Bonkemeyer Millan S, Gan R, Townsend PE. Venous ulcers: diagnosis and treatment. Am Fam Physician 2019;100(5):298–305.

7. Patel SK, Surowiec SM. Venous insufficiency. In: StatPearls [Internet]. Treasure Island (FL): StatPearls Publishing; 2024. Available at: https://www.ncbi.nlm.nih.gov/books/NBK430975/.

8. Donnell O, Allison G, Iafrati M. A systematic review of guidelines for lymphedema and the need for contemporary intersocietal guidelines for the management of lymphedema. J Vasc Surg Venous Lymphat Disord 2020;8(4):676–84.

9. Sleigh BC, Manna B. Lymphedema. In: StatPearls. Treasure Island (FL): StatPearls Publishing; 2023.

10. Dean S, Valenti E, Hock K, et al. The clinical characteristics of lower extremity lymphedema in 440 patients. J Vasc Surg Venous Lymphat Disord 2020;8(5):851–9.

11. Szyber P, Szyber P. Lower limb lymphoedema – therapeutic problem. Therapy 2008;2(1):70–2.

12. Li J, Chen J, Kirsner R. Pathophysiology of acute wound healing. Clin Dermatol 2007;25(1):9–18. https://doi.org/10.1016/j.clindermatol.2006.09.007.

13. Hess CT. Comprehensive patient and wound assessments. Adv Skin Wound Care 2019;32(6):287–8.

14. CliniMed. Phases of Wound Healing. CliniMed website. 2022. Available at: https://www.clinimed.co.uk. Accessed July 26, 2024.

15. Bowden LG, Byrne HM, Maini PK, et al. A morphoelastic model for dermal wound closure. Biomech Model Mechanobiol 2016;15(3):663–81.

16. Hall JE. Guyton and Hall Textbook of medical physiology. Philadelphia, PA: Saunders Elsevier; 2016.

17. Pagano M, Bissacco D, Flore R, et al. Great saphenous vein reflux treatment in patients with femoral valve incompetence, the Excluded Saphenous Vein Technique (ESVT): a pilot study. Eur Rev Med Pharmacol Sci 2018;22(21):7453–7.

18. Weismann K, Krakauer R, Wanscher B. Prevalence of skin diseases in old age. Acta Derm Venereol 1980;60(4):352–3.

19. Kahn SR, Shrier I, Julian JA, et al. Obesity and the risk of venous thromboembolism: a systematic review and meta-analysis. Thromb Haemost 2009;101(5):1000–10.

20. Vivas A, Lev-Tov H, Kirsner RS. Venous leg ulcers. Ann Intern Med 2016;165(3):ITC17–32.

21. Farrow W. Phlebolymphedema-a common underdiagnosed and undertreated problem in the wound care clinic. J Am Col Certif Wound Spec 2010;2(1):14–23.

22. Reddy M, Upton D, Hayes K, et al. A comprehensive review of the treatment of venous leg ulcers. Wounds 2021;33(2):43–53.

23. Moffatt C, Franks P, Doherty D, et al. The role of hemosiderin staining in chronic venous disease: A clinical and histological perspective. J Wound Care 2008; 17(8):335–41.
24. Alavi A, Hafner J, Dutz JP, et al. Atrophie blanche: is it associated with venous disease or livedoid vasculopathy? Adv Skin Wound Care 2014;27(11):518–24. https://doi.org/10.1097/01.ASW.0000455098.98684.95.
25. Nelson EA, Jones J. Venous leg ulcers. BMJ Clin Evid 2008;2008:1902.
26. Rogers AA, Lantis JC, Wylie A, et al. Evidence-based strategies for the management of chronic wounds: a review. Am J Surg 2012;203(2):177–88.
27. Gottrup F, Apelqvist J, Bjansent T, et al. The role of dressings and wound care in wound healing. J Wound Care 2010;19(6):238–45.
28. Edsberg LE, Yee T, Baranoski S, et al. Pressure injury prevention and treatment: a comprehensive review. J Wound, Ostomy Cont Nurs 2016;43(6):564–85.
29. Atkin L, Bućko Z, Conde Montero E, et al. Implementing TIMERS: the race against hard-to-heal wounds. J Wound Care 2019;28(3):1–49. https://doi.org/10.12968/jowc.2019.28.Sup3a.S1.
30. Jull AB, Arroll B, Parag V, et al. Pentoxifylline for treating venous leg ulcers. Cochrane Database Syst Rev 2012;12:CD001733.
31. Kirienko A, Radak D. Clinical acceptability study of once-daily versus twice-daily micronized purified flavonoid fraction in patients with symptomatic chronic venous disease: a randomized controlled trial. Int Angiol 2016;35(4):399–405. 67.
32. Leng F, Yang Z, Long F, et al. Kinesio tape in the treatment of postoperative lymphedema of breast cancer. TMR Non-Drug Therapy 2019;2(2):36–41.
33. Partsch H, Mosti G, ved M. Compression therapy for venous insufficiency: principles and practice. Phlebology 2019;34(7):451–62.
34. Millan S, Can R, Townsend P. Venous ulcers: diagnosis and treatment. Am Fam Physician 2019;100(5):298–305.
35. Partsch H, Clark M. Compression for venous and lymphatic disease: a systematic review of the literature. Phlebology 2014;29(4):169–80.
36. Kuehlmann-Buhler K, Lindner R, Schmelzle R. Lymphedema management: evidence-based guidelines for fitting compression garments and devices. J Vasc Surg 2016;64(1):120–7.
37. Dini M, Partsch H, Moffatt C. Compression therapy for the management of venous disease: an overview of garment design, characteristics, and patient outcomes. Eur J Vasc Endovasc Surg 2015;50(1):35–41.
38. Callam MJ, Harper DR, Allan PL, et al. The effect of compression bandaging on venous ulcer healing: a randomized controlled trial. BMJ 2000;321(7266): 1258–60.
39. O'Donnell TF, Passman MA, Marston WA, et al. Compression therapy for venous insufficiency: a review of the evidence. J Vasc Surg 2014;60(1):24–32.
40. Kuehlmann-Buhler K, Levenson E, Rütten R. A review of garment donning and doffing aids for patients with lymphedema: efficacy and patient experience. J Lymphoedema 2019;14(1):44–55.
41. Meaume S, Couilliet D, Vin F. Prognostic factors for venous ulcer healing in a non-selected population of ambulatory patients. J Wound Care 2005;14(1):31–4.
42. Margolis D, Allen-Taylor L, Hoffstad O, et al. The accuracy of venous leg ulcer prognostic models in a wound care system. J Wound Repair & Regen 2004; 12(2):163–8.
43. Kortenoeven ML, van der Veen K, Heijnen CJ, et al. The lymphatic system: an essential component of fluid homeostasis. J Physiol 2017;595(6):1899–909.

44. Rockson SG. The lymphatic system: anatomy, physiology, and clinical relevance. In: Rook's textbook of dermatology. 9th ed. Blackwell Publishing; 2016. p. 1–23.
45. Földi M, Földi E, Kubik S. Deficiency and insufficiency of the lymphatic system. In: Textbook of Lymphology for physicians and lymphedema therapists. Munich, Germany: Urban and Fisher; 2003. p. 209–15.
46. Moore KL, Dalley AF, Agur AMR. Clinically oriented anatomy. 8th ed. Wolters Kluwer; 2018. p. 338–9.
47. Feldman J, Goudie A, Keith M. Phlebolymphedema: a comprehensive review of its pathophysiology and management. J Vasc Surg 2019;70(4):1285–95.
48. International Society of Lymphology. The diagnosis and treatment of lymphatic disease: a consensus document. Lymphatic Res Biol 2013;11(4):1–16. https://doi.org/10.1089/lrb.2013.0022.
49. The diagnosis and treatment of peripheral lymphedema: 2020 consensus document of the International Society Of Lymphology. Lymphology 2020;53:3–19.
50. International Society of Lymphology. The diagnosis and treatment of peripheral lymphedema: 2013 consensus document of the International Society of Lymphology. Lymphology 2013;46(1):1–11.
51. Schinow SK, Vignes S, Callahan M, et al. Complex decongestive therapy for the management of lymphedema: a comprehensive review. J Lymphoedema 2014; 9(1):34–40.
52. Dunn N, Williams EM, Dolan G, et al. Intermittent pneumatic compression for the treatment of lower limb lymphedema: a pilot trial of sequencing to mimic manual lymphatic drainage versus traditional graduated sequential compression. Lymphatic Res Biol 2022;20(5):514–21.
53. Modaghegh MHS, Soltani E. A newly designed SIPC device for management of lymphoedema. Indian J Surg 2010;72:36–40.
54. Olszewski W.L. and Brunner U. Therapeutics and clinical Risk Management, 2012;8:137-146.
55. Taradaj J, Rosińczuk J, Dymarek R, et al. Comparison of efficacy of the intermittent pneumatic compression with a high- and low-pressure application in reducing the lower limbs phlebolymphedema. Ther Clin Risk Manag 2015;11: 1545–54.

# Intraoperative Pressure Injury Prevention

Lisa Peterson, MSN, RN, CNOR

## KEYWORDS

- Pressure injury • Intraoperative • Operating room • Surgery • Prevention
- Pressure injury prevention • Pressure ulcer

## KEY POINTS

- Surgeries lasting longer than 3 h put patients at risk of an intraoperative acquired pressure injury (PI).
- Patient comorbidities and surgery-specific risk factors should be considered when assessing a patient's risk for a PI.
- Evidence is still growing, so staying up-to-date on the latest evidence-based practice is essential in guiding intraoperative PI prevention care.

## CLINICAL SETTING – OPERATING ROOM

The operating room (OR) is the area *behind the red line*. The goal of this section is to illuminate the role of the OR nurse in pressure injury (PI) prevention, as "proper positioning in the OR is a primary task for OR staff nurses"[1] Surgery-specific needs and patient characteristics, including "health history and body composition," contribute to a patient's risk of an intraoperative PI.[2] PIs that develop within 72 h after a surgical procedure can be attributed to the OR, with stage 3, stage 4, and unstageable pressure injuries considered "never events. This is a billion-dollar issue, as the United States spends over $26 billion annually on PIs.[3,4]

### Learning Objectives

1. Understand OR specific considerations with PI prevention
2. Understand patient-specific risk factors contributing to intraoperative PIs
3. Identify pressure offloading tools to protect patients' skin intraoperatively

### Description of the setting

Pressure offloading devices outside the OR are complex and possibly unsafe to implement intraoperatively. For example, "static devices based on fluid are considered effective"; however, "they have not been indicated for use in the OR, since it is

Children's Surgery Center, UC Davis Health– ATTN, 4301 X Street, Sacramento, CA 95817, USA
*E-mail address:* lapeterson@ucdavis.edu

Nurs Clin N Am 60 (2025) 99–108
https://doi.org/10.1016/j.cnur.2024.07.004
0029-6465/25/Published by Elsevier Inc.

impossible to maintain the surgical position of the patient".[5] This is further complicated by a "lack of research related to the observed PIP (pressure injury prevention)
practices" and, ultimately, a need for "further research".[6]

### Intraoperative Positioning of the Patient

This section focuses on 4 intraoperative patient positions: supine, prone, lithotomy,
and lateral.

*Supine:* Points of concern for a patient in a supine position include the sacrum,
heels, occiput, and scapulae area.[3,7] One study found that the pressure of the sacrum
and occiput ranged from 40 to 60 mm Hg,[7] which exceeds the 32 mm Hg, which "cor-
responds to the capillary filling pressure".[5] When pressure exceeds 32 mm Hg, vessels are occluded, leading to "the development of localized ischemia, tissue
inflammation, tissue anoxia, and necrosis".[8] For heels, the National Pressure Injury
Advisory Panel recommends that the heels are "free of the surface of the operating
table".[9]

*Prone:* Focal points for a patient in the prone position include "facial tissues, the
breasts for females, the lower costal margins, the anterior iliac crests, the genitalia
(particularly for males), the knees, the shins, and the dorsal feet".[10] Prone positioning
can involve the Mayfield skull clamp, which "is a 3-point clamp that is secured to the
skull's outer table," allowing for head stabilization[11] or foam cradles for the head. An
option for the head is Prone View with a "face-contoured polyurethane headrest
covered by a plastic shield," which "reduces facial pressure" while keeping "the
eyes free of any extraocular pressure".[11] Facial tissues are at a higher risk of an intraoperative acquired pressure injury (IAPI) when a head frame is used.[12]

*Lithotomy:* Lithotomy positioning is when the patient is in the supine position, where
"legs are raised and secured" with hip and knee flexion, resulting in elevated pressure
at the sacral and scapular area.[10] A study found that the "standard OR mattress with
the static, air-filled seat cushion placed under the buttocks provided the lowest peak
pressures and the highest skin surface contact area".[2]

*Lateral decubitus:* The patient is kept in this lateral position by positioning tools such
as the beanbag, gel bolsters for smaller patients, and surgical peg boards. Areas of
caution include: "anterior superior iliac spine, the acromion, the underarm chest wall
on the axillary pad, and the auricle".[13]

### Unique characteristics/risk factors

Each patient has varying risk factors (**Fig. 1**), therefore, "individualized interventions
are necessary".[10]

*Length of Surgery:* Surgery is considered the most significant predictor of developing an intraoperative PI. Studies use terminology such as "prolonged surgical
time",[14] "length of surgery",[3] "estimated surgery length greater than or equal to
3.0 h",[12] "surgical time longer than 185 min",[15] and "longer duration of surgery"[16,17]
to express the importance of the length of surgery in PI risk. Research reveals "that
skin pressure increases as the operation time increases".[18] More specifically, a PI
rate was "9% for 4 to 5-h procedures, 10% for 5 to 7-h surgeries, and over 13% for
operations longer than 7 h".[1] The American Perioperative Registered Nurses
(AORN) guidelines state that "surgeries lasting longer than 4 h" put patients at the
highest risk.[7] Additionally, a "2-h (net) surgery can imply 6 or more hours of immobility
for the patient," highlighting the importance of mobility preoperatively and postoperatively.[10] Ultimately, OR nurses know that "the true length of any operation is only
known after surgery is complete," underscoring the value of nursing clinical
judgment.[10]

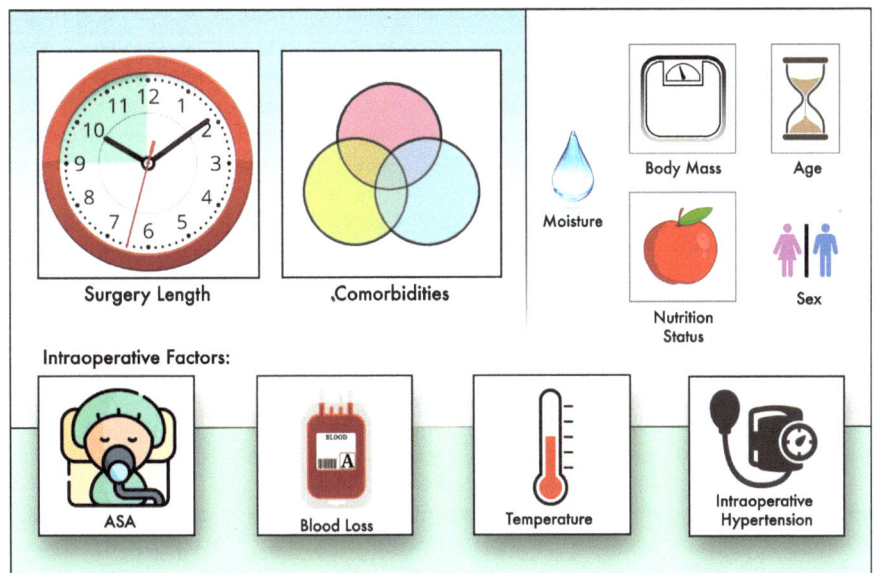

**Fig. 1.** Risk factors for elevated risk of pressure injury. (Image courtesy: Sarah St. Claire.)

*Body Mass Index (BMI):* Patients with a BMI outside normal limits have an increased risk of developing an intraoperative PI.[16] These parameters are not definitive as one study defines the critical ranges as " less than 19.0 or greater than 40.0 kg/m2",[12] while the AORN defines this as BMI greater than or equal to 30 kg/mg2.[9]

### American Society of Anesthesiologists Classification and Type of Anesthetic

The American Society of Anesthesiologists (ASA) classification provides "the relative degree of patient comorbid states".[10] This classification ranges from an ASA I, a completely healthy patient, to an ASA VI, a patient pronounced brain dead. When using the ASA value, "variability exists between anesthesiologists," so this "can contribute to assessing risk and outcomes".[19] Furthermore, one study considers an ASA score of II as a risk factor,[20] whereas a different study found a predictive threshold as an ASA III or higher.[12] Regardless of the exact parameter, ASA is seen as a "significant predictor".[3]

Additionally, "general anesthesia is associated with greater pressure ulcer (PU) incidence than use of regional anesthetic".[10]

*Gender:* The literature is inconclusive on how gender contributes to intraoperative PIs. One study claims the male sex was a "risk",[21] whereas a different study found the female sex as the stronger predictor.[3]

*Hypotension:* Intraoperative hypotension is a risk factor of developing an IAPI[7,14,15,20,22] One study defines critical hypotension as "diastolic blood pressure less than or equal to 60 mm Hg".[23] To combat "prolonged hypotension," vasopressors are used to "increase the arterial pressure," which "reduces microvascular perfusion," placing tissues at risk for cellular death.[10]

*Hyperthermia and hypothermia:* Both hyperthermia and hypothermia "play an active role in forming PIs".[7,16] Vasoconstrictors compound Hypothermia, as narrow microvasculature is further constricted, causing a "decrease in the physiologic heat convection, particularly to the periphery".[10] As little as "a drop of 1.8 C in the core body temperature" elevates the risk of an IAPI by 20%.[10]

*Comorbidities:* Diabetes, obesity, peripheral vascular disease, cancer, and neurologic disease.[24] One study identified critical comorbidities as "cardiovascular disease, respiratory disease, and diabetes mellitus", as well as "low hemoglobin level".[17] The AORN defines comorbidities as "high blood pressure, diabetes mellitus, and vascular, renal, cardiovascular, respiratory problems".[7] More specifically, for patients with diabetes, "the risk of surgery-related pressure ulcers is about 1.5 times more than others".[25]

*Age:* Age is an intraoperative PI risk factor primarily for the geriatric population. Some studies define age as critical over 62 years old[12]; the AORN defines this parameter as 60 years of age.[7]

*Blood Loss:* Blood loss causes a cascading response as "arterial pressures decrease, and lower body temperature, causing vasoconstriction," which makes the patient vulnerable to "ischemic tissue damage".[10] There is statistical significance to the "large amount of bleeding during surgery ($P = .001$),"[26] which the AORN defined as "highest risk if bleeding is more than 400 mL".[7] Finally, additional intraoperative PI risk factors are poor nutrition, moisture, and incontinence.[7] Moisture is a catalyst for PIs because it "significantly reduces blood flow when pressure is applied, causing skin damage".[27] Nutrition contributes as protein levels influence albumin levels.[28] More specifically, hemoglobin and albumin levels both contribute to perfusion efficacy and "were found to be determinant risk factors in the development of PI ($P<.01$)".[15]

### Unique challenges/special populations

Pediatric patients have unique body proportions and "immature skin" based on gestational age.[9] One pediatric study found the prevalence of PIs ranging from 1.4% to 8.2%.[29] These pressure injuries can be from the surfaces these patients are on or the medical devices enhancing their care. Concerning surface-related PIs, "head and face region were most vulnerable to the injury".[30] However, medical device pressure injuries "far surpassed the occurrence of immobility-related pressure injuries".[31] Patients with darker skin tones (DST) are "more likely to develop higher stage PIs," which may be a result of "failure to identify stage 1 pressure damage"[32] accurately. One study found lighter skin was a PI risk factor,[26] which may occur because "current skin assessment protocols are less effective for people with DST"[32] and "subject to misinterpretation".[10] The early signs of PIs in DST "rarely show the blanching response, and erythema may be hard to detect"; thus, "people with DST are more likely to develop higher stage pressure injuries".[32]

### AVAILABILITY OF RESOURCES/PRESSURE OFFLOADING TOOLS

Pressure offloading tools are the "standard care for all patients".[9] The keys to these pressure offloading tools include: "lowest mean interface pressure, lowest peak interface pressure, and highest skin contact area"[33] while being thin enough "to allow x-ray" and maintaining a safe, stable surface for the patient.[10] The "effectiveness of these support surfaces" varies (8), which is compounded by "limited research" assessing the efficacy of these tools.[34]

*Air-Inflated Static Seat Cushion:* The air-inflated static seat cushion has the "best pressure redistribution properties in the sacral region".[33] This cushion is "designed to maximize immersion and envelopment," helping increase surface area and decrease peak pressures.[10] One study found that this device "may reduce pressure injuries in some surgical procedures that last longer than 3 h".[24] Of note is that this cushion is radiopaque and will show artifacts through fluoroscopy.

*Silicone Foam Dressing:* A silicone foam dressing benefits "bony prominences or areas that likely will be exposed to pressure, friction, and shear during procedures".[9]

These dressings protect "specific at-risk sites, especially from tissue shearing".[10] Applying these dressings should be done "during skin assessment, before surgery, while the patient is awake and can move to facilitate placement".[10]

*Alternating Pressure (AP) Overlay:* "An AP overlay mattress has been developed to mimic the practice of cyclical offloading with no perceptible motion".[35] This tool "facilitates the delivery of cyclic micro-motion repositioning, to compensate for the no-repositioning and low immersion and envelopment" of the OR Table.[1]

*Gel Pads:* Gel pads are known for their "good elasticity"; however, "they can be heavy and have poor air permeability".[12] Gel pads can reduce PIs[24] by "enlarging the force area" but "cannot be used for pressure redistribution".[36] Unlike "air cell surgical pads," gel pads were less effective in PI reduction.[34] Aged gel pads are subject to splitting from wear and may "bottom out during OR use".[10]

*Foam pads:* Memory foam padding is known for having a "slow rebound and is soft, comfortable, and skin-friendly".[12] Egg-crate foam padding is "light and soft, but can be easily deformed, resulting in uneven force".[12]

*Pillows, Towels, Sheets, and Blankets:* Pillows, towels, sheets, and blankets are used to elevate a patient to the desired surgical position. These items have "not been designed for conforming to the body contours" and, therefore, "tend to flatten under bodyweight forces".[10]

## TOP WOUNDS FREQUENTLY SEEN IN YOUR CLINICAL SETTING

*Sacral:* When a patient is placed in a supine position, the critical points of pressure include "occiput, scapula, sacrococcyx, and heels," but of these, the "incidence of IAPIs in the sacrococcyx exceeds 85%".[36] A 2020 systematic review found that 37.3% of all intraoperative PIs "developed at the sacrum" when evaluating 9016 PIs.[3] When looking at specific risk factors, "length of surgery and patient's BMI were significant predictors of the peak tissue interface pressure for the sacral area ($P<.001$)".[3]

*Occipital:* While adults "develop more sacral and heel injuries," pediatric patients "experience relatively more occipital pressure injuries".[37] Pediatric patients "up to the age of 5" have a head "proportionally larger than their body," placing their occipital region at risk.[38]

### Risk Assessment Scales

The intraoperative-specific PI risk assessment scales must be used cautiously as "risk assessments alone have little predictive power" and cannot replace "clinical judgment".[10] Additionally, "well-documented risk factors," including length of surgery, are excluded from "tools such as the Norton, Waterlow, or Braden scales".[10] The Braden is less common intraoperatively as it focuses on "risk factors not considered in the OR setting".[39] For hospital-acquired pressure injuries, "there was no significant difference between patients who developed pressure injuries and patients who did not" when evaluating Braden scores.[23] The Braden Q(D) is designed for pediatric patients and includes devices as a PI risk factor. This pediatric assessment "predicts immobility-related and device-related pressure injuries".[31] Scott Triggers includes 4 factors: "age, serum albumin levels or BMI, ASA score, and estimated surgery time".[10,24,40] Serum albumin "maintains the oncotic pressure," which is "the main driving force for vascular refill; thus, lower serum albumin levels might be associated with decreased skin perfusion".[41] Overall, the Scott Triggers tool was more effective than the Braden for the intraoperative setting.[41] The Munro can help perioperative nurses "identify high-risk patients"[39] with "15 items to comprehensively assess the risk factors for PIs during the pre-, intra-, and postoperative phases".[42] Specifically, Munro focuses on "the ASA physical status score, the type of anesthesia, body temperature, hypotension, moisture, surface/motion, and position".[10]

PRAMS includes risk factors such as "diabetes, age, surgical time, the 'conventional' Braden score, previous surgery, and a pre-existing PU".[10] Waterlow focuses on "patient gender, age group, BMI, skin health, mobility, continence, nutrition, and 'special risk' factors".[43] The Norton scale includes: "mental condition, physical activity, mobility, food intake, fluid intake, incontinence, and general physical condition".[44] Lastly, the 3S Intraoperative Risk Assessment Scale is based on the "condition of the skin in the whole body, preoperative activity status, height/weight ratio, stress status of the skin, amount of bleeding in the operation, duration of the operation, stress in the operation, body temperature in the operation, and the position of the operation".[21]

## PREVENTION

The primary forms of intraoperative PI prevention include skin assessments and education. This includes exploring new pressure-offloading resources while engaging in collaborative practice.

- *Skin Assessment:* Skin assessments should be done "at various stages of the patient's perioperative course",[23] specifically, preoperatively, and postoperatively.[9,10,23,24,45] Assessments of skin "cannot detect early damage sub-dermally or identify microscopic signs or predictors" and are "subject to misinterpretation," especially in patients with DST.[10]
- *Education:* As evidence grows, it is vital for OR nurses "to be up-to-date and educated on various devices".[10] This education can come in the form of "evidence-based practice initiatives",[24] "training and education",[46] "educational meetings",[37,] or pressure mapping.[47] Methods such as root cause analysis and fishbone diagrams are "imperative to reducing hospital-acquired PU rates".[10] Education should be curated "based on the actual environment and work characteristics," acknowledging that a Level 1 Trauma Center has different needs than an outpatient surgery center.[46]
- *Collaborative practice:* A collaborative interdisciplinary team is the best way to create buy-in.[9,24,37] The AORN recommends taking an interdisciplinary approach to "develop policies and procedures for the perioperative PI prevention" and work to "standardize practice".[9] Collaboration can include preoperative providers as they are best suited to "apply for skin protection",[37] where "preventative measures begin".[48] Finally, collaboration can include non-health care members such as bioengineers who can "revisit the design of operating tables".[10]

## TREATMENT GOALS

Prevention is the key concerning intraoperative PIs. In a study, the implementation of a PI prevention bundle led to a zero-incidence rate of PIs after potentially 8 intraoperative PIs in the prior year.[49] This bundle was created by an interdisciplinary team focusing on "skin and risk assessments," "protection of all at-risk skin with protocols and products," consistent communication, regular training, audits, and collaboration with the wound care team.[49]

## PROPOSED FORMULARY OF SUPPLIES

When addressing supplies, the location of the supplies needs to be intentional. When supplies are not easily accessible, "it will soon be omitted entirely" as attention will be shifted to other preparation needs.[10] PI prevention supplies "must either be in the pack of surgical supplies or very close to the OR" to limit the time needed to gather items.[10] Supplies that should be readily available include air-inflated static seat cushions, silicone foam dressings, AP overlays, and gel and foam pads.

## SAFETY POLICY AND DOCUMENTATION

Policies and procedures should "align with similar facility documents and be maintained in a location that is readily accessible to perioperative team members.".[9] Skin assessments continue to be a foundational part of prevention and should be documented preoperatively and postoperatively to assess for any intraoperative skin change.[23,24,31,37,38,49] Part of protecting a patient's skin includes following the manufacturer's information for use (IFU). IFUs should be available "for support surfaces and prophylactic dressings, and leaders should monitor staff member compliance".[9] Finally, the operating table pad should be evaluated. This is "frequently overlooked as a worn-out device" as it should be "at least 2 in thick" but preferably up to 5".[10]

## CLINICS CARE POINTS

- Utilize pressure offloading tools that reduce peak pressures and increase the surface area of the patient's skin.
- Not all pressure offloading tools are appropriate for use in the OR.
- Where pressure offloading devices are kept matters because if items are not readily available, they will likely not be used.
- Intraoperative Pressure Injury Prevention risk assessments are available but not all are validated for intraoperative use

## DISCLOSURE

The author has nothing to disclose.

## REFERENCES

1. Gefen A. Minimising the risk for pressure ulcers in the operating room using a specialised low-profile alternating pressure overlay. Wounds International 2020;11(2): 10–6. Available at: https://search.ebscohost.com/login.aspx?direct=true&db=ccm&AN=143369196&site=ehost-live&scope=site. [Accessed 4 February 2024].
2. Teleten O, Prevatt J, Peterson L, et al. Use of pressure mapping to compare two operating room surfaces in the supine with bent knees position and the supine in lithotomy position. Wounds 2021;33(4):86–90.
3. Al MS, Vuncanon B, Kiyohara M, et al. Using continuous intraoperative pressure mapping to describe patterns of tissue interface pressure. AORN J 2022;116(3): 231–47.
4. Bouyer-Ferullo S, O'Connor C, Kinnealey E, et al. Adding a Visual Communication Tool to the Electronic Health Record to Prevent Pressure Injuries. AORN J 2021; 113(3):253–62.
5. Oliveira KF, Nascimento KG, Nicolussi AC, et al. Support surfaces in the prevention of pressure ulcers in surgical patients: An integrative review. Int J Nurs Pract (John Wiley & Sons, Inc) 2017;23(4):n/a–N.PAG.

6. Wang I, Walker R, Gillespie BM. Pressure injury prevention in the perioperative setting: an integrative review. J Perioper Nurs 2018;31(4):27–35.
7. Karahan E, Ayri AU, Çelik S. Evaluation of pressure ulcer risk and development in operating rooms. J Tissue Viability 2022;31(4):707–13.
8. Widiati E, Nurhaeni N, Gayatri D. Medical-Device Related Pressure Injuries to Children in the Intensive Care Unit. Compr Child Adolesc Nurs 2017;40(sup1): 69–77.
9. Speth J. Guidelines in Practice: Prevention of Perioperative Pressure Injury. AORN J 2023;118(1):37–44.
10. Gefen A, Creehan S, Black J. Critical biomechanical and clinical insights concerning tissue protection when positioning patients in the operating room: A scoping review. Int Wound J 2020;17(5):1405–23.
11. Garg B, Bansal T, Mehta N, et al. Patient Positioning in Spine Surgery: What Spine Surgeons Should Know? Asian Spine J 2023;17(4):770–81.
12. Wu Y, Jiang Z, Huang S, et al. Identification of Risk Factors for Intraoperative Acquired Pressure Injury in Patients Undergoing Neurosurgery: A Retrospective Single-Center Study. Med Sci Monit 2021;27:e932340. Published 2021 Sep 29.
13. Zhang Y, Wang L, Song J. Influence of comprehensive nursing cooperation on complications and quality of life in patients with video laryngoscope-guided orotracheal intubation in lateral decubitus position. Am J Transl Res 2023;15(2): 1517–25. Published 2023 Feb 15.
14. Chen Y, He L, Qu W, et al. Predictors of intraoperative pressure injury in patients undergoing major hepatobiliary surgery. J Wound, Ostomy Cont Nurs 2017;44(5): 445–9.
15. Determination of incidence and risk factors of perioperative pressure injury in surgical patients: a descriptive, prospective, and comparative study. Turkiye Klinikleri Journal of Nursing Sciences 2022;14(2):296–303.
16. Retrospective evaluation of the effectiveness of using two different products in preventing the development of pressure injuries in patients undergoing lung lobectomy. J Tissue Viability 2023;32(1):163–7.
17. Haisley M, Sørensen JA, Sollie M. Postoperative pressure injuries in adults having surgery under general anaesthesia: systematic review of perioperative risk factors. Br J Surg 2020;107(4):338–47.
18. Lu X, Yang Q, Zhu L, et al. Correlation analysis of sacrococcygeal pressure and operation time in patients undergoing general anesthesia in the supine position. J Int Med Res 2021;49(7). 300060520984595.
19. Horvath B, Kloesel B, Todd MM, et al. The Evolution, Current Value, and Future of the American Society of Anesthesiologists Physical Status Classification System. Anesthesiology 2021;135(5):904–19.
20. Yılmaz E, Başlı AA. Assessment of pressure injuries following surgery: a descriptive study. Wound Manag Prev 2021;67(6):27–40.
21. Tura İ, Arslan S, Türkmen A, et al. Assessment of the risk factors for intraoperative pressure injuries in patients. J Tissue Viability 2023;32(3):349–54.
22. Chello C, Lusini M, Schilirò D, et al. Pressure ulcers in cardiac surgery: Few clinical studies, difficult risk assessment, and profound clinical implications. Int Wound J 2019;16(1):9–12.
23. Celik B, Karayurt Ö, Ogce F. The effect of selected risk factors on perioperative pressure injury development. AORN J 2019;110(1):29–38.
24. McKenzie RJ, Ramirez C. Preventing pressure injuries in the operating room: Be proactive to avoid perioperative pressure and peripheral nerve injuries. American Nurse Today 2018;19–21. Available at: https://search.ebscohost.com/login.aspx?

direct=true&db=ccm&AN=129885955&site=ehost-live&scope=site.        [Accessed 4 February 2024].

25. Nasiri E, Mollaei A, Birami M, et al. The risk of surgery-related pressure ulcer in diabetics: A systematic review and meta-analysis. Ann Med Surg (Lond) 2021; 65:102336. Published 2021 Apr 17.

26. Özdemir ED, Uslu Y, Karabacak U, et al. Pressure injuries in the operating room: who are at risk? J Wound Care 2023;32(Sup7a). cxxviii-cxxxvi.

27. Choi Y, Kim SR. The effect of uncoated paper application on skin moisture, risk of pressure injury and incidence of pressure injury in neurologic intensive care unit patients: A randomized controlled trial. Int J Nurs Pract (John Wiley & Sons, Inc) 2021;27(4):1–10.

28. Gurun P, Ceylan S, Guner M, et al. Closure of pressure injury and mortality in internal medicine wards. Eur Geriatr Med 2023;14(2):373–80.

29. Pignatti M, D'Arpa S, Roche N, et al. Surgical treatment of pressure injuries in children: A multicentre experience. Wound Repair Regen 2021;29(6):961–72.

30. Rong ZHOU, TANG Xurong, Hong QU, et al. Characteristic of intra-operative pressure injury in children and related influencing factors. Nursing of Integrated Traditional Chinese & Western Medicine 2019;5(6):20–2.

31. Curley MAQ, Hasbani NR, Quigley SM, et al. Predicting pressure injury risk in pediatric patients: the braden QD Scale. J Pediatr 2018;192:189.

32. Oozageer Gunowa N, Hutchinson M, Brooke J, et al. Pressure injuries in people with darker skin tones: A literature review. J Clin Nurs 2018;27(17–18):3266–75.

33. Prado CBC, Machado EAS, Mendes KDS, et al. Support surfaces for intraoperative pressure injury prevention: systematic review with meta-analysis. Rev Lat Am Enfermagem 2021;29:e3493.

34. Guzman S, Allegretti AL, Kormos RL, et al. A comparison of air-cell and gel surgical table pads and an evaluation of the influence of pressure distribution and other factors on pressure injury prevention. J Tissue Viability 2021;30(1):9–15.

35. Allen G. Intraoperative use of a low-profile alternating pressure mattress. AORN J 2020;111(6):711–4.

36. Jin YX, Liu J, Shentu YQ, et al. Effect of "micromovement" in preventing intraoperative acquired pressure injuries among patients undergoing surgery in supine position. Int Wound J 2023. https://doi.org/10.1111/iwj.14408.

37. Ciprandi G, Crucianelli S, Zama M, et al. The clinical effectiveness of an integrated multidisciplinary evidence-based program to prevent intraoperative pressure injuries in high-risk children undergoing long-duration surgical procedures: A quality improvement study. Int Wound J 2022;19(7):1887–900.

38. Nie AM. Pressure injury prevention and treatment in critically ill children. Crit Care Nurs Clin 2020;32(4):521–31.

39. Gül A, Sengul T, Yavuz HÖ. Assessment of the risk of pressure ulcer during the perioperative period: Adaptation of the Munro scale to Turkish. J Tissue Viability 2021;30(4):559–65.

40. Perrenoud B, Maravic P, Delpy P. Pressure injury prevention in the operating unit of a Swiss university hospital: a best practice implementation project. JBI Evid Implement 2023;21(1):46–57.

41. Park SK, Park HA, Hwang H. Development and comparison of predictive models for pressure injuries in surgical patients: a retrospective case-control study. J Wound, Ostomy Cont Nurs 2019;46(4):291–7.

42. Abdi AA, Ali A, El-Ahmed F. Introduction of pressure injury preventive measures and improvement initiatives for patients undergoing prolonged surgery at a

government hospital in the United Arab Emirates. World Counc Enteros Ther J 2020;40(3):24–36.
43. Nayar SK, Li D, Ijaiya B, et al. Waterlow score for risk assessment in surgical patients: a systematic review. Ann R Coll Surg Engl 2021;103(5):312–7.
44. Hultin L, Gunningberg L, Coleman S, et al. Pressure ulcer risk assessment— registered nurses' experiences of using PURPOSE T: A focus group study. J Clin Nurs (John Wiley & Sons, Inc) 2022;31(1/2):231–9.
45. Li N, Cui D, Shan L, et al. The prediction model for intraoperatively acquired pressure injuries in orthopedics based on the new risk factors: a real-world prospective observational, cross-sectional study. Front Physiol 2023;14:1170564.
46. Mao J, Liu G, Zhang M, et al. Summary of the best evidence for prevention of intraopertive pressure skin injury in neurosurgical patients in lateral/prone position. Acta Med Mediterr 2020;36(4):2591–6.
47. Sving E, Bååth C, Gunningberg L, et al. The experiences of operating room teams working with real-time feedback of interface pressure to prevent pressure injuries—a feasibility study. Perioperative Care and Operating Room Management 2020;20:100096.
48. Luo M, Long X-H, Wu J, et al. Incidence and risk factors of pressure injuries in surgical spinal patients: a retrospective study. J Wound, Ostomy Cont Nurs 2019;46(5):397–400.
49. Kimsey DB. A change in focus: shifting from treatment to prevention of perioperative pressure injuries. AORN J 2019;110(4):379–93.

# Tropical Diseases Wounds

Emily Greenstein, APRN, CNP, CWON-AP, FACCWS

## KEYWORDS

- Tropical disease • Ulcer • Wound • Leprosy • Jungle rot • Chagas disease

## KEY POINTS

- Tropical diseases encompass all diseases primarily occurring in the tropic's region (between the latitude lines of the Tropic of Cancer and the Tropic of Capricorn).
- Climate change and global warming may be causing tropical diseases and vectors to spread to areas previously spared.
- Many of these tropical diseases will have symptoms affecting the skin.

## INTRODUCTION

Tropical diseases encompass all diseases primarily occurring in the tropic's region (between the latitude lines of the Tropic of Cancer and the Tropic of Capricorn). This term Is generic and covers all communicable and noncommunicable diseases, genetic disorders, and diseases caused by nutritional deficiencies or environmental conditions. Apart from noncommunicable diseases in tropical countries, a severe disease burden is caused by various microorganisms, parasites, land and sea animals, and arthropods. Skin disease manifestations are common in tropical regions, and 20% to 40% of new consults at primary care levels have skin problems in countries with tropical climates.[1] Tropical diseases are not restricted to the tropics, and we have seen an emergency of many of these diseases in the United States. Increasing migration, international travel, tourism, and work visits to the tropical regions have contributed to the increase.[2] Climate change and global warming may be causing tropical diseases and vectors to spread to areas previously spared. The last decade has shown a resurgence in tropical diseases in the United States, including Chagas disease, a chronic systemic parasitic infection caused by a protozoan *Trypanosoma cruzi*, and vector-born viral encephalitides[3] (**Fig. 1**). Other previously rare but emerging diseases include leprosy, cutaneous leishmaniasis, and tropical ulcers.[3]

### Fungal Disease

Many fungal infections occur more frequently in tropical zones or areas restricted to the tropics. According to the literature, the dominance of skin infections in tropical countries is due to the climate and overcrowding.[1] In the tropics, tinea capitis and

Vibra Health Fargo, 4425 168th Avenue Southeast, Horace, ND 58047, USA
*E-mail address:* egreenst8@gmail.com

Nurs Clin N Am 60 (2025) 109–118
https://doi.org/10.1016/j.cnur.2024.08.006
0029-6465/25/© 2024 Elsevier Inc. All rights reserved, including those for text and data mining, AI training, and similar technologies.
nursing.theclinics.com

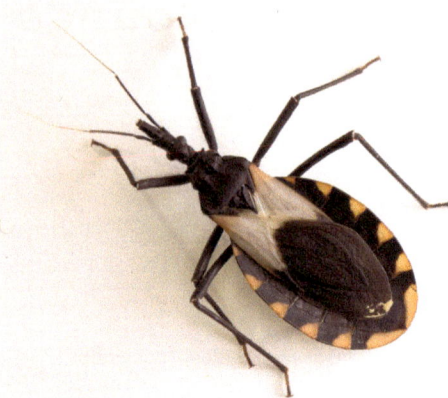

**Fig. 1.** Chagas disease is spread through contact with the feces of infected triatomine bugs.

tinea corporis are much more common. This is subject to variation in different areas. For example, in Saharan Africa, tinea capitis is endemic in school children, and prevalence rates in schools can exceed 20%.[4] Treatment for fungal diseases includes oral antifungal therapy, which is costly and inaccessible to most.

### Bacterial Infections

In the tropics, patterns of skin infections can be seen, with the most common being Group A streptococcal and streptococcal skin infections. Based on epidemiology in scabies-endemic tropical locations, scabies is a critical underlying factor for high rates of complicated skin-borne infections and other complications.[5] Scabies is a contagious skin disease caused by a parasitic mite *Sarcoptes scabiei*. Scabies mites burrow under the skin, resulting in intense itching. Scabies include the web spaces of the fingers and toes, wrists, buttocks, breasts in females, and genitals.[5] Treatment for scabies consists of a topical scabicide such as 5% permethrin, 0.5% malathion in aqueous base, 10% to 25% benzyl benzoate emulsion, or 5% to 10% sulfur ointment.[6] Oral ivermectin has also been found to be highly effective and is approved for treatment in several countries.[7]

### Neglected Tropical Diseases

#### Chagas disease

Chagas disease can be transmitted by the consumption of food or beverages that are contaminated with *T cruzi* during pregnancy or childbirth through blood transfusion and organ transplant. Signs and symptoms are usually present in two phases. During the acute phase, symptoms may be mild and nonspecific (headache, fever, enlarged lymph nodes, muscle pain, and abdominal or chest pain). If bitten by a triatomine bug, the first signs may include a skin lesion or a purplish swelling of the eyelids. During the chronic phase, the parasites are hidden in the digestive and heart muscles, and symptoms can include destruction of the nervous system, cardiac arrhythmias or progressive heart failure, and sudden death.

Chagas disease rates in the United States were estimated at 238,091 cases in 2012.[8] Previous estimates from 2005 showed 62,070 cases. The states that showed the most significant levels of disease were California, Texas, Florida, and New York.[3] Treatment for Chagas disease includes medications such as benznidazole or nifurtimox, which kill the parasite. Treatment also includes supportive measures. Public health recommends the control and prevention of the *T cruzi* parasite. This includes spraying dwellings and surrounding areas with insecticides, good hygiene practices in food handling, screening of blood donors, and house improvements and cleanliness to prevent vector infestation.[3]

### Leprosy

Leprosy, or Hansen's disease, is a chronic infection caused by the *Mycobacterium leprae* bacteria. Common symptoms include red, thickened patches on the skin, reduced sensation, numbness, weakness in hands or feet, and nonhealing wounds, blisters, and cracks in the skin of the hands or feet[9] (**Fig. 2**). If untreated, leprosy can cause extensive and destructive damage, and nerve damage leads to progressive sensory loss. Leprosy is spread from person to person through respiratory droplets. In the United States, there have been around 180 cases diagnosed annually, which is a slow increase from less than 100 in 1999.[10] Leprosy affects different people in different ways according to their immune response. The current classification of leprosy by the World Health Organization (WHO) is based on an assessment of the number of skin lesions; patients with less than 5 lesions are classified as paucibacillary (PB) and those with more than 5 as multibacillary (MB) forms of leprosy.[7] However, literature has found flaws in this scheme; for example, acid-fast bacilli have been detected in cases classified as PB.[7] Such cases presumably provide a risk of onward transmission of the infection. Many initiatives have been made to help improve detection rates and simplify the diagnosis process. Increased access to laboratory-based testing methods with slit skin smear and histopathology of skin biopsies as well as the development of some point-of-care molecular antigen detection kits have been initiated to decrease the risk of transmission.[11] Leprosy treatment includes antibiotics and topical supportive care. Sometimes, surgical amputations are needed to treat nonhealing wounds and infections. Prevention includes early diagnosis and treatment, good hygiene, and the preventative use of rifampicin in areas of high occurrence.[9]

### Cutaneous Leishmaniasis

Cutaneous leishmaniasis (CL) is caused by the parasite *Leishmania* and is transmitted through the bites of infected female phlebotomine sand flies (**Fig. 3**). Transmission has been identified in the United States in Texas and Oklahoma.[7] Clinical manifestations range from small and localized skin lesions to large nodules or plaques covering multiple body surfaces. They can mimic other skin conditions such as squamous cell

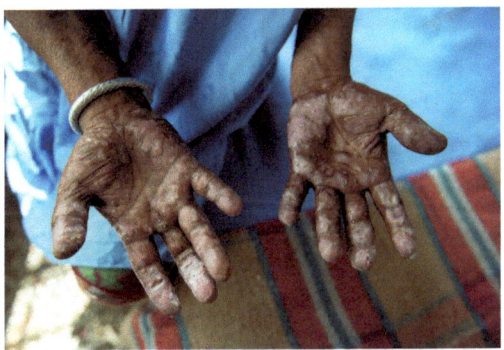

**Fig. 2.** Elderly lady with leprosy spots on her hands.

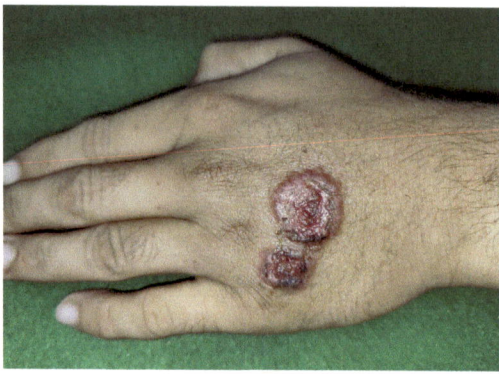

**Fig. 3.** Cutaneous leishmaniasis on a patient's hand. CL is spread by the bite of sandflies.

cancer, leprosy, or fungal skin infections.[12] The primary treatment is to prevent morbidity. The oral agent miltefosine is approved to treat CL. Prevention includes using personal protective measures to avoid sandfly contact, avoiding outdoor activities, especially from dusk to dawn, applying insect repellant, and spraying sleeping quarters with insecticide.

### Tropical Ulcer

Tropical ulcer, also known as jungle rot, is a chronic ulcerative lesion thought to be caused by a variety of *Mycobacterium ulcerans*. Although not as common today as it was during the Vietnam War, jungle rot is still something that can occur today. Ulcers occur on exposed body parts, primarily the anterolateral aspect of the lower limbs (**Fig. 4**). Tropical ulcers are excruciating and often begin with inflammatory papules that rupture. For an ulcer, the ulcers may eventually develop into squamous cancer after 10 or more years.[13] Treatment for tropical ulcers includes penicillin or metronidazole, improved nutrition, debridement, moist wound healing, compression, limb elevation, and, in extreme cases, amputation.[14] Prevention includes good hygiene, using shoes and socks to avoid trauma, and improving nutritional access.

### Mycetoma

Mycetoma is an infection that presents as localized swelling with the development of papules and sinus tracts on the skin surface. It is caused by either actinomycetes,

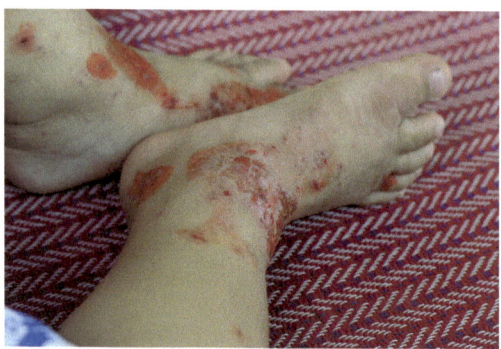

**Fig. 4.** Young man with tropical ulcers or jungle rot on his feet.

filamentous bacteria (antinomycetoma), or fungi (eumycetoma).[15] The countries with the highest prevalence are Mexico and Sudan.[16] If uncontrolled, the disease can proceed to cause severe limb deformities and osteomyelitis.[14] In Sudan, it has been found that there is an increased risk of infection in communities where cattle are grazed close to houses.[15] Treatment includes many antibiotics, including imipenem, moxifloxacin, and Linezolid, in addition to more traditional dapsone and co-trimoxazole.[17]

### Cutaneous Tuberculosis

Cutaneous tuberculosis (TB) is a skin infection that results from the bacterium *Mycobacterium tuberculosis*.[18] Cutaneous TB is less common than pulmonary TB. Even in areas where TB is common, such as India and sub-Saharan Africa, cutaneous TB occurs in less than 0.1% of the population.[18] Direct exposure of the skin or mucous membranes with tubercle bacilli results in a tuberculous chancre. The chancre appears 1 to 4 weeks after inoculation, presenting as a firm red papule, becoming a painless shallow ulcer with a granular base.[19] Diagnosis of cutaneous TB is usually made by skin biopsy. Tubercle bacilli can be detected by tissue stains such as Ziehl-Neelsen, polymerase chain reaction (PCR), and culture.[20] Treatment of patients with cutaneous TB usually involves a combination of isoniazid, rifampicin, pyrazinamide, and ethambutol given over a period of 6 months for a standard course.[20]

### Dengue Fever

Dengue fever is a viral illness transmitted by the bite of a mosquito. Patients present with fever, headache, rash, nausea, vomiting, and pains. In some severe cases, plasma leakage with or without hemorrhage or severe organ impairment can occur.[21] Each year, an estimated 400 million infections are caused by dengue fever. Dengue fever belongs to the Flavivirus family, including yellow fever and Zika. Patients who are already infected can transmit the virus via mosquitoes after the first symptoms appear until up to 2 weeks later. Blood samples enable diagnosis during the first 5 days of symptoms. The presence of immunoglobulin (Ig)M against the dengue virus or an increase in the IgG titers against the dengue virus in 2 different blood samples confirms a diagnosis.[22] Unfortunately, there is no specific treatment for dengue fever. Treatment focuses on supportive measures, including acetaminophen, aspirin, or other anti-inflammatories, to reduce fever and joint pains, rest, and plenty of fluids.[22]

### Zika Virus

Zika virus causes an infection that is spread by mosquitoes. It presents with flu-like symptoms and an itchy rash and can cause neurologic symptoms.[23] Zika virus is a small spherical single-stranded RNA virus belonging to the family Flaviviridae. Clinical features of Zika include a rash which is either morbilliform or scarlatiniform.[23] The rash starts on the face on day 1 and spreads to the trunk and limbs. The rash may affect palms and soles and may be accompanied by swelling. The rash begins to fade within 2 to 3 days. Petechiae may be observed inside the mouth on the palate.

Clinical symptoms were diagnosed with the Zika virus, and Igs were repeated 2 to 3 weeks with cross-reactivity with tests for dengue viruses. There is no specific treatment available against the Zika virus. The infection is usually self-limiting with supportive care. However, there can be some complications from the Zika virus, such as Guillain-Barre syndrome.[24] Guillain-Barre is a rare, rapid-onset form of paralysis that an infection can trigger. Zika virus has also been found to replicate and persist for several months in the placenta and the brain tissue of a fetus.[24] This results in an increased risk of fetal loss, growth retardation, and birth defects such as fetal microcephaly.

## Pinta

Pinta, also called puru-puru, is a skin disease caused by bacteria called *Treponema carateum*. Other species of *Treponema* are responsible for yaws and syphilis. Pinta is mostly found scattered in Central and South America.[25] It is primarily transmitted by direct skin or mucous membrane contact. Clinical features of pinta usually occur in 3 stages.[25] Primary pinta, or the early phase, occurs after an incubation period of 2 to 3 weeks. Clinical presentation includes 1 or more papules that slowly enlarge to become itchy, red, and scaly plaques. The areas most affected are exposed skin, such as the top of the feet, legs, hands, and forearms. Secondary pinta, or the second phase, occurs when a more widespread skin eruption occurs. This happens after 6 months to 3 years, with abnormal pigmentation and lesions. Lesions may appear red, white, blue, violet, or brown. Tertiary pinta, or the late phase, occurs when the skin becomes achromic and atrophic. The diagnosis of pinta is made based on the appearance of the lesions.[25] Serologic blood tests will be positive for syphilis. Skin biopsies using silver stain may reveal characteristics of treponemes in early lesions. Treatment of pinta includes antibiotics such as penicillin, tetracycline, or erythromycin.[25]

## Syphilis

Syphilis is a sexually transmitted infection caused by the spirochete *Treponema pallidum*. Syphilis has symptomatic and asymptomatic stages and, if left untreated, can have significant long-term neurologic and cardiac complications. Syphilis is transmitted from person to person by direct contact with syphilitic ulcers or by infected blood through microtrauma during sexual intercourse. Syphilis ulcers occur most commonly on the genitals and anal area but can also appear on the lips or mouth. Reported cases of syphilis have been on the rise. Syphilis is a plague that continues to affect millions of people worldwide, and incidence is increasing.[26] Clinical features of syphilis usually start to occur between days 10 and 90, averaging 21 days. Syphilis can be classified into 3 stages: primary, secondary, and tertiary.[27] Chancres at the point of entry of the *T pallidum* spirochete characterize primary syphilis. This usually results in a painless ulcer, a small, firm red papule on the genital area. The ulceration may go unnoticed; the ulcer usually heals within a few weeks without treatment. Secondary syphilis is a generalized infection characterized by a rash and systemic symptoms. If untreated, these symptoms eventually resolve over several weeks but can reoccur. Systemic symptoms may include fever, headache, malaise, myalgia, arthralgia, and lymphadenopathy. Cutaneous features of secondary syphilis include a nonitchy rash, which is present in about 90% of cases.[27] The rash might appear subtle or rough, red, or as reddish-brown papules. The rash usually occurs on the trunk and frequently can affect the palms and soles of the feet. Rarely does the rash present as a cluster of erythematous papules resembling a flower, and this morphology is described as "corymbose" syphilis. Grayish-white plaques can occur in the groin, inner thighs, armpits, and under the breasts. Latent syphilis occurs many years later and can be divided into 2 subgroups: early latent and late latent.[27] In the early latent phase, the patient is very contagious, and infection can easily be passed to sexual partners and pregnant women can pass it to the fetus. In the late latent syphilis, usually 2 years after infection, the patient becomes noninfectious to sexual partners but can still pass from a pregnant woman to her fetus. Tertiary syphilis develops decades after the initial infection. Late signs and symptoms can develop up to 20 to 40 years after infection. Untreated infection can lead to endarteritis and complications, including cardiovascular and neurologic disorders.

Syphilis is diagnosed through history and physical examination along with PCR testing.[28] Skin biopsies may or may not show characteristic histopathological features. Serologic testing to detect antibodies from treponemal infection is the most common test. However, the test cannot distinguish between types of treponemal infections such as yaws or pinta.[28] After high-risk sexual encounters, repeat screening is advised at both 6- and 12-weeks postexposure. False-positive tests can occur, particularly in autoimmune disease, intravenous drug use, pregnancy, and older age patients. The treatment for syphilis includes penicillin injections, tetracyclines, or cephalosporins.[28] Treatment failures can occur at any stage of the infection, so close monitoring and follow-up are essential. All sexual activity should be refrained from until all syphilis lesions are completely healed and treatment is completed. Partner notification and management are fundamental to prevent reinfection and spread.

## Yaws

Yaws is a chronic bacterial infection caused by the spiral bacteria of the genus *Treponema*. The organism is closely related to the subspecies *pallidum*, which causes syphilis and pinta.[29] The disease is primarily found in poor communities in tropical climates. About 75% to 80% of people affected by yaws are children under 15 years. Transmission occurs through person-to-person contact. The initial lesions of yaws occur most commonly on the limbs. The incubation period is about 9 to 90 days, averaging 21 days.[29] Yaws initially presents as a papilloma along with bacteria.

Without treatment, the papilloma will ulcerate. Papillomas and ulcers are very infectious and can quickly spread to others.[30] Diagnosis of yaws is made based on serologic tests, PCR testing, and clinical presentation. Treatment of yaws includes either azithromycin or benzathine ponicillin.[30]

## Lymphatic Filariasis

Lymphatic filariasis, also known as elephantiasis, is an infection that occurs when filarial parasites are transmitted to humans through mosquitoes. The infection is usually acquired in childhood and causes hidden damage to the lymphatic system. The global estimate of people affected by lymphatic filariasis was 25 million men with hydrocele and over 15 million people with lymphedema.[31] Lymphatic filariasis is caused by parasites classified as nematodes (roundworms) in the Filariodidea family. There are 3 types of these worms: *Wuchereria bancrofti*, responsible for 90% of the bases; *Brugia malayi*, which causes the other 10%; and *Brugia timori*, which has been linked to the disease.[31] Adult worms invade the lymphatic vessels and disrupt the normal function of the lymph system. The worms can live for approximately 6 to 8 years, producing millions of microfilariae circulating in the blood.[31] Lymphatic filariasis infection symptoms include asymptomatic, acute, and chronic conditions. Most infections are asymptomatic, contributing to the transmission of the parasite.[32] Even though the host is asymptomatic, the infection can still cause damage to the lymphatic system and the kidneys and alter the body's immune system. When lymphatic filariasis develops into a chronic condition, it leads to lymphedema of the limbs or hydrocele, which is scrotal swelling. Such deformities can lead to isolation, loss of income, and decreased mental health. Acute episodes of local inflammation involving the skin, lymph nodes, and lymphatic vessels often accompany chronic lymphedema.[32] Patients are also at higher risk for developing secondary bacterial skin infections due to underlying lymphatic damage.

The WHO-recommended treatment for prevention includes mass drug administration (MDA) of chemotherapy agents.[33] The recommendation is an annual dose of medications to at-risk populations. The medicines used have a limited effect on adult parasites but can effectively reduce the density of microfilariae in the bloodstream and prevent the spread of the parasites from mosquitoes.[33] The MDA regimens include albendazole twice a year for areas with loiasis, ivermectic with albendazole in countries with onchocerciasis, diethylcarbamazine citrate (DEC), and albendazole in countries without onchocerciasis; and ivermectin together with DEC and albendazole in countries without onchocerciasis and where other programmatic conditions are met.[33]

Surgical treatments for debulking the skin and creating lymphovenous anastomosis to improve drainage can be performed. Some studies have shown that topical coumarins and flavonoids effectively reduce lymphedema.[34] Strategies for long-term management include working with patients on skin hygiene, wearing comfortable footwear, using compression bandages and pneumatic compression devices, regularly washing with soap and water, limb elevation, and the use of antibiotic creams to prevent flares of lymphagitis.[35]

## SUMMARY

In conclusion, many diseases in the United States were previously thought to only occur in tropical regions. Severe poverty, climate changes and warming, human migrations, and changing global shipping patterns have contributed to the ongoing transmission of tropical diseases on the Gulf Coast. Efforts are urgently needed to detect, treat, and manage these infections.

## CLINICS CARE POINTS

---

- Tropical diseases are on the rise in the United States.
- Clinicians need to be familiar with diseases they may not treat daily.
- Early detection and treatment of neglected tropical diseases can prevent loss of life.
- Some tropical diseases can present as skin lesions or ulcers.

---

## DISCLOSURE

The author has nothing to disclose.

## REFERENCES

1. Hay RJ, Nicols R, Williams HE, et al. The global burden of skin disease in 2010: an analysis of the prevalence and impact of skin conditions. J Invest Dermatol 2014;134:1527–34.
2. Semenza JC, Ebi KL. Climate change impact on migration, travel, travel destinations, and the tourism industry. J Trav Med 2019;26(5):taz026.
3. World Health Organization. Chagas disease (also known as American trypanosomiasis). April 4, 2024. Retrieved from: Chagas disease (also known as American trypanosomiasis) (who. int) on May 10, 2024.
4. Coulibaly O, L'Ollivier C, Piarroux R, et al. Epidemiology of human dermatophytoses in Africa. Med Mycol 2018;56:145–61. View article.
5. Marks M, Romani L, Sokana O, et al. Prevalence of scabies and impetigo 3 years after mass drug administration with ivermectin and azithromycin. Clin Infect Dis 2020;70(8):1591–5.

6. Bergström FC, Reynolds S, Johnstone M, et al. Scabies mite inactivated serine protease paralogs inhibit the human complement system. J Immunol 2009;182: 7809–17.

7. WHO, Available at: https://www.who.int/lep/leprosy/en/. Accessed May 10, 2024.

8. Manne-Goehler J, Umeh CA, Montgomery SP, et al. Estimating the burden of chagas disease in the United States. PLoS Neglected Trop Dis 2016;10(11):e0005033.

9. Centers for Disease Control and Prevention. "Hansen's Disease (Leprosy)." 2017. Available at: https://cdc.gov/leprosy. Accessed May 23, 2024.

10. Domozych R, Kim E. "Increasing incidence of leprosy and transmission from armadillos in Central Florida: a case series.". JAAD Case Rep 2016;2(3):189–92.

11. Tatipally S, Srikantam A, Kasetty S. Polymerase chain reaction (PCR) as a potential point of care laboratory test for leprosy diagnosis – a systematic review. Trop Med Infect Dis 2018;3. pii: E107.

12. Markel W, Makhoul K. Cutaneous leishmaniasis: recognition and treatment. Am Fam Physician 2004;69(6):1455–60.

13. Odom RB, Davidsohn I, James WD, et al. Clinical diagnosis by laboratory methods. In: Elston DM, editor. Andrews' diseases of the skin: clinical dermatology. Saunders Elsevier; 2006. 276–267. ISBN 978-0-7216-2921-6.

14. G-Beiras C, Ubals M, Corbacho-Monné M, et al. Yaws, haemophilus ducreyi, and other bacterial causes of cutaneous ulcer disease in the South Pacific Islands. Dermatol Clin 2021;30(1). 25-22. ISSN 0733-8635.

15. Fahal AH. Mycetoma: a thorn in the flesh. Trans R Soc Trop Med Hyg 2004; 98:3–11.

16. de Hoog GS, van Diepeningen AD, Mahgoub el-S, et al. New species of Madurella, causative agents of black-grain mycetoma. J Clin Microbiol 2012;50:988–94.

17. Welsh O. Response to newer therapeutic modalities for actinomycetoma by Nocardia species. Int J Dermatol 2018;57:65–6.

18. Dias MF, Bernardes Filho F, Quaresma MV, et al. Update on cutaneous tuberculosis. An Bras Dermatol 2014;89(6):925–38.

19. Flavin RJ, Gibbons N, O'Briain DS. Mycobacterium tuberculosis at autopsy–exposure and protection: an old adversary revisited. J Clin Pathol 2007;60(5): 487–91.

20. Patterson JW. Weedon's skin pathology. 5th edition. Netherlands: Elsevier; 2020. p. 687–91.

21. Thomas E, John M, Kanish B. Mucocutaneous manifestations of Dengue fever. Indian J Dermatol 2010;55(1):79–85.

22. Low J, Ooi E, Vasudevan S. Current status of Dengue therapeutics: research and development. J Infect Dis 2017;215(S2):S96–102.

23. Lucey DR, Gostin LO. The emerging zika pandemic: enhancing preparedness. JAMA 2016. https://doi.org/10.1001/jama.2016.0904.

24. Parry GJ, Peacey M, Buenz EJ. Little risk of severe complications associated with Zika infection in New Zealand. N Z Med J 2016;129(1440):108–13.

25. Lupi O, Madkan V, Tyring SK. Tropical dermatology: bacterial tropical diseases. J Am Acad Dermatol 2006;54(4):559–78.

26. Kamat S, Vaghasia A, Dharmender J, et al. Syphilis: is it back with a bang? Indian Dermatol Online J 2024;15(1):73–7.

27. Tsuboi M, Evans J, Davies EP, et al. Prevalence of syphilis among men who have sex with men: a global systematic review and meta-analysis from 2000-20. Lancet Global Health 2021;9(8):e1110–8.

28. Whiting C, Schwartzman G, Khachemoune A. Syphilis in dermatology: recognition and management. Am J Clin Dermatol 2023;24(2):287–97.

29. Kazadi WM, Asiedu KB, Agana N, et al. Epidemiology of yaws: an update. Clin Epidemiol 2014;6:119–28.
30. Asiedu K, Amouzou B, Dhariwal A, et al. Yaws eradication: past efforts and future perspectives. Bull World Health Organ 2008;86(7):499.
31. Rebollo MP, Bockarie MJ. Can lymphatic filariasis be eliminated by 2020? Trends Parasitol 2017;33(2):83–92.
32. Chandy A, Thakur AS, Singh MP, et al. A review of neglected tropical diseases: filariasis. Asian Pac J Tropical Med 2011;4(7):581–6.
33. Bjerum CM, Ouattara AF, Aboulaye M, et al. Efficacy and safety of a single dose of ivermectin, diethylcarbamazine, and albendazole for treatment of lymphatic filariasis in Côte d'Ivoire: an open-label randomized controlled trial. Clin Infect Dis 2020;71(7):e68–75.
34. Shenoy RK. Clinical and pathological aspects of filarial lymphedema and its management. Kor J Parasitol 2008;46(3):119–25.
35. Stocks ME, Freeman MC, Addiss DG. The effect of hygiene-based lymphedema management in lymphatic filariasis-endemic areas: a systematic review and meta-analysis. PLoS Neglected Trop Dis 2015;9(10):e0004171.

# Wounds in the Unhoused Population

Beth Gall, MSN, RN, PHN, WOCN, FNP-BC[a],
Holly Kirkland-Kyhn, PhD, FNP-c, GNP-c, CWCN[b],*,
Tuba Sengul, PhD, CWON Nurse[c]

## KEYWORDS

• Homelessness • Wound care • Low-resource settings • Nursing care

## KEY POINTS

• *Prevalence and Impact*: The number of homeless individuals has risen significantly, with many facing severe health challenges due to unmet health and housing needs.
• *Unique Wound Characteristics*: Wounds in the unhoused population can be both acute and chronic, often exacerbated by environmental exposure and lack of consistent care.
• *Challenges in Care*: Substance abuse, poor nutrition, and lack of access to clean water and health care services hinder effective wound healing.
• *Resource Management*: Utilizing both basic and advanced wound care products effectively is crucial in low-resource settings.
• *Role of Nurses*: Nurses must provide continuous education, regular follow-ups, and adapt care plans to meet the unique needs of homeless individuals to promote.

## DESCRIPTION OF THE SETTING

Homelessness is a persistent issue globally, posing significant challenges to society.[1] Providing health care to this population can be difficult; however, wound care, a prevalent issue among the homeless, can serve as an initial step in building trust and relationships.[1] Homeless individuals often require specialized attention from compassionate caregivers but frequently lack access to professional care, advice, or necessary supplies.[1] In 2017, more than 188,000 people were experiencing homelessness in California.[2] By 2020, the number of people experiencing homelessness (PEH) had risen to over 255,000.[2] When health and housing needs go unmet, it becomes challenging for individuals to access health care services and stabilize their lives.[2] The consequences of this can be severe.[2] Untreated health issues become

[a] Betty Irene Moore School of Nursing, UC Davis, 2845 48th street, Sacramento, CA 95817, USA; [b] Health Sciences, UC Davis Betty Irene Moore School of Nursing, 2845 48th street, Sacramento, CA 95817, USA; [c] Koç University School of Nursing, Davutpaşa St. No: 4, Topkapı, Istanbul 34010, Turkey
* Corresponding author.
*E-mail address:* kirklandwalsh@ucdavis.edu

Nurs Clin N Am 60 (2025) 119–127
https://doi.org/10.1016/j.cnur.2024.07.007      **nursing.theclinics.com**

more complex when considering social determinants of health, such as health literacy, education level, environment, occupation, and recreation.[2] Homeless individuals are more likely to experience trauma, exposure, overdoses, and chronic conditions compared to housed persons; this leads to more frequent emergency department visits, more extended hospital stays, and earlier deaths.[2]

This article will discuss wound assessment, treatment, and documentation concerning nurses in low-resource settings.[3] While patients may have access to multiple assessment and treatment modalities in hospitals, once they are discharged to home (or the street/shelter) or their primary care provider, resources for assessment and treatment are limited to 4 to 5. For this article, we will focus on the assessment, treatment, and documentation of PEH, their skin, and their wounds.

## UNIQUE CHARACTERISTICS

Wounds that occur in low-resource settings may be either acute from trauma or associated with chronic co-morbidities or manifestations of chronic illnesses.[4–6] Within the population of PEH, patients experience trauma from dog bites, burns, and falls.[6] Unhoused individuals may have chronic untreated illnesses such as diabetes, congestive heart failure, and venous and vascular diseases.[6] However, they are also exposed to extreme weather conditions, repeated trauma, and infectious diseases.[6] In addition to exposure to extreme weather conditions, current data have found that the number of aging PEH has increased.[6] Current estimates show that over 6% of PEH are over age 65% and 40% report disabling severe health conditions.[2] As people age, their skin becomes drier and thinner, losing the rete ridges that keep the superficial layer attached to deeper layers.[6] Consequently, PEH over age 65 often develop skin tears from trauma and falls.[7]

## UNIQUE CHALLENGES

Substance abuse issues, including the use of tobacco and stimulants, interfere with healing.[8] Exposure to extreme cold or heat and prolonged sun exposure exacerbates these problems.[8] Additionally, unhoused individuals often lack access to clean water, proper bedding, clothing, and healthy diets.[8] They also have limited access to dressings or home health nurses for hands-on care.[8] Many unhoused individuals have uncontrolled diabetes with chronically high blood sugars, leading to poor healing.[8] Poor diets, often high in sodium from fast food, contribute to these health issues.[8] Furthermore, sleeping in cars while sitting up causes chronic lower extremity edema and skin breakdown.[8] The use of tobacco, alcohol, and other drugs not only impacts wound healing but also increases the risk of developing abscesses and other complications.[8] Poor health literacy further complicates these issues.[8] In many cases, individuals may undergo emergency surgery and be discharged back to the streets before their surgical wounds can fully heal.[8]

## AVAILABILITY OF RESOURCES

Basic medical supplies for patients covered by Medicaid can be sourced through specialized online pharmacies[9] Health care providers must become familiar with these pharmacies to ensure the timely ordering and delivery of necessary supplies to a specified address.[9] To justify the provision of supplies, documentation must include detailed wound descriptions, including type, measurements (length, width, depth), and the amount of drainage.[9] This information is crucial to determining the monthly dressings required.[9] Given the transient nature of many patients, who may not have a fixed address, arrangements can be made for supplies to be delivered to a hostel or the patient's case manager.[9] Advanced wound care products, although expensive, can extend the wear time of dressings.[9] However, over-the-counter alternatives that necessitate more frequent changes might be sufficient throughout the healing process.[9] Nurses should explore local discount stores to identify available products that can be adapted for wound care.[3] This approach can be cost-effective and practical in resource-limited settings, providing essential patient care without incurring significant expenses.[3]

## CASE STUDIES: EXAMPLES AND MANAGEMENT IN THE UNHOUSED POPULATION

The following case studies illustrate wound care's diverse and complex nature in the unhoused population. These examples provide practical insights into assessment, treatment, and documentation strategies that can be adapted for low-resource settings.

### 37-Year-Old Unhoused Male with Degloving Injury to Penis

*Essential identifying characteristics*: The nearly circumferential degloving appearance of the wound (**Fig. 1**). Clean with open wound edges with minor surrounding skin trauma or damage with undermining present, no purulence.

*Prevention and Education*: Outer genitalia wound repair occurs faster than wounds on other body parts without almost no scarring.[10] Avoid placing rings, cords, bottles, or other constricting objects on the penis for either sexual gratification or urination purposes.[11] It is especially important to exercise caution while using drugs and alcohol, as these can impair judgment and safe sex practices.[11] Instead of urinating into narrow-mouthed bottles, use wide-mouthed paper cups.[11]

*Treatment goals*: Regular hygiene and education on seeking treatment if infection or cellulitis develops are essential.[11] A product that maintains wound moisture is recommended.[11] Additionally, it is crucial to educate patients on the importance of follow-up visits with their provider or nurse every 1 to 2 weeks to monitor the wound status.[11]

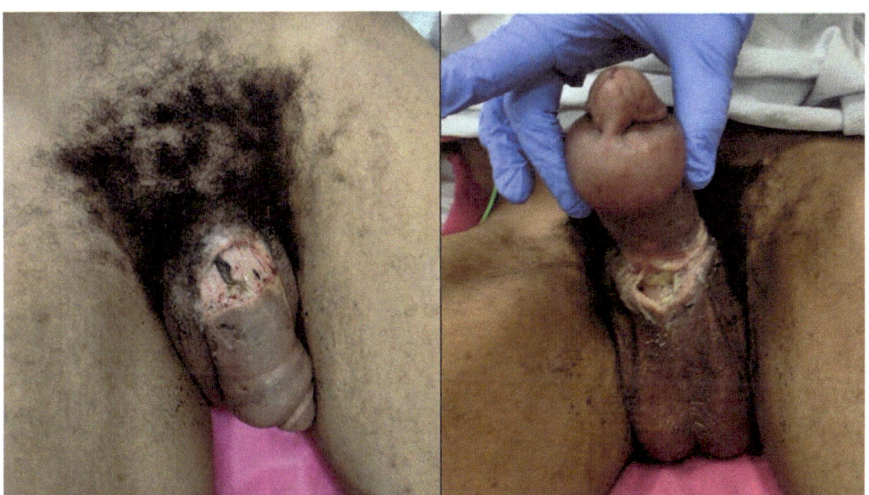

**Fig. 1.** 37-Year-old unhoused male with degloving injury to penis.

*Proposed formulary*: Antimicrobial wound ointments such as Medical grade Honey and bacitracin should be used with non-adherent gauze (eg, oil emersion, Vaseline gauze, Adaptic).[11] Alginate or hydrofiber impregnated with silver may also be used but will likely need to be moistened with sterile water or saline to adhere correctly and maintain wound moisture.[11] Additional supplies include Kerlix, tubular elastic gauze netting (size 2 or 311), tape, and scissors.[11]

*Safety policy and documentation*: Education on regular hygiene and wound cleansing, product use, and frequency of dressing changes. The dressing needs to be durable and keep the glans of the penis exposed and be removable by the patient.[12] Caution when wrapping is to avoid a tight, circumferential dressing, which can cause vascular compromise and tissue necrosis.[11] Instruct patient on seeking emergency treatment or follow-up for newly developed black or brown tissue indicating necrosis, increasing redness, swelling, fever, and other systemic signs of infection such as lightheadedness, racing heart, fever, and shortness of breath: document wound care and precautions/instructions.[11]

### 36-Year-Old Unhoused Female with Multiple Stab Wounds

*Essential identifying characteristics*: Stab wounds are puncture wounds that are deeper than they are wide[13] (**Fig. 2**). They typically have clean edges without surrounding skin trauma or damage that can be caused by blunt force trauma.[13] Stab wounds may have a deep wound bed and open wound edges without undermining or purulence if uninfected.[13] These wounds can be challenging to manage due to depth, risk of infection, and large amounts of exudate.[13] A few millimeters of redness, swelling, warmth, tenderness, and exudate surrounding open wounds are expected and should not be confused with infection.[14]

*Prevention*: Trust your instincts and be attentive to your surroundings.[15] If you sense danger or are being followed, stop, and ask someone for help or go to the nearest public place.[15] Use a 24-h convenience store, police station, or emergency room in the early morning as fewer people are out.[15] Carry yourself confidently (head held high, eyes alert).[15] Travel, camp, and use drugs with a buddy that you trust to avoid assault;

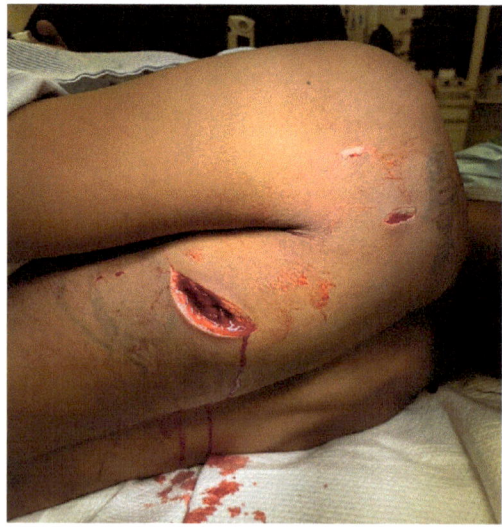

**Fig. 2.** 36-Year-old unhoused female with multiple stab wounds.

use shelters with security for nighttime, and carry mace or pepper spray.[15] Do not inject drugs while you have an open wound; instead, use rectal or inhaled forms.[15]

*Treatment goals*: Daily dressing changes will initially be required due to large amounts of exudate.[11] Dressing changes can gradually be decreased as wound size and exudate decrease.[11] Regular hygiene is needed to treat and prevent infection and cellulitis if it develops.[11] Use an agent with antimicrobial properties for cleansing and a dressing will keep the wound moist and absorb exudate.[11] Due to hard to reach locations, bring a family member or friend willing to learn to perform wound care.[11] Follow-up visits with the provider or nurse are made every 1 to 2 weeks to monitor wound status.[11]

*Proposed formulary*: Gauze, foam, hydrofiber, alginate (can be impregnated with silver, methylene blue, gentian violet, or other antimicrobial products), tape.

*Safety policy and documentation*: Education on hygiene and wound cleansing, product use and frequency of dressing changes, seeking emergency treatment or follow-up for purulence, increasing redness, swelling, fever, and other systemic signs of infection such as lightheadedness, racing heart, and shortness of breath.[11] Document wound care and precautions/instructions.[11]

### 55-Year-Old Unhoused Male with a Hand Abscess

*Essential identifying characteristics*: open wound with exposed subcutaneous tissue and open wound edges, typically associated with hand swelling (**Fig. 3**). Look for surrounding skin cellulitis, purulence from the wound, or undermining of wound edges.

*Prevention*: Use alcohol, wipe or clean skin before injecting drugs, use clean needles, and do not inject drugs while you have an open wound; instead, use rectal or inhaled forms.[11] Wear gloves when moving belongings or setting up campsites to avoid cuts/trauma to hands.[11]

*Treatment goals*: Prevent infection with through cleansing and promote healing through a moist environment, absorb exudate, and perform wound care 2 to 3 times weekly until the wound closes.[11]

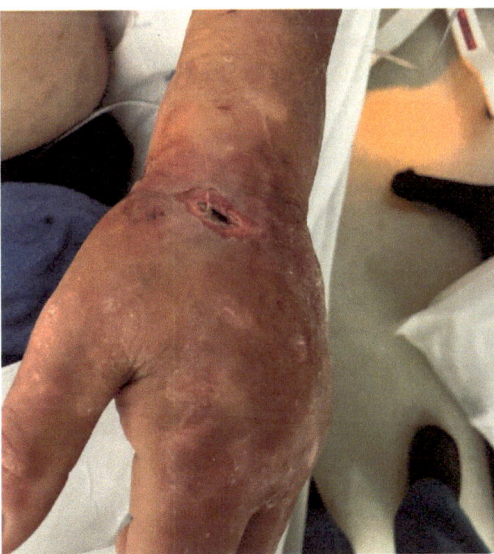

**Fig. 3.** 55-Year-old unhoused male with a hand abscess.

*Proposed formulary*: Strip cotton ribbon packing or gauze with wound gel such as triad/zinc oxide, medical grade honey, or iodoform.[11] It can also be used with antiseptic solutions such as Dakins or acetic acid; however, it must be changed every 24 hours.[11] Alginates or hydrofiber dressings are also an option and can be changed twice weekly, but scissors may be required to cut the product.[11] Tape.[11]

*Safety policy and documentation*: Education on hygiene and wound cleansing, product use and frequency of dressing changes, seeking emergency treatment of follow-up for increasing redness, swelling, fever, and other systemic signs of infection such as lightheadedness, racing heart, and shortness of breath.[11] Document wound care and precautions/instructions.[11]

### R Calf Injury from Bike Accident

*Essential identifying characteristics*: Lacerations from blunt trauma causes abraded edges.[13] Subcutaneous tissue and fascia can be exposed to early necrosis on a skin flap (**Fig. 4**).[13] A few millimeters of redness, swelling, warmth, tenderness, and exudate surrounding open wounds are expected and should not be confused with infection.[14] Look for surrounding skin cellulitis, purulence from the wound, and undermining at the skin flap.[14]

*Prevention*: During biking, wear long pants, socks, and shoes. Helmet. Avoid biking after using drugs or alcohol to prevent bike accidents. Do not inject drugs while you have an open wound; instead, use rectal or inhaled forms.

*Treatment goals*: Treat infection and cellulitis, use a dressing with antimicrobial properties that will promote wound healing using a moist environment, and absorb exudate, preferably a dressing that can be changed 2 to 3 times per week instead of daily.[11] Weekly monitoring is done to ensure the skin flap does not necrose.[11] Potential referral to emergency department (ED) or Surgeon for increasing necrosis or once skin flap declares itself non-viable (gray or black color without granulation tissue formation underneath).[11] Perform wound care as instructed until the wound closes.[11]

*Proposed formulary*: A wound gel or ointment used with gauze such as Medical grade ihoney, Iodosorb, Zinc Oxide/Triad.[11] The alternative is an alginate or hydrofiber

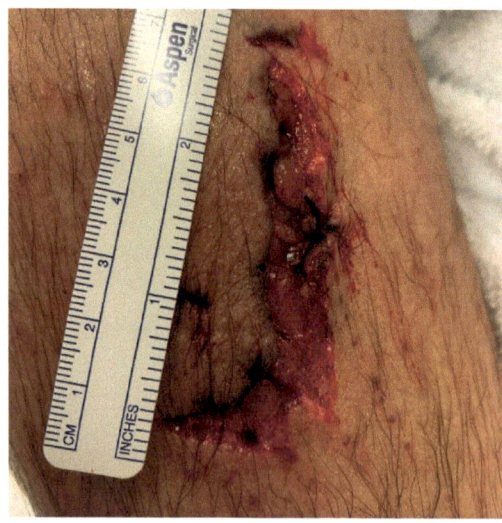

**Fig. 4.** R calf injury from bike accident.

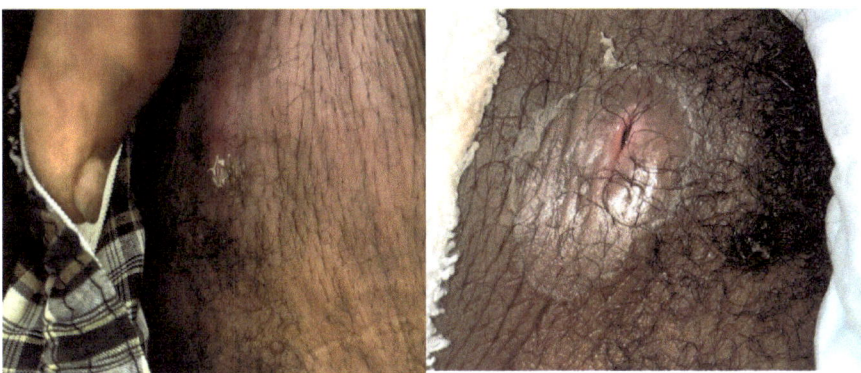

**Fig. 5.** 67-Year-old unhoused male with mons pubis abscess.

with or without silver impregnation, which can be changed twice weekly if the exudate is mild/moderate.[11] Dakin solution or acetic acid with gauze can also be used and is inexpensive to make at home-downside if this needs to be changed every 24 hours[11] and secured with Tape.[11]

*Safety policy and documentation*: Education on regular hygiene and wound cleansing, product use, and frequency of dressing changes.[11] Seek emergency treatment or follow-up for increasing redness, fever, chills, purulent drainage, or pain.[11] Monitor the wound for increasing gray or blackened tissue areas, indicating the peri-wound skin is no longer viable.[11]

### 67-Year-Old Unhoused Male with Mons Pubis Abscess

*Essential identifying characteristics*: Erythema, fluctuance, induration, purulence, cellulitis, pain, fever, chills, signs of systemic infection (**Fig. 5**).

*Prevention*: Regular hygiene, cleansing skin before drug injection, using clean needles, and using rectal or inhaled forms until an open wound heals. Do not puncture, pick, or pop boils or large pimples. Instead, use warm compresses or seek medical care.

*Treatment goals*: Maintain regular hygiene, keep the wound site clean, and change outer dressing when wet.[11] Current evidence-based practice makes no specific guidelines for or against packing skin abscesses.[16] Seek care immediately if the abscess recurs or the wound closes and re-develops, increasing purulent drainage, pain, redness, swelling, or induration.[11]

*Proposed formulary*: Cover the wound with gauze, which can absorb drainage. Secure the dressing using tape, tight socks, or underpants.[11] If a cavity is being packed, use a plain or iodoform packing strip or piece of gauze.[11] You can also use a packing strip coated with wound gel or ointment such as Zinc oxide/triad, medical grade honey, or an antiseptic solution such as Dakin's or acetic acid.[11] Gauze or packing strips with Dakin's solution or acetic acid need to be changed every 24 hours at a minimum since gauze provides no antimicrobial defense but does leave the wound open to drain once end of dressing is left out as a wick.[17]

*Safety policy and documentation*: Education on hygiene and wound cleansing, product use and frequency of dressing changes, seeking emergency treatment or follow-up for increasing redness, swelling, purulence, fever, and other systemic signs of infection such as lightheadedness, racing heart, and shortness of breath.[11] Document wound care and precautions/instructions.[11]

## SUMMARY

In conclusion, wound care in the unhoused population presents unique challenges due to the lack of resources, high prevalence of chronic conditions, and increased risk of trauma and infection. Effective management requires a comprehensive approach, including detailed assessment, appropriate treatment, and diligent documentation. Basic and advanced wound care products must be utilized judiciously to maximize healing outcomes while being cost-effective. Case studies highlight this population's diverse and complex nature of wounds and underscore the importance of tailored care plans. Nurses are crucial in providing education and continuous support to ensure proper wound management in these vulnerable individuals.

## CLINICS CARE POINT

- Keep wound base moist to allow for healing and surrounding skin dry and clean to prevent further breakdown.

## DISCLOSURE

The authors have nothing to disclose.

## REFERENCES

1. Kirkland-Kyhn H. The nurse practitioner role in treating the homeless and rough-sleeper population. J Am Assoc Nurse Pract 2020;32(4):287–9. Available at: https://journals.lww.com/jaanp/fulltext/2020/04000/the_nurse_practitioner_role_in_treating_the.2.aspx. [Accessed 4 July 2024].
2. Liu CY, Chai SJ, Watt JP. Communicable disease among people experiencing homelessness in California. Epidemiol Infect 2020;148.
3. Smith F, Sharp A. Undertaking a person-centred assessment of patients with chronic wounds. Nurs Stand 2019;34(10):77–82.
4. Johnson BZ, Stevenson AW, Prêle CM, et al. The Role of IL-6 in Skin Fibrosis and Cutaneous Wound Healing. Biomedicines 2020;8(5):101.
5. Valdivielso-Ramos M, Martin-Santiago A, Azaña JM, et al. Capillary malformation–arteriovenous malformation syndrome: a multicentre study. Clin Exp Dermatol 2021;46(2):300–5.
6. Kirkland-Kyhn H, Zaratkiewicz S, Teleten O, et al. Caring for aging skin. Am J Nurs 2018;118(2):60–3.
7. Van Tiggelen H, LeBlanc K, Campbell K, et al. Standardizing the classification of skin tears: validity and reliability testing of the International Skin Tear Advisory Panel Classification System in 44 countries. Br J Dermatol 2020;183(1):146–54.
8. Jain NP, Shao K, Stewart C, et al. The effects of alcohol and illicit drug use on the skin. Clin Dermatol 2021;39:772–83.
9. Rouvinez-Bouali N. In the skin of a "worldly" female doctor manager. In: Leadership and power in international development (building leadership bridges). Emerald Publishing Limited; 2018. p. 231–46.
10. Mirastschijski U, Jiang D, Rinkevich Y. Genital wound repair and scarring. Med Sci 2022;10(2):23.
11. Doctors Without Borders. Wound care protocol. OCB; 2018. Available at: https://www.doctorswithoutborders.org/wound-care-protocol. [Accessed 11 July 2024].

12. Bishoff JT, Peretsman SJ, Sabanegh ES, et al. Dressing for surgical wounds of the penis. Urology 1996;47:250–1.
13. Smock WS, Stack LB. Sharp-force-pattern injuries. In: Knoop KJ, Stack LB, Storrow AB, et al, editors. The Atlas of Emergency Medicine, 5e. McGraw Hill; 2021. Available at: https://accessemergencymedicine.mhmedical.com/content.aspx?bookid=2969&sectionid=250461275.
14. Zitelli JA. Secondary intention healing: An alternative to surgical repair. Clin Dermatol 1984;2(3):92–106.
15. Women's Violence Prevention Project Alliance. Keeping Safe on the Streets. [Brochure]. Available at: https://nhchc.org/wp-content/uploads/2019/08/FOSS_Keeping_Safe.pdf.
16. Evenocheck J, Olmschenk A. After incision and drainage for skin abscesses, does packing of the wound with gauze lead to better healing outcomes? Evid Based Pract 2022;25(3):27–8.
17. Tantillo TJ, Klein B, Wilson M, et al. Orthopaedic surgical dressings. Orthoplastic Surgery 2021;5:9–17.

# Innovative Approaches and Collaborative Strategies in Wound Care

# Common Oncologic Wounds

Salomé M. Loera, DNP, ACCNS-AG, PCCN, CCRN-CMC, SCRN[a,b,*]

## KEYWORDS

- Oncology • Wounds • Wound care • Radiation dermatitis • Extravasation

## KEY POINTS

- Cancer is a leading cause of morbidity and mortality worldwide. Care of patients with oncologic disorders spans the care continuum, with cancer patients accounting for 15% of intensive care unit admissions and 10.5% of hospitalizations overall. Skin conditions associated with oncology treatment include radiation dermatitis and chemothrapy-induced extravasation.
- Radiation therapy is commonly employed to eradicate cancerous cells or reduce tumor burden. Acute radiation dermatitis is a common complication of radiation therapy. Specialty dressings and other evidence-based interventions may reduce the risk and severity of radiation-related dermatitis.
- Chemotherapy centers and oncology nursing units should have established protocols, training, and supplies for the management of extravasation, including ready access to extravasation kits.

## INTRODUCTION

Cancer is a leading cause of morbidity and mortality worldwide.[1] Care of patients with oncologic disorders spans the care continuum, with cancer patients accounting for 15% of intensive care unit admissions and 10.5% of hospitalizations overall.[2] Given the prevalence of cancer, clinicians may anticipate encountering oncologic complications, including wounds, in a variety of specialties and care settings. Clinicians caring for patients with cancer diagnoses are often not directly involved in delivering oncologic treatment but must recognize and manage wounds related to treatment. Unique attributes of this patient population include skin hypersensitivity, palliative considerations, and impaired wound healing secondary to nutritional deficit and effects of chemotherapy or radiation.[3] Care settings with limited access to expert clinicians or specialty wound care supplies may pose additional challenges. In such scenarios, exchanging brand names for generic products may be necessary. Wounds commonly associated with oncologic disease and treatment include dermatitis secondary to radiation, skin toxicity associated with chemotherapy, and extravasation of chemotherapy agents.[3–5]

<sup>a</sup> Conway School of Nursing, The Catholic University of America, Washington, DC, USA; <sup>b</sup> Inova Health System, Falls Church, VA, USA
* 615 Alumni Lane #337, Washington, DC 20064.
E-mail addresses: loera@cua.edu; salome.loera@inova.org

Nurs Clin N Am 60 (2025) 129–141
https://doi.org/10.1016/j.cnur.2024.07.008
0029-6465/25/© 2024 Elsevier Inc. All rights reserved, including those for text and data mining, AI training, and similar technologies.

nursing.theclinics.com

## RADIATION-RELATED DERMATITIS
### Identification

Radiation therapy is commonly employed to eradicate cancerous cells or reduce tumor burden. Radiation causes the death of rapidly dividing cells, including cancer cells, directly and indirectly by damaging structures, DNA, and chemicals within the cell. External beam radiation (the most common form of radiation therapy) affects rapidly dividing epidermis cells, sebaceous glands, and hair follicles, triggering an inflammatory cascade.[3,5] Acute skin toxicity may occur of because of radiation therapy, resulting in areas of severely impaired tissue regeneration, delaying wound healing.[3] Despite specific protocols to reduce the risk of injury to surrounding skin and tissues, up to 95% of individuals undergoing radiation therapy experience radiation-related skin reactions, such as dermatitis.[3,5] Factors that increase the risk of radiation-related skin injury include concurrent treatment with chemotherapy and having skin or connective tissue disorders.[3,5] Skin injuries related to radiation are often dose-specific. Doses of 30 Gy units of ionizing radiation can lead to permanent damage of the sweat and sebaceous glands, resulting in pruritis and dry skin, while $\geq$ 50 Gy of radiation is associated with development of moist desquamation or peeling of skin.[5] Acute radiation dermatitis (ARD) occurs within 90 days of radiation exposure.[6,7] Presentation ranges in severity from slight erythema to peeling skin (desquamation) and even skin necrosis and ulceration.[5–7] Approximately 36% of patients develop moderate to severe acute dermatitis characterized by moist desquamation.[8] The National Cancer Institute Common Terminology Criteria for Adverse Events (NCI CTCAE) scale may be used to grade the severity of ARD[5,9,10] (**Table 1**).

Clinicians should consider ARD in patients with possible pressure injury/ulcer (PU/I) who have received radiation within the past 90 days, especially if the involved areas are not typically exposed to pressure. Grade 1 ARD may be wrongly ascribed to a Stage 1 or 2 PU/I, while Grade 4 ARD may be incorrectly diagnosed as a Stage 4

**Table 1**
**National Cancer Institute Common Terminology Criteria for Adverse Events acute radiation dermatitis grading scale[5,9,10]**

| National Cancer Institute Common Terminology Criteria for Adverse Events Grade | 0 | No Change |
|---|---|---|
| | 1 | Mild dermatitis is characterized by mild, blanchable erythema or peeling, dry, scaly skin (dry desquamation) (**Fig. 1**). Onset is typically within days to weeks of initiating therapy. Pruritus, hair loss, and decreased sweating are common associated symptoms. Symptoms may fade within a month. |
| | 2 | Moderate dermatitis is characterized by moderate to brisk erythema and patchy, moist desquamation confined to skin folds and creases. It may be associated with moderate edema. Moist desquamation is due to radiation exposure, resulting in skin thinning and weeping due to the loss of integrity in the epithelial barrier and decreased oncotic pressure. It is characterized by epidermal necrosis, exudate, and often severe pain. |
| | 3 | Moderate dermatitis with moist desquamation in areas other than skin folds and creases (**Fig. 2**). Bleeding in the regions of dermatitis may be induced by minor trauma or abrasion. |
| | 4 | Severe dermatitis characterized by skin necrosis or ulceration of full-thickness dermis with life-threatening consequences. Spontaneous bleeding at the involved area can occur, and a skin graft may be indicated. |

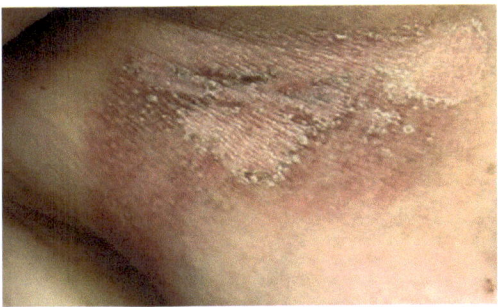

**Fig. 1.** Acute radiation dermatitis with erythema (National Cancer Institute Common Terminology Criteria for Adverse Events [NCI CTAE] Grade 1).[11]

PU/I or deep tissue injury. Chronic dermatitis may develop from 15 days to years after the beginning of radiation therapy. It is an extension of the acute process and involves additional inflammatory changes in the skin.[5,6] Characteristics of chronic dermatitis include the disappearance of follicular structures such as pores, fragile skin, and small, dilated blood vessels on the surface of the skin (telangiectasia or spider veins).[5,6] Secondary skin cancers may also develop following exposure to radiation therapy.

### Prevention and Treatment

Preventing, treating, and mitigating the symptoms of ARD is an essential element of care for patients undergoing radiation therapy. Common strategies for preventing and ameliorating ARD include wearing loose clothing, using electric razors rather than wet shaving, and avoiding applying cosmetic products or sun exposure to the radiation site.[5,7] Typically, patients may be advised to wash the radiation site with lukewarm water and pH-neutral soap daily.[5] Among patients with head and neck or breast cancer receiving radiation, colonization with *Staphylococcus aureus* was found to be a

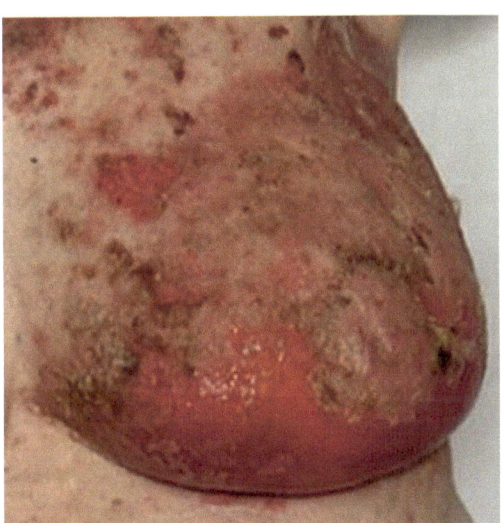

**Fig. 2.** Acute radiation dermatitis with moist desquamation (NCI CTAE Grade 3).[12]

significant factor associated with the development of Grade 2 ARD as compared to those who only developed Grade 1 ARD.[13] An associated randomized controlled trial found a significant reduction in the development of Grade 2 ARD among patients who received prophylactic decolonization with intranasal mupirocin ointment twice daily and chlorhexidine body cleanser once daily for 5 days before radiation therapy and every 5 days for 2 weeks during radiation therapy.[14] The care team must be alert to subtle signs and symptoms of infection, mainly if the patient is immunocompromised. Wound cultures should be obtained if there are concerns for cutaneous infection at the site of dermatitis.

There is limited high-quality, consistent evidence on the prevention and treatment of ARD, and the majority of interventions lack consistent evidence.[15] The Multinational Association of Supportive Care in Cancer (MASCC) has developed consensus-based clinical practice guidelines for preventing and managing acute ARD based on a Delphi study of international experts' evaluation of available evidence[15] (**Boxes 1** and **2**).

---

**Box 1**

**Multinational Association of Supportive Care in Cancer recommendations for prevention of acute radiation dermatitis[15]**

Multinational Association of Supportive Care in Cancer (MASCC) Recommendations by Intervention Type and Patient Population

- Photo biomodulation therapy and Mepitel film are recommended for patients with breast cancer, although there is evidence that both interventions may benefit those receiving radiation therapy for head and neck cancer.[15] Photo biomodulation therapy (non-invasive low-level laser therapy) affects stem and progenitor cells, enhancing cell differentiation, which in turn improves the healing rate of tissues, reduces inflammation, and may decrease pain.[16] Side effects are typically mild and involve skin itching, redness, and irritation.[16] Associated time, costs, and lack of availability may limit the use of this treatment.[15]
- Mepitel-brand (silicone-based polyurethane) film is shown to significantly reduce moist desquamation when prophylactically applied before and throughout radiation therapy.[15,17] Mepitel dressing is associated with reduced trauma and pain during removal as compared to other dressings, and so may be preferable for patients with sensitive or fragile skin.[17,18] This dressing has limited absorptive properties, which can result in fluid accumulation at the site, posing risk for microbial growth.[17]
- Hydrofilm-brand (polyurethane) film is another film-type dressing demonstrated to prevent moist desquamation and reduce overall severity of ARD when applied prophylactically.[15,19] This dressing has also been shown to reduce radiation treatment-related symptoms, including itching, burning, and pain, resulting in improved quality of life.[18] Hydrofilm has greater adhesive properties than Mepitel and may be preferable in areas subject to greater mechanical strain, such as skin folds, or perspiration.[18] Allergic reaction or skin irritation may be a side effect of Hydrofilm dressing.[19]
- Topical, highly potent corticosteroids mometasone and betamethasone are recommended for the prevention of ARD.[15] No recommendations were made for other topical corticosteroids, such as hydrocortisone, due to lack of expert consensus.[15] Mometasone cream has been shown to reduce the severity of ARF when applied at the beginning and throughout radiation therapy, thereby improving patients' quality of life.[15,20] Similarly, patients treated with betamethasone cream at the onset of radiation therapy and twice daily during treatment had reduced onset and severity of ARD.[12,21] Side effects of these steroid creams are typically mild and may include burning or stinging pain.
- Olive oil is a naturally derived agent recommended for effective prevention of ARD as it has been shown to reduce intensity of ARD.[15,22,23] Studies demonstrating benefits of olive oil in reducing severity of ARD involved application of olive oil 3 times a day.[22] Turmeric (curcumin)-based topical applications also have some evidence of preventing ARD but did not achieve consensus recommendation by experts.[13] Experts caution that oil-based formulations can lead to increased erythema.[13]

---

**Box 2**

**Multinational Association of Supportive Care in Cancer recommendations for management of acute radiation dermatitis[15]**

MASCC Recommendations by Type of Intervention
- Mepilex Lite-brand foam dressings are recommended for the treatment of ARD and have been shown to reduce radiation-related erythema.[15,24]
- There is an expert near-consensus on the use of using Mepitel-brand (silicone-based polyurethane) film to manage ARD.[15]
- Two topical nonsteroidal agents, doxepin and hydroactive colloid gel, also achieved expert near-consensus agreement on their potential benefit for the treatment of ARD.[15]
- Doxepin HCL cream is a topical variation of doxepin, a tricyclic antidepressant believed to relieve pruritus by blocking histamine.
- Hydroactive colloid gel, such as CovaTec DuoDERM-brand gel, supports moisture retention and is demonstrated to delay the onset and prevalence of ARD among patients undergoing radiation therapy.[25]

---

MASCC notes that evidence is limited to absent for most potential interventions for ARD.[13] However, specific dressings and non-steroidal agents have expert consensus or near-consensus regarding their efficacy in managing ARD.

Several topical anti-inflammatory agents have also been evaluated for their potential ability to decrease ARD severity and symptoms. While many of these agents may not reduce the severity or duration of ARD, they may improve patients' quality of life by relieving or reducing symptoms such as pruritis and pain.[26] Topical agents for symptom management of ARD include beta-sitosterol, *Calendula officinalis*, hyaluronic

---

**Box 3**

**Suggested formulary of supplies for prevention and management of acute radiation dermatitis**

Dressings
- Molnlycke Mepitel brand (silicone-based polyurethane) film dressing for prophylactic treatment prior to and throughout radiation therapy, particularly for patients with delicate skin.
- Hartmann-Conco Hydrofilm brand (polyurethane) film dressing for prophylactic management of ARD and related symptoms, ideal for areas prone to moisture or mechanical stress.
- Molnlycke Mepilex Lite brand foam dressing for ARD and radiation-induced erythema treatment.

Topical Agents
- CovaTec DuoDERM brand hydroactive colloid gel to support skin moisture retention and delay the onset and prevalence of ARD.
- Mometasone furoate ointment, a topical corticosteroid, for application at the beginning and throughout radiation therapy to reduce severity of ARF.
- Betamethasone dipropionate, a topical corticosteroid available in cream, gel, lotion, and ointment forms, to reduce onset and severity ARD.
- Doxepin HCL cream for treatment of ARD-induced pruritis.
- Olive oil for topical use to reduce intensity of ARD.
- Skin cream or spray for ARD symptom relief that contains *Calendula officinalis*, hyaluronic acid, comfrey extract, or turmeric.

Anti-Microbial Agents
- Intranasal mupirocin ointment, United States Pharmacopeia (USP) 2%, and chlorhexidine gluconate wash, such as Molnlycke Hibiclens, for prophylactic decolonization of *S. Aureus*, which is associated with increased risk for development of Grade 2 ARD.[13,14]

**Table 2**
**Skin/tissue damage and presentation associated with extravasation of chemotherapy**

| Type of Damage and Potential Presentation[28–31] | Chemotherapy Agent[28,31] |
|---|---|
| Vesicant:<br>• Blistering with local or extensive tissue necrosis<br>• Ulceration with or without tissue necrosis<br>• Complete loss of skin thickness and injury to underlying structures, including tendons, ligaments, and nerves | • Actinomycin D<br>• Amsacrine<br>• Carmustine<br>• Cisplatin (concentrations above 0.4 mg/dL)<br>• Dactinomycin<br>• Daunorubicin<br>• Doxorubicin<br>• Epirubicin<br>• Idarubicin<br>• Mitomycin<br>• Mitoxantrone<br>• Paclitaxel<br>• Trabectedin<br>• Vinblastine<br>• Vincristine<br>• Vindesine<br>• Vinflunine<br>• Vinorelbine |
| Exfoliant (may have limited vesicant actions):<br>• Blistering without necrosis (**Fig. 3**)<br>• Superficial skin shedding or peeling (desquamation) | • Aclacinomycin<br>• Cisplatin (concentrations above 0.4 mg/dL)<br>• Docetaxel liposomal<br>• Doxorubicin mitoxantrone<br>• Oxaliplatin paclitaxel |
| Irritant (does not have vesicant actions or cause blistering):<br>• Local irritation, inflammation, pain, or burning sensation at the extravasation site without blister formation, ulceration, or necrosis<br>• Pain or a burning sensation may occur with an infusion at the IV site and along the vein | • Arsenic trioxide<br>• Bendamustine<br>• Bleomycin<br>• Busulfan<br>• Cabazitaxel<br>• Carboplatin<br>• Cisplatin (concentrations below 0.4 mg/dL)<br>• Dacarbazine<br>• Daunorubicin liposomal<br>• Dexrasoxane<br>• Docetaxel<br>• Doxorubicin liposomal<br>• Etoposide<br>• Fluorouracil<br>• Fotemustine<br>• Gemcitabine<br>• Ifosfamide<br>• Irinotecan<br>• Ixabepilone<br>• Melphalan<br>• Oxaliplatin<br>• Paclitaxel (albumin-bound)<br>• Streptozocin<br>• Teniposide<br>• Topotecan<br>• Trastuzumab emtansine |

*(Reprinted with permission from* Elsevier. The Lancet Oncology, 2023; 24(4): e172-e185.)

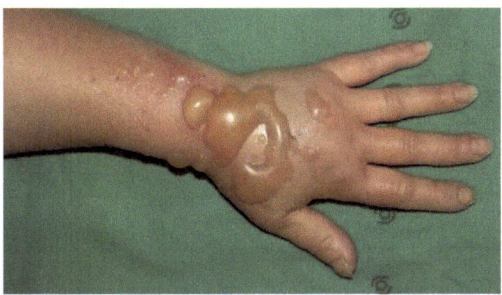

**Fig. 3.** Chemotherapy extravasation with blistering.[32]

acid, comfrey extract, olive oil, and turmeric.[7,26] Commercially available creams or sprays for treatment of ARD symptoms often contain 1 or more of these agents.[7] Patients should be cautioned to evaluate creams or sprays for irritating or drying components such as alcohol[7] (**Box 3**).

### *Safety Policy and Documentation*

Patients undergoing radiation therapy should be evaluated for ARD throughout and after treatment, including during any hospitalization. Erythema, desquamation, or any other skin reaction at the radiation site should be noted and documented.[27] Treatment of ARD is complex, and it is advisable to consult a wound care nurse or clinician with experience in the management of oncologic conditions.[27] Nurses and other clinicians caring for patients receiving radiation therapy should be aware that ARD can be prevented or mitigated with prophylactic interventions. There should be documentation of patient education and counseling regarding the potential adverse effects of radiation therapy and any ARD-related interventions.

## CHEMOTHERAPY-INDUCED EXTRAVASATION
### *Identification*

Pharmacologic therapy with antineoplastic agents, also known as chemotherapy, is a cornerstone of cancer treatment. Most commonly, chemotherapy is administered intravenously (IV).[28] Extravasation, defined as the unintentional infiltration of a drug into subcutaneous or sub-dermal tissue surrounding the vein receiving an infusion, is a relatively rare but serious risk associated with chemotherapy[28] and reported incidences of extravasation range from 0.1% to 6%, with greater incidences reported for peripheral infusions compared to implanted ports.[28,29] However, extravasation may

| Table 3 | | |
|---|---|---|
| **National Cancer Institute Common Terminology Criteria for Adverse Events infusion site extravasation grading scale**[9,32] | | |
| NCI CTCAE Grade | 0 | No Change. |
| | 1 | Painless edema. |
| | 2 | Erythema with associated symptoms such as edema, pain, induration, or phlebitis (**Fig. 4**) |
| | 3 | Ulceration or necrosis; severe tissue damage; surgical intervention indicated (**Fig. 5**). |
| | 4 | Life-threatening consequences; urgent surgical intervention indicated. |

*(Reprinted with permission from* Elsevier. The Lancet Oncology, 2023; 24(4): e172-e185.)

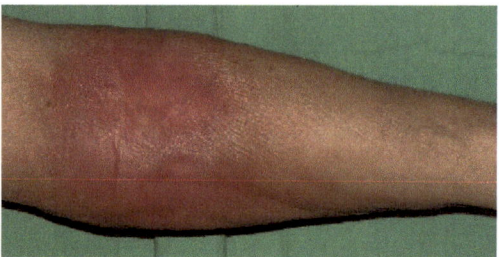

**Fig. 4.** Chemotherapy extravasation with erythema (NCI CTCAE Grade 2).[32]

be underreported or underrecognized, particularly with chemotherapy agents that are non-vesicants or in cases of delayed reaction.[29]

Presentation and severity of chemotherapy-induced extravasation (CIE) varies depending on the type of damage induced by a chemotherapeutic agent, the time before intervention, and the amount of infiltration.[28,29] Extravasation of a vesicant agent poses a significant risk for long-term skin and tissue injury, including tissue necrosis, if extravasation occurs.[28,30,31] Conversely, extravasation of non-vesicant agents generally does not cause persistent tissue damage, although irritant agents induce inflammatory reactions.[29] Chemotherapy-induced extravasation may be categorized according to the type of damage caused by infiltration (eg, vesicant vs irritant) and associated presentation (**Table 2**).

Like ARD, chemotherapy-related extravasation may be graded using a National Cancer Institute Common Terminology Criteria for Adverse Events (NCI CTCAE) scale (**Table 3**).

Inflammatory skin or vascular reactions to injections of antineoplastic or immune-modulating agents can be differentiated from extravasation-related symptoms and injury. Examples of these inflammatory conditions may include flare-type allergic reactions or vascular irritation.[28] Transient, painless streaking erythema along the vein and swelling at the time of injection is characteristic of flare reaction.[28,29,33,34] Burning or itching at the injection site may also develop with a flare reaction but typically resolves within a few hours and lasts no longer than 24 hours.[28,29,33,34] Vascular irritation commonly results in transient pain and erythema or discoloration along the vein.[28] Conversely, sustained erythema and swelling surrounding the injection site are typically seen with extravasation.[28]

### Prevention and Treatment

Identification of risk factors associated with CIE and timely, appropriate treatment of extravasation are essential to prevent and mitigate CIE-related skin and tissue injury

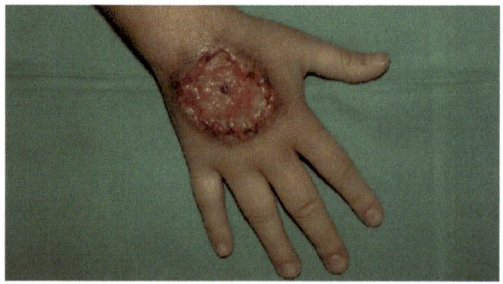

**Fig. 5.** Chemotherapy extravasation with ulceration (NCI CTCAE Grade 3).[32]

---

**Box 4**
**Prevention of chemotherapy-induced extravasation**[28,29,32,34]

Preventative Measures for CIE
- Appropriate selection of vascular access for chemotherapy administration:
  - Use of central venous access devices (CVADs), such as implanted ports or peripherally inserted central catheters, is preferable, as they are associated with reduced risk for extravasation. Infusions of vesicants lasting greater that 1 hour should be administered via central venous access.[29] During infusion of vesicants, the CVAD should be assessed at least once per hour for patency and any local signs of extravasation.[29]
  - Avoid peripheral catheters in the dorsum of the hand, antecubital fossa, the radial and ulnar aspects of forearm, near joints, or in veins that are superficial, small, or fragile.
  - Select the smallest bore IV cannula deemed appropriate for the chemotherapy agent and use the largest peripheral vein available or central venous access. Never utilize a butterfly needle-type IV catheter.
  - Cover IV site with transparent dressing so the site may be monitored for any possible extravasation.
- Consider patient-specific factors that may warrant placement of central venous access, including, but not limited to the following:
  - Lymphedema/swelling or history of local lymph node dissection.
  - Alterations in level of consciousness or sensation that may limit the patient's ability to report discomfort or maintain proper positioning and compliance with the presence of IV access during infusion.
  - Conditions or treatments associated with impaired endothelium or healing, such as diabetes, vascular disease, or corticosteroid therapy.
- Provide patient education on the risk for extravasation, including signs, symptoms, and the need to minimize movement or manipulation of the IV site during infusion. Instruct patients to report any symptoms of discomfort, pain, and changes in sensation or appearance surrounding the infusion site.
- Closely monitor the IV site and surrounding area during infusion and ask the patient about any new pain or changes in sensation. Assess the IV site, including blood return and patency, every 5 to 10 minutes during infusion and immediately upon any signs or symptoms consistent with CIE.[28,29]

---

(**Boxes 4** and **5**). Patient-specific risk factors for CIE include conditions associated with impaired circulation, vasculature, sensation, or cognition.[28,29,32] Infusion-related risk factors include cannulation sites, multiple IV starts, and duration of the infusion.[28,29,32] Education and training of clinicians is essential to ensure appropriate practice related to chemotherapy administration.[28] Institutional policies that guide individual clinical practice should be based upon the most current international guidelines and literature.[28,29,32,34,35]

Nurses and other clinical team members should be aware that extravasation of vesicants can initially present without any symptoms ("silent extravasation") or with less severe symptoms, such as erythema, pain, and swelling, before progressing to tissue necrosis and ulceration if the actions of the vesicant are not interrupted.[32] Therefore, close monitoring during infusion and expedient interventions to address potential CIE, regardless of initial presentation, is imperative (**Box 5**). Overall, there is limited evidence and consensus regarding the treatment of CIE.[28,29,32] Best practice management of CIE may be guided by recommendations made by oncologic organizations, including the Oncologic Nursing Association, and outcomes of relevant clinical research.[28,29,31,32,34,35]

Novel approaches to the management of extravasation-associated wounds include hyperbaric oxygen therapy, and negative pressure wound therapy.[28] However, evidence for these approaches to managing CIE is limited, and consensus on related treatment regimens has not been established[28] (**Box 6**).

**Box 5**

**Treatment of chemotherapy-induced extravasation[28,29,31,32,34,35]**

Initial Response and Non-Pharmacologic Interventions
- Immediately stop the infusion.
- Maintain the IV catheter and attempt to aspirate chemotherapy agent back out of the catheter using a 10 -mL syringe. Aspiration of the vesicant may also be attempted using percutaneous needle aspiration or a simple squeezing maneuver.
- Remove the IV catheter unless it will be used to administer antidote or other necessary medications.
- Elevate the involved extremity and apply warm or cold packs for at least the first 24 to 48 hours of the potential CIE. Cold therapy should be avoided in cases of CIE involving vincristine or other vinca alkaloids. Warm therapy may be applied in all cases of CIE, unless otherwise indicated by the chemotherapy manufacturer, ideally 4 times daily for 20 minutes during the first 48 hours.
- Mark boarders of erythema, obtain photography of the site to monitor progression, and document all findings, including symptoms and interventions.

Pharmacologic and Surgical Interventions
- Subcutaneous injection of sterile saline at the extravasation site, with volume dependent on the site (20–30 mL, hand; 20–50 mL, forearm; 40–90 mL, antecubital fossa), and application of a steroid cream, every 2 to 3 days, depending on the severity of the extravasation.[32]
- Dexrazoxane hydrochloride systemic IV infusion as an antidote for extravasation of anthracycline. Dexrazoxane may also be considered as an antidote for doxorubicin and epirubicin-related extravasation.
- Hyaluronidase subcutaneous injections as an antidote for vinca-alkaloids, etoposide, and taxane-related extravasation.
- Dimethyl sulfoxide (DMSO) topical application as an adjunctive antidote for anthracycline-related extravasation.
- Sodium thiosulfate subcutaneous injection as an antidote for extravasation of doxorubicin, epirubicin, vinblastine, and mitomycin C.
- Surgical debridement of necrotic tissue and skin grafting may be necessary in cases of full-thickness skin necrosis and chronic ulceration.

**Box 6**

**Suggested formulary of supplies for prevention and management of chemothrapy-induced extravasation[28,31,32,34,35]**

Initial Response and Non-Pharmacologic Management of CIE
- Extravasation kits containing syringes, IV cannulas, hot/cold packs, gauze pads, adhesive plaster, gloves, and antidotes. These kits should be readily accessible in all nursing units and outpatient settings where chemotherapy is regularly administered.[28]
- Extra supplies, including 10 mL syringes for aspiration, sterile saline for injection or subcutaneous infusion, hot/cold packs, and chemotherapy-resistant gloves.

Pharmacologic Management of CIE
- Sterile saline and corticosteroid cream to implement subcutaneous infusion and topical cream regimen to treat CIE.
- Dexrazoxane hydrochloride IV infusion as an antidote for extravasation of anthracycline, doxorubicin, and epirubicin.
- Hyaluronidase for subcutaneous injection as an antidote for extravasation of vinca-alkaloids, etoposide, and taxanes.
- Dimethyl sulfoxide (DMSO) topical preparation for adjunctive treatment of anthracycline-related extravasation.
- Sodium thiosulfate for subcutaneous injection as an antidote for extravasation of doxorubicin, epirubicin, vinblastine, and mitomycin C.

## Safety Policy and Documentation

Chemotherapy centers and oncology nursing units should have established protocols, training, and supplies for the management of extravasation, including ready access to extravasation kits.[28,34,35] Institutional policies should address IV site assessment frequency during chemotherapy infusion, initial management of extravasation, and documentation of potential CIE.[28,35] Preventative or routine care measures and interventions with organizational policy should be documented, including the type of venous access used, number and location of venipuncture attempts, initial and ongoing assessment of line patency, and patient education.[29] Critical documentation elements for potential CIE include the name of the drug involved, estimated amount extravasated, IV access and location, description of signs/symptoms, photographs of the site, and interventions taken.[29]

## CLINICS CARE POINTS

- ARD is a common complication of oncologic radiation therapy and approximately 36% of all patients develop moderate to severe ARD with moist, peeling skin (desquamation).
- Mepitel and Hydrofilm brand polyurethane film-type dressings are shown to significantly prevent and reduce severity of ARD with moist desquamation when applied prophylactically prior to, and throughout, radiation therapy.
- There is limited to poor evidence for the majority of topical agents commonly employed to prevent and manage ARD. Olive oil, hydroactive colloid gel, and doxepin topical cream have been demonstrated to reduce the prevalence and severity of ARD.
- Extravasation of chemotherapy agents is a relatively rare but potentially serious complication of oncology treatment, particularly if the agent is a vesicant that causes skin and tissue necrosis.
- Nurses and other clinicians must recognize that extravasation may initially present with minimal initial signs and symptoms, but can result in serious adverse outcomes, including tissue necrosis, especially if extravasation is not rapidly addressed.

## DISCLOSURE

The authors have nothing to disclose.

## REFERENCES

1. World Health Organization. WHO. Cancer. 2022. Available at: https://www.who.int/news-room/fact-sheets/detail/cancer?gad_source=1&gclid=Cj0KCQjw8J6w BhDXARIsAPo7QA8yBhHb1eSzDEyfPF4-exYQNtgtoEF8ixijHUWAw4cMUZSTBk W55FEaAhsYEALw_wcB.
2. Martos-Benítez FD, De Dios Soler-Morejón C, Lara-Ponce KX, et al. Critically ill patients with cancer: a clinical perspective. World J Clin Oncol 2020;11(10):809–35. https://doi.org/10.5306/wjco.v11.i10.809.
3. Deptuła M, Zieliński J, Wardowska A, et al. Wound healing complications in oncological patients: perspectives for cellular therapy. Postępy Dermatologii i Alergologii 2019;36(2):139–46. https://doi.org/10.5114/ada.2018.72585.
4. Kreidieh F, Moukadem H, Saghir NSE. Overview, prevention and management of chemotherapy extravasation. World J Clin Oncol 2016;7(1):87. https://doi.org/10.5306/wjco.v7.i1.87.

5. Bauer C. Understanding radiation dermatitis. Wound Care Advisor. 2020. Available at: https://woundcareadvisor.com/understanding-radiation-dermatitis/.

6. Spałek M. Chronic radiation-induced dermatitis: challenges and solutions. Clin Cosmet Invest Dermatol 2016;9:473–82. https://doi.org/10.2147/ccid.s94320.

7. Ranaweera A. DermNet. Available at: https://dermnetnz.org/topics/radiation-dermatitis#: ~ :text=Acute%20radiation%20dermatitis&text=The%20patient%20may%20have%20skin,the%20severity%20of%20the%20reaction. Published 2012.

8. Behroozian T, Goldshtein D, Wolf JR, et al. MASCC clinical practice guidelines for the prevention and management of acute radiation dermatitis: part 1) systematic review. EClinicalMedicine 2023;58:101886. https://doi.org/10.1016/j.eclinm.2023.101886.

9. National Cancer Institute. Common Terminology Criteria for adverse Events (CTCAE) version 5.0. U.S. Department of Health and Human Services; 2017. Available at: https://ctep.cancer.gov/protocoldevelopment/electronic_applications/docs/CTCAE_v5_Quick_Reference_8.5x11.pdf. [Accessed 16 March 2024].

10. National Cancer Institute. Patient-Reported Outcomes version of the Common Terminology Criteria for Adverse Events. PRO-CTCAE) 2023. Available at: https://healthcaredelivery.cancer.gov/pro-ctcae/. [Accessed 16 March 2024].

11. Ramseier JY, Ferreira M, Leventhal JS. Dermatologic toxicities associated with radiation therapy in women with breast cancer. International Journal of Women's Dermatology 2020;6(5):349–56. https://doi.org/10.1016/j.ijwd.2020.07.015.

12. Crocker C. Radiation-induced pemphigus in a patient with an invasive ductal carcinoma of the breast: a case report. Oxford Medical Case Reports 2020;2020(1). https://doi.org/10.1093/omcr/omaa001.

13. Kost Y, Rzepecki AK, Deutsch A, et al. Association of Staphylococcus aureus colonization with Severity of acute radiation dermatitis in patients with breast or head and neck cancer. JAMA Oncol 2023;9(7):962. https://doi.org/10.1001/jamaoncol.2023.0454.

14. Kost Y, Deutsch A, Mieczkowska K, et al. Bacterial decolonization for prevention of radiation dermatitis. JAMA Oncol 2023;9(7):940. https://doi.org/10.1001/jamaoncol.2023.0444.

15. Behroozian T, Bonomo P, Patel P, et al. Multinational Association of Supportive Care in Cancer (MASCC) clinical practice guidelines for the prevention and management of acute radiation dermatitis: international Delphi consensus-based recommendations. Lancet Oncology/Lancet Oncology 2023;24(4):e172–85. https://doi.org/10.1016/s1470-2045(23)00067-0.

16. Dompe C, Moncrieff L, Matys J, et al. Photobiomodulation—underlying mechanism and clinical applications. J Clin Med 2020;9(6):1724. https://doi.org/10.3390/jcm9061724.

17. Tayyib NA. Prophylactic use of Mepitel® film to prevent radiation-induced moist desquamation in cancer patients. Curēus 2023. https://doi.org/10.7759/cureus.42186.

18. Dejonckheere CS, Dejonckheere E, Layer JP, et al. Barrier films for the prevention of acute radiation dermatitis in breast cancer: a systematic review and meta-analysis of randomised controlled trials. Breast 2023;71:31–41. https://doi.org/10.1016/j.breast.2023.07.001.

19. Schmeel LC, Koch D, Schmeel FC, et al. Hydrofilm polyurethane films reduce radiation dermatitis severity in hypofractionated whole-breast irradiation: an objective, intra-patient randomized dual-center assessment. Polymers 2019;11(12):2112. https://doi.org/10.3390/polym11122112.

20. Hindley A, Zain Z, Wood LJ, et al. Mometasone furoate cream reduces acute radiation dermatitis in patients receiving breast radiation therapy: results of a randomized trial. Int J Radiat Oncol Biol Phys 2014;90(4):748–55. https://doi.org/10.1016/j.ijrobp.2014.06.033.
21. Sunku R, Kalita AK, Bhattacharyya M, et al. Effect of corticosteroid ointment on radiation induced dermatitis in head and neck cancer patients: A prospective study. Indian J Cancer 2021;58(1):69. https://doi.org/10.4103/ijc.ijc_790_18.
22. Cui Z, Xin M, Yin H, et al. Topical use of olive oil preparation to prevent radiodermatitis: results of a prospective study in nasopharyngeal carcinoma patients. Int J Clin Exp Med 2015;8(7):11000–6. Available at: https://pubmed.ncbi.nlm.nih.gov/26379896.
23. Kao Y, Sheng-Kai K, Wu MY, et al. Topical prevention of radiation dermatitis in head and neck cancer patients: a network Meta-analysis. In Vivo 2022;36(3):1453–60. https://doi.org/10.21873/invivo.12851.
24. Diggelmann KV, Zytkovicz A, Tuaine JM, et al. Mepilex Lite dressings for the management of radiation-induced erythema: a systematic inpatient controlled clinical trial. Br J Radiol 2010;83(995):971–8. https://doi.org/10.1259/bjr/62011713.
25. Censabella S, Bollen H, Orlandini M, et al. Efficacy of a hydroactive colloid gel versus historical controls for the prevention of radiotherapy-induced moist desquamation in breast cancer patients. Eur J Oncol Nurs 2017;29:1–7. https://doi.org/10.1016/j.ejon.2017.04.003.
26. Iacovelli NA, Torrente Y, Ciuffreda AR, et al. Topical treatment of radiation-induced dermatitis: current issues and potential solutions. Drugs in Context 2020;9:1–13. https://doi.org/10.7573/dic.2020-4-7.
27. Feight D, Baney T, Bruce SD, et al. Putting evidence into practice. Clin J Oncol Nurs 2011;15(5):481–92. https://doi.org/10.1188/11.cjon.481-492.
28. Kreidieh FY. Overview, prevention and management of chemotherapy extravasation. World J Clin Oncol 2016;7(1):87. https://doi.org/10.5306/wjco.v7.i1.87.
29. Sauerland C, Engelking C, Wickham R, et al. Vesicant extravasation Part I: Mechanisms, pathogenesis, and nursing care to reduce risk. Oncol Nurs Forum 2006;33(6):1134–41. https://doi.org/10.1188/06.onf.1134-1141.
30. NCI Dictionary of Cancer Terms. Available at: Cancer.gov. https://www.cancer.gov/publications/dictionaries/cancer-terms/def/vesicant-extravasation.
31. Doolittle D, Albert-Mari M. Closing the knowledge gap on extravasation. Pharm Pract News 2019. Available at: https://www.pharmacypracticenews.com/Clinical/Article/04-22/Closing-the-Knowledge-Gap-On-Extravasation/66553. [Accessed 2 June 2024].
32. Onesti MG, Carella S, Fioramonti P, et al. Chemotherapy extravasation management. Ann Plast Surg 2017;79(5):450–7. https://doi.org/10.1097/sap.0000000000001248.
33. Mini Gill J, Frost J, Park R, et al. Venous flare reactions: A case report of reactions following etoposide infusion. Clin J Oncol Nurs 2018;22(6):597–9. https://doi.org/10.1188/18.cjon.597-599.
34. Wickham R, Engelking C, Sauerland C, et al. Vesicant Extravasation Part II: evidence-based management and continuing controversies. Oncol Nurs Forum 2006;33(6):1143–50. https://doi.org/10.1188/06/onf.1143-1150.
35. Kim SS, Holcombe RF. Development of chemotherapy-induced extravasation management algorithm to facilitate and improve care of cancer patients. J Clin Oncol 2014;32(30_suppl):224. https://doi.org/10.1200/jco.2014.32.30_suppl.224.

# Surgical Site Infection Arising from the Operating Room

Asiye Gul, RN, PhD[a],*, Tuba Sengul, PhD, CWON[b],
Holly Kirkland-Kyhn, PhD, FNP-c, GNP-c, CWCN[c]

## KEYWORDS

- Surgical site infection • Infection control • Operating room • Intraoperative practices
- Patient safety

## KEY POINTS

- *High Risk of surgical site infections (SSIs)*: SSIs are a significant threat to patient safety, increasing mortality, morbidity, and health care costs.
- *Primary Causative Agents*: *Staphylococcus aureus* is a leading cause of SSIs, with other common pathogens including coagulase-negative staphylococci and gram-negative bacteria.
- *Infection Control Advances*: Effective infection control practices, such as proper hand hygiene, surgical techniques, and antimicrobial prophylaxis, reduce SSIs rates.
- *Operating Room Environment*: Maintaining a clean and controlled operating room environment, including air quality and minimal traffic, is essential to prevent SSIs.
- *Comprehensive Prevention*: A multi-faceted and continuous approach is necessary to prevent SSIs, involving both patient and procedural factors.

## INTRODUCTION

Each year, millions of surgical procedures are performed worldwide. Patients are at a high risk of developing surgical site infections, especially during the intra-operative period.[2] These infections, which occur either at the surgical incision site[3] or in deeper tissues,[2] are therefore termed surgical site infections (SSIs).[4] SSIs represent a significant challenge in surgery due to their association with increased mortality, morbidity, hospital length of stay, and cost,[5,6] and they are among the most common reasons for readmissions[7] while significantly threatening patient safety and decreasing quality of life.[2] The use of implant material during surgery can result in inflammation and

[a] Istanbul Kültür University, Faculty of Health Science, Nursing Department, Istanbul, Turkey;
[b] Koç University School of Nursing, Istanbul, Turkey; [c] Betty Irene Moore School of Nursing at UC Davis, CA, USA
* Corresponding author.
*E-mail addresses:* a.gul@iku.edu.tr; asiyegul2003@yahoo.com

Nurs Clin N Am 60 (2025) 143–152
https://doi.org/10.1016/j.cnur.2024.07.003
0029-6465/25/© 2024 Elsevier Inc. All rights reserved, including those for text and data mining, AI training, and similar technologies.

rejection, necessitating additional surgical procedures or implant removal.[8] *Staphylococcus aureus* is often found to be the primary cause of SSIs, accounting for a significant proportion of cases (40%–70%), with coagulase-negative staphylococci and gram-negative bacteria also commonly identified as causative.[9]

In recent years, significant advances have taken place in the implementation of infection control practices, standardized routine hand and skin cleansing, surgical techniques, operating theater air conditioning and heating, cleanliness and sterilization/disinfection procedures, and the appropriate use of antimicrobial prophylaxis (ie, selection, dosage, and duration of perioperative prophylaxis).[10] A major focus of global health care is the prevention of SSIs.[2] Evidence-based guidelines for preventing SSIs indicate that successful reductions in SSIs rates have been achieved with effective interventions.[3] A multi-faceted, continuous approach is needed to prevent and reduce surgical site infections.[10] Because SSIs are primarily acquired during surgery when the wound is open, several infection prevention practices in the operating theater must be examined.[7] This article addresses the risk factors for SSIs in the operating room and preventive measures.

## INCIDENCE

SSIs constitute at least 15% of healthcare-associated infections acquired by hospital patients. However, measuring the incidence is challenging as many infections may occur after the patient has been discharged.[4] A total 2% to 5% of patients undergoing surgical procedures are exposed to SSIs.[2] This rate is approximately 1% in the United States, with approximately 8000 deaths directly related to the condition.[2] The frequency of occurrence can vary between 0.1% and 50%, depending on the nature and conditions of the surgical procedure.[11] Guest and colleagues (2023) examined data from 50,000 adult patients undergoing open surgical procedures and found an incidence of SSIs to be 11%. They also determined that the incidence varied significantly across different surgical categories, ranging from 0.4% to 15.4%. They also found that the incidence differs to a lower degree according to the patient's underlying risk and the nature of the procedure, such as whether it was elective or required.[3] Surgical site infection incidence rates are significantly higher in low-income and middle-income countries due to inadequate infection prevention practices.[3] Data on the global and regional prevalence rates need to be improved.[12] In developing countries, SSIs occur annually in over 30% of surgical patients.[2] A systematic review and meta-analysis conducted by Mengistu and colleagues (2023) found that the incidence of SSIs ranged from 7.2% in the African region, which was the highest, to a global average of 2.5%.[12] According to the 2017 data from the National Healthcare-Associated Infections Surveillance Network in Turkey, the overall SSIs rate is 0.72%.[13]

The existing data on SSIs costs are rising and need to be improved.[14] Estimated costs of SSIs treatment vary widely, ranging from $400 to $30,000 depending on the type and site of the infection.[15] In a retrospective study conducted by Guest and colleagues (2023), SSIs increased the surgical wound healing time by an average of 15 days per wound, and the total health care cost of surgical wound treatment was determined to be an average of £3537 per wound.[3] In the United States, health care-associated infections are the most costly of all hospital-acquired infections, estimated to cost $3.3 billion annually and increase the length of hospital stay by 9.7 days.[2]

## RISK FACTORS IN THE OPERATING ROOM

Most infections are acquired during surgery.[4] Knowing the risk factors contributing to SSIs and intervening to prevent them can decrease their development.[5] There are numerous known factors related to the risk of SSIs.[2] Risk factors can be classified into patient-related and surgery-related characteristics.[5] For the development of SSIs, preoperative patient-related risk factors can be non-modifiable (such as age and exposure to radiation in the surgical area) or modifiable (such as glucose control, to-bacco use, and obesity).[14] Individuals at high risk include the elderly and those with diabetes, peripheral vascular disease, chronic obstructive pulmonary disease, nutri-tional disorders or fluid-electrolyte imbalances, previous radiation exposure, intrao-perative blood loss of more than 500 mL, or those undergoing medical treatments (chemotherapy, corticosteroids, or immunosuppressive drugs).[16] Awareness of un-derlying factors predisposing patients to infection can help identify those at highest risk and potentially enhance their resistance to infection before surgery by improving nutrition, controlling blood sugar, and closely monitoring them for early signs of infec-tion postoperatively.[4] It has been shown that prolonged surgical duration increases the risk of SSIs. The increase occurs when surgery duration exceeds the 75th percen-tile.[9] Cheng and colleagues (2017) found that the incidence of SSIs increased by 13%, 17%, and 37% for each 15, 30, and 60 minutes of surgery, depending on the proced-ure.[11] Among the modifiable risk factors for SSIs, procedural aspects such as the probability of instrument contamination, the number of personnel involved in the sur-gery, and intraoperative traffic are included.[6] Any event during surgery that induces vasoconstriction, such as hypothermia or mild hypovolemia, alters tissue oxygenation, leading to higher infection rates.[7]

Surgical wounds have a high risk of contamination with pathogenic microorgan-isms from the patient's skin or the environment.[2] The microorganisms that cause SSIs can be endogenous or exogenous.[2,9] Exogenous microorganisms are carried by air particles, personnel (hands, skin, and mucosal areas), or, less commonly, inanimate objects (instruments, materials, furniture, or solutions).[9] Most SSIs origi-nate from the patient's endogenous flora, and this flora contaminates the wound through direct contact during the procedure.[4,7] Bacterial load, bacterial virulence, and the patient's ability to resist infection all contribute to developing surgical site infections.[2–4]

## PRECAUTIONS THAT CAN BE TAKEN TO PREVENT SURGICAL SITE INFECTIONS IN THE OPERATING ROOM

An integral component of infection control is the prevention of SSIs.[9] Members of the intraoperative team have several roles to play in reducing the risk of SSIs to patients.[17] Wearing appropriate surgical attire, following sterile technique, applying surgical skin antisepsis, increasing patient oxygenation, and minimizing the opening of operating room doors are some of the ways to contribute.[10,17] Besides prophylactic antibiotics, SSIs prevention includes ensuring an aseptic environment and strict operating room discipline for all staff.[9]

### Operating Room Environment

*Operating Room Air:* Contamination caused by microorganisms in the air plays a sig-nificant role in the pathogenesis of SSIs.[9] The spread of dust laden with live micro-organisms (including *Staphylococcus aureus*) by surgical team members has been demonstrated. Patients settle on surfaces, including surgical wounds, instruments, textile fibers, skin flakes, and respiratory aerosols.[18] The amount of live bacteria in the operating room air is highly related to the risk of SSIs, especially in surgical patients susceptible to infections.[2,15,19] Contamination of the surgical area due to airborne par-ticles occurs in 30% of cases due to particles settling directly on the incision site and in

70% of cases due to particles settling on instruments and the surgeon's hands and then being transferred to incision site.[9]

While no specific universal standard exists for airborne microbial contamination in the operating room, it is perceived that the risk increases when microbial counts in sampled air exceed a unit, forming 36 to 150 colonies per $m^3$ of air (CFU).[20] During a moderate level of physical activity, an individual releases about 10 million particles per day. During walking, about 5% to 10% of these particles carry bacteria, and the emission rate increases to $10^4$ per minute.[15] Perioperative personnel can shed microbial particles, textile fibers, and skin cells from their clothing into the operating room air as they move around.[14] The microbial load in the operating room air can increase due to conditions such as dermatitis and upper respiratory tract infections among operating room staff.[7,15,18] The amount of airborne microbial particles in an operating theater depends on the number of people present and their activity levels.[4] Covering the patient's body leads to the highest level of airborne particle count at the beginning of the operation as it necessitates personnel movement and other activities.[9] Sadri Zadeh and colleagues (2014) found that airborne particles accumulate as the number of individuals in the room increases.[15]

During surgery, dust particles, textile fibers, and microorganism-laden respiratory aerosols in the operating team and surrounding environment can enter surgical instruments or directly into the surgical site, leading to SSIs.[19] Dalstrom and colleagues (2008) recorded contamination rates on open trays in the operating room as 4% at 30 minutes, 15% after 1 hour, 22% after 2 hours, 26% after 3 hours, and 30% after 4 hours.[21] Covering the surgical tray with a sterile surgical towel greatly reduces the risk of contamination, so the time the tray is opened should be as close to the start of surgery as possible.[7,21]

Maintaining a clean surrounding environment and sufficient airflow to remove particulates from the sterile area is crucial to preventing surgical site infections.[14,15] The ventilation of operating rooms should provide a minimum of 20 air changes per hour, with 4 changes being clean air.[22] Where possible, high-efficiency particulate air (HEPA) filters should filter this air.[7] A laminar airflow system, a unidirectional, positive-pressure air flow, is recommended for high-risk procedures such as orthopedic surgery, cardiac surgery, and organ transplantation.[22] Placing implant materials during surgery may make the wound susceptible to infection even if only a few bacteria enter.[4] Operating room cleanliness and disinfection are crucial to prevent SSIs. All horizontal surfaces must be wiped with a damp cloth at the beginning of the day, and after each procedure, the operating room must be cleaned and disinfected with detergent and water.[4,14] It is reasonable to clean walls and ceilings twice yearly, as they are rarely heavily soiled.[7] Immediate action should be taken to address specific blood or bodily fluid spills,[7] which may require cleaning with chlorine solutions.[4] The surface integrity should be assessed while cleaning and disinfecting environmental surfaces. Tears or holes in surgical mattresses and arm boards can create a conducive environment for microbial growth by allowing fluid entry.[14] As inanimate objects and surfaces rarely cause SSIs, it is unnecessary to perform routine cultures in the operating theater environment.[7]

*Operating Room Traffic:* To minimize the risk of contaminating the operating theater, the number of persons should be limited, as personnel can shed cells and microorganisms from their skin, and the number of aerosol particles in the operating room is directly related to the number of people present.[22] Besides limiting the operating room staff, all necessary equipment, materials, and instruments should be prepared and kept inside the operating room before the procedure to restrict entry and exit traffic.[14] Operating room doors should remain closed to maintain a positive pressure atmosphere during surgical procedures.[22] There is a common consensus that numbers should not exceed 5 or 6 people in the operating theater to ensure that the airborne bacterial level does not exceed 10 CFU/m$^3$.[9] Minimizing unnecessary personnel movement during surgical procedures and frequent opening of the operating room door is recommended.[23]

The entry of any computer, laptop, radio, and, most importantly, mobile phone into the operating room is a possible source of cross-contamination. These types of equipment contain resistant microorganisms, with percentages ranging from 44% to 98% (gram-negative rods and *Staphylococcus aureus*).[9] Qureshi and colleagues (2020) found that 93 out of 100 mobile phones in an orthopedic surgical operating room were contaminated, with *Coagulase-negative Staphylococcus* (62%), *Micrococcus* (41%), and *Bacillus* (26%) frequently isolated. They also noted a reduction in contamination after cleaning the phone cracks and mobile covers.[24] The best practice is the avoidance of the use of portable electronic devices in the operating theater. If they need to be used, they must be cleaned carefully with an alcohol-based solution before entering the operating theater.[9]

*The sequence of patients entering the operating room:* The practice of scheduling dirty case toward the end of the day should be abandoned.[7] No evidence suggests an increase in the risk of SSIs when a clean surgical operation follows a contamination operation, provided that the operating room is thoroughly decontaminated between patients using a well-standardized protocol and/or procedure.[7,9] However, contaminated procedures are most appropriately carried out at the end of the operating theater schedule, and surgical staff should follow personalized decontamination techniques to prevent transmission of microorganisms from staff to patients.[9]

### Patient Preparation

*Skin preparation:* The skin is a source of the body's microbes, so it is essential that the skin is optimally prepared before surgery.[2,7,9] Inadequate skin antisepsis, including failure to follow the manufacturer's instructions (eg, application and drying time), can create opportunities for contaminated skin flora to enter the incision site.[14] Current data suggest the use of chlorhexidine instead of povidone-iodine.[10] Chlorhexidine also maintains efficacy in the context of any blood or serum and is the antiseptic of choice for patients colonized with *Staphylococcus aureus*.[7] Wang and colleagues (2023) revealed in their meta-analysis that compared to patients undergoing skin disinfection with povidone-iodine, those undergoing chlorhexidine disinfection had lower incidences of SSIs, superficial SSIs rates, and deep SSIs rates. For the prevention of SSIs, the evidence available to date suggests that chlorhexidine is superior to povidone-iodine.[25]

The day or morning before the surgery, a full-body shower or bath with antimicrobial or non-antimicrobial soap, without shaving the surgical site hairs, is recommended.[9,14] Taking a bath or shower with an antiseptic (chlorhexidine or povidone-iodine) before surgery reduces the bacterial count on the skin. A clear correlation between preoperative bathing and a reduction in wound infection rates has not been established.[4] However, such baths are strongly recommended by the Centers for Disease Control and Prevention.[14]

If the hair needs to be removed, it must be done outside the operating room, preferably just before the intervention, using clippers or a depilatory agent, as shaving with a razor blade is associated with an increased risk of SSIs.[7,10] Bacteria, especially if the skin has been shaved a few hours before surgery, proliferate in micro-abrasions caused by the razor blade on the skin surface.[4]

*Body temperature:* Hypothermia is defined as a body temperature of less than 36 °C (96.8°F) and is linked to an increased risk of SSIs, increased bleeding, cardiac morbidity, and prolonged hospital stay.[10,26] Moderate-quality evidence suggests that maintaining normothermia during the preoperative period significantly reduces the risk of SSIs compared to not warming at all.[27] Active warming for at least 30 minutes before incision is more beneficial.[4,7] If the procedure does not require active patient warming, the patient should remain warm with blankets.[4] For procedures lasting longer than 30 minutes, maintaining the patient's body temperature above 36°C throughout the perioperative period is recommended.[26] Warm intravenous fluids during surgery have been shown to maintain patients at a warmer body heat than room temperature fluids.[28] Solutions used for body cavities during surgery should also be heated to between 39°C and 40°C.[4]

### Surgical Process

*Hand hygiene of surgical personnel:* Hand hygiene, surface cleaning, and disinfection should be performed according to the institution's policies and procedures.[14] All members of the surgical team who will be working in the surgical field should scrub their arms and hands with an antiseptic solution for 2 to 5 minutes.[26] The first scrub of the day should involve using an antiseptic soap solution for 5 minutes and thoroughly cleaning the subungual areas.[5,7] Between procedures, consecutive washes with antiseptic soap or alcohol solutions for 2 minutes each can also be performed.[26] Although surgical hand scrubbing has been used in the past, it is not currently recommended due to its association with microtrauma and colonization. Instead, brushless washing and double gloving are recommended.[5] All jewelry should be removed during hand hygiene, and artificial nails should not be worn as they are associated with increased hand colonization by bacteria and yeasts. The relationship between the application of nail polish by surgical team members and the risk of SSIs has not yet been proven.[7] However, it is recommended that operating room personnel do not wear artificial nails.[23] Hand hygiene suggests that chlorhexidine reduces bacterial counts compared to traditional scrubbing with povidone-iodine, and alcohol-based hand rubs, when used with other antiseptic agents, can reduce bacterial populations on hands compared to wet scrubbing.[10] Alcohol-based hand rubs are equally effective on clean hands and can be used as an alternative to surgical scrubbing in repeated washings. Hands should be dry as the effectiveness of alcohol-based hand rubs may decrease on wet hands.[4]

*Surgical dressing:* The use of caps, masks, gowns, and shoes in the operating room is essential for protecting health care workers from infectious blood and other fluids and ensuring patient safety.[5] While there is no clinical study proving that the use of these barriers in the operating room leads to a decrease in SSIs rates, they are recommended as part of standard precautions.[7] Operating room attire should be covered appropriately with elastics at the waist, ankles, neck, and wrists to prevent shedding of skin flakes.[9] Sterile surgical dressings and gowns minimize contamination but lose their effectiveness when wet.[26] Tears and scratches in surgical gowns, especially in the arm or abdomen area, can be potential sources of contamination, so waterproof gowns or more durable gowns should be worn.[7] The World Health Organization (WHO) asserts that disposable and reusable drapes and gowns are equivalent.[27] Because shredded paper on disposable garments can be a source of lint on reusable woven fabrics, such paper products should not be placed in the same bin as fabric clothing.[22] It is recommended that staff stay in the operating room attire to prevent contamination and infection risk for the patient.[29]

*Surgical Mask and Hair Cover Usage:* Masks must be worn to cover the nose and mouth in all restricted areas.[22] This has been found to reduce aerosol droplet contamination by 98.48% compared to not wearing a face mask.[30] Edmiston and colleagues

(2005) noted that the barrier properties of standard tie-on surgical masks were most effective in the first 90 minutes compared to longer use intervals.[20] Kelkar and colleagues (2013) found that masks significantly reduced bacterial dispersion initially but became almost ineffective after 2 hours.[31] Zhiqing and colleagues (2018) concluded that surgical masks could potentially be a source of SSIs, primarily when used for long hours, notably exceeding 2 hours. They recommended changing the surgical mask after each procedure, especially those lasting longer than 2 hours.[32] Coughing and sneezing release droplets into the environment; therefore, people with respiratory infections should not be allowed into the operating room.[22] It is emphasized that unnecessary talking should be avoided to minimize the contamination risk of surgical masks, and double-layer masks could be an effective measure to reduce contamination.[30] Additionally, it should be noted that tight masks and headgear increase the shedding of contaminated skin particles due to friction on the skin.[9] Hair is the main source of staphylococci and can cause contamination. Therefore, the hair covers should cover all hair, neck, and ears. The extent to which the microbial population is attracted to the hair is directly related to the length and cleanliness of the hair. Hair should be shampooed frequently.[22]

During surgery, good-quality gloves must be worn.[9] Wearing double gloves is recommended, especially during orthopedic surgeries, as approximately 50% of gloves may be perforated. Double gloving increases the barrier against contaminants from the patient to the surgical staff and vice versa.[26] However, wearing double gloves has not reduced the risk of SSIs associated with decreased perforation.[4] Gloves should be changed immediately after accidental perforation.[7,27] The rate of glove perforation with direct contact with the skin is 15% in single-glove cases compared to only 5% in double-glove cases.[9] Gloves should be changed when contaminated or perforation is suspected, and after any surgical procedure that has been contaminated, such as anastomosis, before the prosthesis is inserted and incisions are closed.[26]

There are no studies that measure the effect of shoe covers on the bacterial count on the floor, and since there is no direct contact between an open wound and the floor, there is no logical reason for their use.[4] To reduce SSIs, it is recommended that people discontinue wearing plastic/paper shoe covers and use easily washable shoes dedicated solely to the operating room. This is because there is no noticeable difference in the floor contamination between personnel wearing shoe covers and those wearing normal shoes in the operating theater.[7]

*Surgical technique:* To minimize the risk of SSIs, adherence to aseptic principles is essential.[4] Good surgical technique reduces SSIs risk. Surgeons should handle tissues gently whenever possible, limit the use of electrocautery, and remove all devitalized tissues before closure.[7,9] A correlation has been observed between the duration of intraoperative hypotension and the SSIs rate and between compromised vascularization and oxygenation at intestinal anastomoses. Therefore, maintaining normovolemia is crucial.[26]

*Materials used in surgery:* For infection to occur, it has been found that 6.5 million bacteria are required when no sutures are used, whereas only 100 bacteria are sufficient when silk sutures are used.[4] Despite debates about their utility, antiseptic-coated sutures reduce in vitro bacterial colonization.[26] Using antibiotic-coated sutures has resulted in approximately a 30% reduction in SSIs.[10] To reduce SSIs risk independent of the type of surgery, the use of triclosan-coated sutures is recommended.[27] However, the Society of Healthcare Epidemiology of America/Infectious Diseases Society of America guidelines do not recommend their use as a strategy for preventing SSIs.[10,27] Antiseptic-impregnated sutures can reduce SSIs rates when SSIs rates remain high despite implementing all basic infection control measures.[7,27] During surgery, transparent, adhesive, and sterile surgical drapes are used to maintain the sterility of environmental surfaces, equipment, and the patient's surroundings.[27] A Cochrane review conducted in 2018 comparing adhesive drapes with non-adhesive drapes (5 studies, 3082 participants) found that using adhesive drapes was associated with increased SSIs risk.[1] The Infectious Diseases Society of America and the Guidelines Development Group have decided that plastic adhesive incision drapes (whether antimicrobial or not) should not be used.[27]

## SUMMARY

Many intraoperative risk factors contribute to the development of SSIs. Infection prevention interventions are the most critical way to reduce surgical site infections. Preventing SSIs will reduce associated morbidity, mortality, and health care costs. Prevention of SSIs in operating rooms should be a top priority. All surgical team members should prioritize taking preventive measures to reduce the risk of infection for every surgical patient.

## CLINICS CARE POINTS

- *Sterile Techniques*: Ensure strict adherence to sterile techniques during surgical procedures to minimize contamination and infection risks.
- *Environmental Control*: Maintain optimal air quality and cleanliness in the operating room, using HEPA filters and regular cleaning protocols.
- *Prophylactic Antibiotics*: Administer appropriate prophylactic antibiotics based on surgical procedures and patient risk factors to prevent SSIs.
- *Minimize Operating Room Traffic*: Limit the number of personnel and movement in the operating room to reduce airborne contamination.
- *Hand Hygiene*: Emphasize the importance of proper hand hygiene practices for all surgical team members, including using alcohol-based hand rubs and double gloving.

## DISCLOSURE

The authors have nothing to disclose.

## REFERENCES

1. Liu Z, Dumville JC, Norman G, et al. Intraoperative interventions for preventing surgical site infection: an overview of Cochrane Reviews. Cochrane Database Syst Rev 2018;2. https://doi.org/10.1002/14651858.CD012653.pub2.
2. Markström I, Bjersä K, Bachrach-Lindström M, et al. Prerequisites for infection prevention interventions during the intraoperative phase from the perspective of operating room nurses: An integrative review. Research Square 2023;1–37. https://doi.org/10.21203/rs.3.rs-3082832/v1.
3. Guest JF, Fuller GW, Griffiths B. Cohort study to characterize surgical site infections after open surgery in the UK's National Health Service. BMJ Open 2023; 13(12). https://doi.org/10.1136/bmjopen-2023-076735.
4. Wilson J. Preventing wound infection. In: Wilson J, editor. Infection control in clinical practice. 3rd Edition. Poland: Elsevier Health Sciences (US); 2019. p. 279–306. ISBN 978-0-7020-7696-1.

5. Balkan A, Çelebi C. Surgical site infections. Black Sea. J Health Sci 2020;3(2): 45–60.
6. Calò P, Catena F, Corsaro D, et al. Optimisation of perioperative procedural factors to reduce the risk of surgical site infection in patients undergoing surgery: a systematic review. Discov Health Systems 2023;2(6):6.
7. Roy MC. The Operating Room. In: Guide to Infection Control in the Healthcare Setting. G Bearman (Ed). By International Society for Infectious Diseases. Chapter last updated: August 2023. Accessed March 30, 2024. Available at: https://isid.org/guide/infectionprevention/the-operating-room/.
8. Zhu D, Luo Q. Effectiveness of nursing intervention in the operating room to prevent wound infections in patients undergoing orthopaedic surgery: A meta-analysis. Int Wound J 2023;20(10):4103–11.
9. Chauveaux D. Preventing surgical-site infections: Measures other than antibiotics. Orthop Traumatol Surg Res 2015;101(1 Suppl).
10. Rosa R, Sposato K, Abbo LM. Preventing surgical site infections: Implementing strategies throughout the perioperative continuum. AORN J 2023;117(5):300–11.
11. Cheng H, Chen BP, Soleas IM, et al. Prolonged operative duration increases risk of surgical site infections: A systematic review. Surg Infect 2017;18(6):722–35.
12. Mengistu DA, Alemu A, Abdukadir AA, et al. Global incidence of surgical site infection among patients: Systematic review and meta-analysis. Inquiry 2023; 60. 469580231162549.
13. Hekimoğlu CH, Batır E. Cerrahi Alan Enfeksiyonu Sürveyansı. T.C. Sağlık Bakanlığı Halk Sağlığı Genel Müdürlüğü Bulaşıcı Hastalıklar Dairesi Başkanlığı, Ankara. 2018. Available at: https://hsgm.saglik.gov.tr/depo/birimler/bulasici-hastaliklar-ve-erken-uyari-db/Dokumanlar/Rehberler/CERRAHI_ALAN_ENFEKSIYONU_SURVEYANSI. pdf. [Accessed 29 March 2024].
14. Murphy LW. Preventing surgical site infections. AORN J 2023;117(2):126–30.
15. Sadrizadeh S, Tammelin A, Ekolind P, et al. Influence of staff number and internal constellation on surgical site infection in an operating room. Particuology 2014; 13:42–51.
16. Snyder JS, Sump CA. Managing Wound Care. In: Snyder JS, Sump CA, editors. Swearingen's all-in-one nursing care planning resource. 6th Edition. St. Louis, Missouri: Elsevier; 2024. p. 536–44.
17. Reese SM. Optimizing the relationship between perioperative personnel and infection preventionist to reduce surgical site infections. AORN J 2023;118(4): 224–31.
18. Parvizi J, Barnes Sue, Shohat Noam, et al. Environment of care: Is it time to reassess microbial contamination of the operating room air as a risk factor for surgical site infection in total joint arthroplasty? Am J Infect Control 2017;45(11):1267–72.
19. Colella Y, Valente AS, Rossano L, et al. A fuzzy inference system for the assessment of indoor air quality in an operating room to prevent surgical site infection. Int J Environ Res Publ Health 2022;19(6):3533.
20. Edmiston CE, Seabrook GR, Cambria RA, et al. Molecular epidemiology of microbial contamination in the operating room environment: Is there a risk for infection? Surgery 2005;138(4):573–82.
21. Dalstrom DJ, Venkatarayappa I, Manternach AL, et al. Time-dependent contamination of opened sterile operating-room trays. J Bone Joint Surg Am 2008;90(5): 1022–5.
22. Phillips N, Hornacky A. Principles of aseptic and sterile techniques. In: Fourteenth Edition, Phillips N, Hornacky A, editors. Berry & Kohn's operating room technique. St. Louis, Missouri: Elsevier; 2021. p. 251–65.

23. Humphreys H, Bak A, Ridgway E, et al. Rituals and behaviours in the operating theatre - joint guidelines of the Healthcare Infection Society and the European Society of Clinical Microbiology and Infectious Diseases. J Hosp Infect 2023;140: 165.e1–28.
24. Qureshi NQ, Mufarrih SH, Irfan S, et al. Mobile phones in the orthopedic operating room: Microbial colonization and antimicrobial resistance. World J Orthoped 2020;11(5):252–64.
25. Wang P, Wang D, Zhang L. Effectiveness of chlorhexidine versus povidone-iodine for preventing surgical site wound infection: A meta-analysis. Int Wound J 2023;21(2).
26. Badia JM, Rubio Pérez I, Manuel A, et al. Surgical site infection prevention measures in general surgery: Position statement by the surgical infections division of the Spanish Association of Surgery. Cir Esp 2020;98(4):187–203.
27. World Health Organization. Global Guidelines for the Prevention of Surgical Site Infection (2nd Edition). Geneva, Switzerland: 2018. Accessed March 08, 2024. Available at: https://apps.who.int/iris/rest/bitstreams/1168437/retrieve.
28. Campbell G, Alderson P, Smith AF, et al. Warming of intravenous and irrigation fluids for preventing inadvertent perioperative hypothermia. Cochrane Database Syst Rev 2015;(4). https://doi.org/10.1002/14651858.CD009891.pub2.
29. Hafiani EM, Cassier P, Aho S, et al. Guidelines for clothing in the operating theatre. Anaesth Crit Care Pain Med 2021;41(3):101084.
30. Ogo N, Foran P. The effectiveness and compliance of surgical face mask wearing in the operating suite environment: An integrated review. J Perioper Nurs 2020; 33(4):11–8.
31. Kelkar US, Gogate B, Kurpad S, et al. How effective are face masks in operation theatre? A time frame analysis and recommendations. Int J Infect Control 2013; 9(1):1–6.
32. Zhiqing L, Yongyun C, Wenxiang C, et al. Surgical masks as source of bacterial contamination during operative procedures. J Orthop Translat 2018;14:57–62.

# Transition of Care Challenges and Opportunities for Chronic Wounds

Ron Billano Ordona, DNP, FNP-BC, GS-C, WCC[a,b,c,d,*]

## KEYWORDS

- Transition of care • Chronic wounds • Skilled nursing facilities
- Community-based care • Wound management

## KEY POINTS

- Challenges in transition of care: Effective communication and standardized discharge planning are critical to prevent readmissions and adverse events from acute to community-based care settings.
- Role of skilled nursing facilities (SNFs): SNFs are crucial in managing patients with acute and chronic wounds, particularly older adults with multiple chronic conditions.
- Interdisciplinary team approach: Involving providers, wound care-trained nurses, physical therapists, and caregivers in care planning is essential for preventing pressure injuries and managing chronic wounds.
- Caregiver training and support: Educating and supporting both formal and informal caregivers are vital to improve wound care management and enhance patient outcomes in home and community settings.

## BACKGROUND AND INTRODUCTION

The movement of patients from one level of care or care setting to another is commonly termed transition of care (TOC).[1] This may mean a transfer within a healthcare facility, such as when a patient is transferred from an intensive care unit to a telemetry floor or vice versa. In other scenarios, a TOC happens when patients move from one healthcare facility to another, such as from an acute level of care (ie, the hospital) to post-acute care, commonly referred to in general terms as post-acute care services. This typically involves discharging patients from the hospital to

[a] Senior Care Clinic House Calls, Sacramento, CA, USA; [b] Care Home by RNs, Sacramento, CA, USA; [c] Care Home by RNs, Houston, TX, USA; [d] Betty Irene Moore School of Nursing, University of California, Davis, Sacramento, CA, USA
* 4970 Walnut Avenue, Sacramento, CA 95841.
*E-mail address:* rbordona@ucdavis.edu

Nurs Clin N Am 60 (2025) 153–163
https://doi.org/10.1016/j.cnur.2024.07.014 **nursing.theclinics.com**
0029-6465/25/© 2024 Elsevier Inc. All rights are reserved, including those for text and data mining, AI training, and similar technologies.

a community care environment, whether short-term rehabilitation care, such as in a skilled nursing facility (SNF), or custodial care, normally a long-term stay.[2]

Open communication in healthcare[3] becomes one of the key factors that make a successful transition from one level of care to another or from one care facility to another. A common example is in scenarios such as when patients within an acute care setting move from the emergency department (ED) to one of the units in the main hospital, such as the intensive care unit (ICU), or from the ICU to the general medical-surgical (M-S) floors.[4] These transitions, in themselves, are challenging because of competing priorities. The ED staff's competing priority is treating more critically ill patients as they triage and progress through the care continuum. At the other end of this spectrum are the M-S unit staff members of the primary hospital, who may also be juggling the priorities for that staff member's patient load. This staff member may perceive a patient's admission from the ED to the M-S unit as disrupting the flow, making it a non-priority.

## CHALLENGES AND VARIATIONS IN THE TRANSITION OF CARE

This scenario is an example of a challenging aspect of the TOC within the auspices of the same hospital structure. Picture this in a setting of a patient moving from a separate healthcare entity (ie, the acute care facility) to a community-based facility such as a SNF. In this case, the movement of patients, hence, the exchange of information, happens not within the same geographic location, such as in the same hospital building, but in separate buildings, often without electronic health record interoperability.[5] Because of the relative need for more standardization in discharge planning,[6] the transition period from one care setting to another carries a high risk of an inadequate transfer of information, such as wound conditions and wound care management.[7] Thus, adverse events can occur because of the relative fragmentation of communication, partly due to the lack of warm hand-offs from one care provider to the next.[8] The transition from acute care settings to skilled nursing care settings for patients with chronic wounds presents similar, if not more, challenges to those undergoing an internal TOC (ie, moving from one hospital unit to another), as exemplified by the ED to ICU and regular hospital unit transfers.

The advantage of that internal TOC is that healthcare professionals (HCPs) in those same settings work with the same electronic health record and can, therefore, peruse shared-documentation[5] and information to gather more data should the communication between the providers is not adequate. In the case of acute care to SNF or other community-based care facility transfers, it is challenging to share documents effectively and efficiently. Electronic health records so far, except for some particular and rare settings, do not communicate with each other.[5] This adds to the complexity of the TOC between these healthcare settings. There is an impetus between organizations and home-based and community-focused healthcare systems and providers to integrate during this care transition. This period is especially crucial because Medicare has implemented the Hospital Readmission Reduction Program[9] and imposes penalties on hospitals for high readmission rates. For instance, a 2015 study in a Northern California county revealed that more than half of patients discharged without a primary care provider (PCP) experienced readmission within 7 days and up to 30 days after discharge.[10] An estimated 20% of hospitalized patients were readmitted to the hospital for the same condition they were discharged with between 30 days after discharge, and approximately 30% were readmitted within 90 days. Studies find that at least one medical error occurs in readmitted patients who ineffectively transitioned from the hospital to community settings and 20% experience 1 or more adverse events.[2]

## Settings

The TOC varies widely due to the significant differences in the continuum of care[11] between states, counties, and healthcare settings. For example, the continuum of care in California is expansive, so the care transitions have added complexities. Two divergent factors determine the variations in the level of care on the continuum: the intensity of patient care needs and the severity of the illness (**Fig. 1**). Acute care facilities provide high intensity of care and high severity of disease. On the other end of the spectrum is the home or an independent living space where the severity of illness is low or, in some cases, may be absent; thereby, the intensity of patient care is also low.

As a step-down from acute care settings, long-term acute care hospitals (LTACHs),[12] sub-acute care facilities (typically a dedicated unit within some SNFs), or stand-alone congregate living health facilities (CLHFs)[13] manage patients or residents on long-term tracheostomies or respiratory ventilators. Neurologic insults such as cerebrovascular accidents, traumatic events resulting in traumatic brain injuries, end-stage multiple sclerosis, end-stage amyotrophic lateral sclerosis, and other similar conditions usually cause these patients or residents who are typically on long-term percutaneous intragastric tube feedings, to be more susceptible to developing stage 3 or 4 pressure wounds and other related higher-complexity conditions. These facilities typically have respiratory therapists who co-manage residents with tracheostomies or are on a ventilator machine. The bed capacity in this spectrum of care varies from 50 to 100 beds for LTACHs, 10 to 15 beds for subacute care units within SNFs, and 6 to 25 beds for CLHFs, depending on county population. **Fig. 1** illustrates the continuum of care that may be unique to California. However, this approximates the continuum of care across the United States. Each state may have variances based on local regulations, local coverages, and benefits such as Medicaid (MediCal in California) reimbursements.

California's continuum of care[11] is unique to the state because aside from the federally recognized facilities such as acute care facilities, SNFs,[14] which may be short-term rehabilitation following Medicare guidelines, and assisted living facilities (ALFs),[15] California has other facilities in the continuum that serves patients or

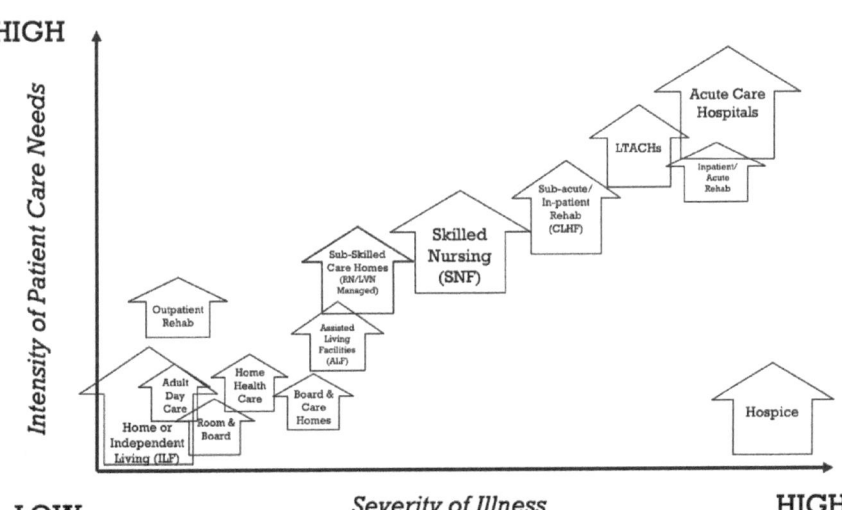

**Fig. 1.** Continuum of care in California.

residents at varying degrees of care and illness intensity. Some of the services may be covered by the California state-funded MediCal, which covers some qualifying stays for transitional housing such as in subacute units, CLHFs if patients or residents require more complex care, or the smaller independent living facilities (ILFs)[16] also known as "room and board" (R&B) facilities. Thus, ILFs, the larger versions of the R&B homes, are where the severity of illness and the intensity of patient care needs are low. Individuals living at home are independent in their daily activities (ADLs). Primary care focuses on preventing hospital readmissions for patients with stable chronic conditions like hypertension and diabetes. The goal is more preventive care rather than treating acute illnesses.

### *Acuity of Care*

The spectrum of care within this continuum ranges from low acuity, more chronic care with little to no professional care provider involvement, or the other end of the spectrum, where high acuity with a high level of professional care provider involvement.[17] In acute care settings, HCPs typically refer to individuals admitted as patients, whereas in long-term care settings, HCPs may refer to them as residents. When an individual is not able to go back home because of the higher need for assistance with ADLs, they may transition into residential care facilities for the elderly (RCFEs),[18] which is the official name for ALFs regulated by the California Department of Social Services. This level of care is further differentiated based on size, such as medium to large facilities with more than 6 bedrooms are considered ALFs, and those that have 6 bedrooms or less are more commonly referred to as residential assisted living or "care homes" or "board and care" homes.

These smaller settings tend to accept residents who need extensive assistance with daily activities, such as transfers from bed to wheelchair. Heavier care residents may require more one-on-one care or assistance with Hoyer lifts for transfers. HCPs manage some of these residential care homes, referred to as "sub-skilled care homes," which are a step down from SNFs. With state licensing approvals, these homes can care for residents with conditions typically restricted in ALFs due to HCPs involvement in care planning, management, and caregiver training.[19] Adult daycare centers support the continuum of care by providing respite for family caregivers. They help with ADLs, incontinence care, and medication assistance during the individual's stay. However, they do not provide higher acuity care, such as wound or behavioral care.

Depending on the severity of the illness, hospice agencies[20] provide end-of-life care for patients discharged to a lower level of care, such as homes or ALFs. Alternatively, home health agencies[20] cater to patients requiring a period of rehabilitation, where a team of physical therapists (PTs), occupational therapists, speech therapists, social workers, and others provide rehabilitative therapy in the homes or places of residence. Outpatient rehabilitation facilities offer an option for individuals who can leave their residences, providing access to rehabilitation equipment that is not feasible to bring home, for individuals with comorbidities requiring more extensive rehabilitation, inpatient, or acute care rehabilitation hospitals provide suitable rehabilitation modalities.

### *The Most Common Chronic Wounds in Community-based Care*

For patients with chronic wounds, especially deep wounds such as stage 3 or 4 pressure ulcers/injuries, there are some limitations due to regulations for options in the continuum of care. RCFEs, by regulation, must get an exception[19] approved by state licensing with a clear plan of care and the involvement of licensed professionals such as registered nurses or licensed vocational nurses/licensed practical nurses to manage these wounds. This leaves few options for patients with chronic wounds to transition to community-based care. CLHFs are often adept at managing deep wounds, but the number of CLHFs in the state is limited, and this care model has yet to catch on to payers and health plans. SNFs are crucial in caring for patients with acute and chronic wounds or those who are recovering from recent hospital stays, such as hip or knee surgeries. They also care for long-term patients who cannot adequately be cared for at home. According to the Johns Hopkins Bloomberg School of Public Health, managing wounds in SNFs is challenging.[21] Medicare covers SNF care, primarily for older adults with multiple chronic conditions such as diabetes, heart failure, and chronic kidney disease.

Chronic wounds in post-acute, community-based care, including those in SNFs, are protracted[22] and, therefore, costly to the healthcare system. Aside from that, chronic wounds do affect the quality of life (QOL) of individuals affected, be it in their physical, emotional, social, or functional aspects of living. The quality improvement[23] project at an academic medical center found that pressure ulcers/injuries happen primarily from home, owing to the less skilled care in the homes. In contrast, wounds in nursing homes were this study's second source of ED visits.[3] Wound management in SNFs traditionally falls under a nurse's responsibility for daily dressing changes. Still, chronic wounds can become non-healing for a myriad of reasons, requiring specialized medical knowledge and training to diagnose and treat these chronic wounds adequately. Nurses sometimes have no choice but to send patients to the ED, resulting in the revolving door syndrome of admission and readmissions.[21] Skin tears[24] occur in any setting. However, the 3 most common chronic wounds in SNFs include pressure ulcers/injuries, vascular ulcers, which may be venous or arterial, and diabetic foot ulcers.[25]

### Pressure injury

Pressure injuries (PIs) are among the most common chronic wounds managed by home health, community-based care facilities, SNFs, and CLHFs. PIs are localized skin and soft tissue injuries from prolonged pressure and shear, usually exerted over bony prominences.[26] PIs are staged between 1 and 4 depending on the thickness and extent of the wound.[27] Deep tissue (DT) and unstageable PIs are not assigned a stage or depth. Vulnerable population groups, such as those with conditions of hypo-perfusion[28,29] that highly predispose them to develop DTPIs that evolve into PIs, include neurologic disease, cardiovascular disease, prolonged anesthesia, dehydration, malnutrition, hypotension, or postoperative patients.[26] The main objective in care planning for this susceptible population is to prevent the development of PIs. This requires an interdisciplinary team approach involving providers, wound care-trained nurses, PTs, certified nursing assistants (CNAs), and caregivers. Nurses plan, manage, monitor, and document care. CNAs handle most bedside care tasks, such as turning, repositioning, and incontinence care.

The caveat to identifying PIs is awareness of PI mimics, such as skin changes at the end of life.[30] Even though the healthcare team provides adequate care, skin failure at the end of life is unavoidable. This and other mimics are common in this community-based, long-term care setting. The proper diagnosis is of utmost importance and must be done by a trained or wound-certified advanced practice provider.[3]

### Vascular ulcers

Vascular ulcers, a type of PI mimic, must be considered in differential diagnoses. They include arterial, neurotrophic, and venous ulcers, each distinguished by specific locations and appearances. Chronic and recurrent, these ulcers often lead to a higher risk of lower leg amputation. Mislabeling of vascular wounds as PIs is common due to a lack of wound specialists in community settings, highlighting the need for re-education.

## TYPES OF VASCULAR ULCERS

1. Arterial Ulcers:
   - *Location:* Distal areas, dorsum of the foot or toes.
   - *Appearance:* Initially, the edges are irregular, but they progress to be well-defined. Grayish, unhealthy granulation tissue with minimal bleeding upon debriding.
   - *Symptoms:* Pain, especially at night, relieved by extremity dependency. Signs of chronic ischemia like hairlessness, pale skin, and absent pulses.[31]
2. Neurotrophic Ulcers:
   - *Appearance:* Punched-out with a deep sinus, often under calluses or pressure points (eg, first or fifth metatarsophalangeal joint).
   - *Symptoms:* Surrounded by chronic inflammatory tissue, brisk bleeding upon probing or debriding. Typically painless due to neuropathy causing hypesthesia and diminished positional sense.[31]
3. Venous Ulcers:
   - *Location:* "Gaiter" region of the legs (mid-calf to below the medial and lateral malleoli).
   - *Appearance:* Larger, shallower, moist granulating base with irregular borders. Surrounding tissue may show stasis dermatitis.
   - *Symptoms:* Mild pain, relieved by elevation.[31]
4. Diabetic Ulcers:
   - *Cause:* Result from diabetic pathophysiology affecting the bone structure, particularly the foot.
   - *Symptoms:* Well-established neuropathy leads to decreased or lost sensation, common in poorly controlled diabetics.[31]

## CHALLENGES OF WOUND CARE IN COMMUNITY-BASED SETTINGS

The causes of delayed wound healing come from many different factors. These factors include wound site situation (local) or an underlying disease process (systemic) that can contribute to the etiology of chronic wounds. Local factors include a lack of oxygen supply to the skin and wound infections. Systemic factors include obesity, smoking, malnutrition, diabetes, and others. Another factor associated with chronic wounds is mobility, particularly pressure ulcers/injuries. Functional impairment, such as immobility, is one of the most common risk factors for geriatric syndromes, such as PIs or falls, to mention a few. Furthermore, cardiovascular and neurologic disease patients are more susceptible to impaired wound healing.[25,32]

Wound care in primary settings can be complicated in multiple co-morbidity patients with an ineffective discharge process. Home health nurses often work independently, making it critical to provide support to guide clinical decision-making through education, development of guidelines and protocols, or care pathways. Current health plans' coverage limits the number of weekly visits for nurses and providers, leaving homebound patients to rely on non-professional help or family caregivers.

## OPPORTUNITY IN COMMUNITY AND HOME-BASED CARE IN MANAGING CHRONIC WOUNDS

Community and home-based care programs can effectively care for patients discharged from hospitals with chronic wounds in a home setting, shelters, homeless encampments, or assisted living or residential care facilities. Home-based care, as defined by the World Health Organization,[33] is a series of services provided to people in their homes that may include physical, psychosocial, or palliative care activities.[34] Home-based care effectively extends medical services beyond the hospital using evidence-based practices. Custodial care, the largest segment, often involves unpaid family caregivers who may face burnout without proper training. Formal home health care includes licensed nurses, aides, and therapists, while physicians and advanced practice providers provide home-based primary care.[2]

Opportunities exist to simplify and cascade training on wound management to family caregivers, formal caregivers, nurses, and advanced practice providers.[11] There is value in teaching and learning about identifying wound types, such as vascular wounds, compared to pressure ulcer/injury wounds. A look at a local level 1 trauma academic medical center in 2019[10,28] revealed that among the multiple-visit patients with chronic wounds present on admission, those who came from home outnumbered those who came from SNFs. It can be postulated that there is a knowledge deficit or care deficit regarding wound care among family and informal caregivers. Prevention is key, and patient and caregiver engagement, which can be initiated during the discharge process from acute care, becomes of utmost importance. There is an opportunity to tighten the post-discharge communication between discharge planners and the patient or caregivers. American Association of Retired Person and the Betty Irene Moore of Nursing at the University of California in Davis produced simplified instructional videos that are accessible to the public for free, published by the American Journal of Nursing,[35] including topics such as general wound care, pressure ulcer prevention, treatment of skin tears, and diabetic foot care among others.

### Interdisciplinary Team Planning and Communication

Naylor[36] demonstrated that successful TOC considers nurse-led and interdisciplinary team approaches. Communication includes sharing information in a warm hand-off with shared photos and discussion strategies with home-based care providers and home health nurses, outpatient clinics, and family caregivers, which can improve communication between care transitions. Furthermore, future partnerships can mentor skin care and wound management with the community and home-based caregivers. Collaboration between transition-of-care sites should aim to identify hospital-to-community TOC modalities for chronic wound management. HCPs need to incorporate caregiver education as part of the TOC. Community-based professionals, caregivers, and family members can identify innovative approaches to providing access to care for a vulnerable population, including the homeless or the homebound, with chronic wounds.[37,38]

Assessment of caregivers' (whether formal or informal caregivers) ability to manage skin and chronic wounds is done by way of knowledge and skills. Collaboration with community resources, healthcare vendors, and private entities with shared goals to deliver education and provide hands-on training for family caregivers and others in the home or community.[37]

### Safety Policy and Advocacy

The interprofessional team in TOC approaches must prioritize patient safety, advocate for patient and family independence, and prevent unnecessary ED visits or hospital readmission.[2] The continued development of educational modules to educate community-based providers such as home health nurses, PCPs, and community-based wound care clinics must be emphasized. One of the biggest challenges to this initiative is the lack of support and funding so that programs such as these can be sustainable. In recent years, the refocusing toward value-based care[39] for both Medicare and Medicaid/MediCal recipients is gaining traction, which can potentially help push forward this safety advocacy, which will bring community-based providers toward effective delivery of care where patients with chronic wounds live.

## SUMMARY

Effective management of chronic wounds during the TOC from acute to community settings is crucial to prevent readmissions and improve patient outcomes. Addressing communication challenges, standardizing discharge planning, and educating caregivers can enhance the quality of care. Interdisciplinary team approaches and integrating advanced wound care practices are essential in managing chronic wounds in community settings.

## CLINICS CARE POINTS

- TOC presents a challenge to healthcare settings across the continuum of care.
- Readmission reduction is a focus in acute, SNF and home health care settings.
- Standardization of the discharge process can enhance TOC and the quality of care.
- Incorpotating advanced wound care and caregiver education is one way to address TOC for patients with chronic wounds.

## DISCLOSURE

The author is in private practice, providing home-based primary and advanced wound care and consulting for community-based care facilities.

## REFERENCES

1. Chartbook on care Coordination: Transitions of care. Agency for Healthcare Research and Quality. Available at: https://www.ahrq.gov/research/findings/nhqrdr/chartbooks/carecoordination/measure1.html. (Accessed July 1, 2024).
2. Post-Acute Transitional Services: Safety in Home-Based Care programs. PSNet, Available at: https://psnet.ahrq.gov/primer/post-acute-transitional-services-safety-home-based-care-programs, (Accessed July 1, 2024). 2024.
3. Schnipper J., Fitall E., Hall K., et al., Approach to improving patient safety: communication. PSNet Annual Perspective, Available at: https://psnet.ahrq.gov/perspective/approach-improving-patient-safety-communication. (Accessed July 1, 2024). 2021.
4. Santhosh L., Cornell E., Rojas C., et al., Diagnostic Safety across Transitions of care throughout the healthcare System: Current state and a call to action. AHRQ Agency for Healthcare Research and Quality, Available at: https://www.ahrq.gov/diagnostic-safety/resources/issue-briefs/dxsafety-care-transitions.html. (Accessed July 1, 2024). 2023.
5. HealthIT.gov, Available at: https://www.healthit.gov/faq/what-ehr-interoperability-and-why-it-important. (Accessed July 1, 2024).
6. Bajorek S. and McElroy V., Discharge planning and transitions of care. PSNet Patient Safety Network, Available at: https://psnet.ahrq.gov/primer/discharge-planning-and-transitions-care. (Accessed July 1, 2024). 2020.

7.  Earlam A., Woods L. and Lind K., American Nurses Association, Transitioning wound care patients to post-acute care. American Nurse, Available at: https://www.myamericannurse.com/wound-care-post-acute-care/. (Accessed July 1, 2024). 2018.

8.  Novy TK, Woith WM. Standardized hospital discharge communication for patients with pressure injuries. J Wound, Ostomy Cont Nurs 2022;47(3). https://doi.org/10.1097/WON.0000000000000644.

9.  Hospital Readmissions Reduction Program (HRRP). CMS.gov, Available at: https://www.cms.gov/medicare/payment/prospective-payment-systems/acute-inpatient-pps/hospital-readmissions-reduction-program-hrrp. (Accessed July 1, 2024).

10. Ordona R, Kirkland-Kyhn H. Transition of care: wound management innovative collaboration with home health and primary care. Presented at the CAHSAH Annual Conference & Expo: May 20, 2024; Palm Springs, CA, United States of America.

11. About continuum of care. California Hospital Association, Available at: https://calhospital.org/issue/continuum-of-care/#:~:text=About%20Continuum%20of%20Care&text=Hospital%20case%20managers%20help%20support,home%20and%20community%2Dbased%20services. (Accessed July 1, 2024).

12. Muldoon S., Know the differences: LTACHs vs SNFs. HealthLeaders, Available at: https://www.healthleadersmedia.com/clinical-care/know-differences-ltachs-vs-snfs#:~:text=SPONSORED%20%7C%20By%20Sean%20R.,hospital%2C%20thereby%20increasing%20total%20cost. (Accessed July 1, 2024).

13. CA Health & Safety Code Section 1250. California.Public.Law, Available at: https://california.public.law/codes/ca_health_and_safety_code_section_1250. (Accessed July 1, 2024).

14. Skilled nursing facilities. California Department of Aging, Available at: https://www.aging.ca.gov/Care_Options/Skilled_Nursing_Facilities/. (Accessed July 1, 2024).

15. Assisted living facilities. California Department of Aging, Available at: https://www.aging.ca.gov/Care_Options/Assisted_Living_Facilities/. (Accessed July 1, 2024).

16. Lauretta A. and Heyn P., What is independent living?. Benefits, types and costs. Forbes Health, Available at: https://www.forbes.com/health/senior-living/independent-living/. (Accessed July 1, 2024).

17. Ordona R, Geiss J. Home-based primary care and senior living synergies. Presented at the CALA Summer Symposium: June 23, 2020; Virtual.

18. Department of Social Services, Residential Care Facility for the Elderly (RCFE): Manual of Policies and Procedures. Department of Social Services, Available at: https://www.cdss.ca.gov/ord/entres/getinfo/pdf/rcfeman1.pdf. (Accessed July 1, 2024).

19. Cal. Code Regs. tit. 22, § 87615 - Prohibited health conditions. LII/Legal Information Institute, Available at: https://www.law.cornell.edu/regulations/california/22-CCR-87615. (Accessed July 1, 2024).

20. Home health agency and hospice utilization, California Department of Health Care Access and Information (HCAi), Available at: https://hcai.ca.gov/data/healthcare-utilization/home-health-agency-and-hospice-utilization/. (Accessed July 1, 2024).

21. Ebot J. Managing complex wounds in skilled nursing facilities (SNFs). Cureus 2023. https://doi.org/10.7759/cureus.47581.

22. Weigelt MA, Lev-Tov HA, Tomic-Canic M, et al. Advanced wound diagnostics: toward transforming wound care into precision medicine. Adv Wound Care 2022; 11(6):330–59.
23. Ordona, Kirkland-Kyhn. Opportunity for 104 NPS: Transition of care in chronic wound management. Presented at the CANP 46th Annual Educational Conference: March 19-21, 2024. Anaheim, CA, United States of America.
24. LeBlanc K, Campbell KE, Wood E, et al. Best practice recommendations for prevention and management of skin tears in aged skin. Journal of Wound, Ostomy, and Continence Nursing/Journal of WOCN 2018;45(6):540–2.
25. Raeder K, Jachan DE, Müller-Werdan U, et al. Prevalence and risk factors of chronic wounds in nursing homes in Germany. Int Wound J 2020;17(5):1128–34.
26. Zaidi S.R.H. and Sharma S., Pressure ulcer. StatPearls - NCBI Bookshelf, Available at: https://www.ncbi.nlm.nih.gov/s/NBK553107/#:~:text=Pressure%20injuries%2C%20also%20termed%20bedsores%2C%20decubitus%20ulcers%2C,and%20shear%2C%20usually%20exerted%20over%20bony%20prominences. (Accessed July 1, 2024). 2024.
27. Kottner J, Cuddigan J, Carville K, et al. Prevention and treatment of pressure ulcers/injuries: The protocol for the second update of the international Clinical Practice Guideline 2019. J Tissue Viability 2019;28(2):51–8.
28. Kirkland-Walsh H. and Teleten O., Hypoperfusion major contributor to deep tissue injury in ICUs. CHPSO-Division of the Hospital Quality Institute Newsletter, Available at: http://www.chpso.org/post/hypoperfusion-major-contributor-deep-tissue-injury-Icus'?utm_campaign=November%20-%20December%20Newsletter & utm_medium=email&utm_source=bundle_and_blast. (Accessed July 1, 2024).
29. Kennerly SM, Sharkey PD, Horn SD, et al. Nursing assessment of pressure injury risk with the braden scale validated against sensor-based measurement of movement. Healthcare 2022;10(11):2330.
30. Dalgleish L, Campbell J, Finlayson K, et al. Acute skin failure in the critically ill adult population: a systematic review. Adv Skin Wound Care 2020;33(2):76–83. https://doi.org/10.1097/01.asw.0000617844.69248.92.
31. Facs A.G.M., Vascular ulcers: practice essentials, epidemiology, etiology, Available at: https://emedicine.medscape.com/article/1298345-overview#:~:text=Overview,vascular%20disease%2C%20including%20work%20incapacity. (Accessed July 1, 2024).
32. Lumbers M. Challenges in wound care for community nurses: a case review. Br J Community Nurs 2019;24(Sup3):S25–7.
33. The Growing Need for Home Health Care for the Elderly: Home Health Care for the Elderly as an Integral Part of Primary Health Care Services. World Health Organization (WHO), Available at: https://iris.who.int/handle/10665/326801. (Accessed July 1, 2024).
34. Wolff-Baker D, Ordona RB. The expanding role of nurse practitioners in Home-Based Primary Care: Opportunities and challenges. J Gerontol Nurs 2019; 45(6):9–14.
35. The American Journal of Nursing (AJN), Available at: https://journals.lww.com/ajnonline/pages/videogallery.aspx. (Accessed July 1, 2024).
36. Naylor M.D. and Sochalski J.A., Scaling up: bringing the transitional care model into the mainstream, PubMed, 103, 2010, 1–12, Available at: https://pubmed.ncbi.nlm.nih.gov/21053533. (Accessed July 1, 2024).
37. Oyesanya TO, Loflin C, Harris G, et al. "Just tell me in a simple way": A qualitative study on opportunities to improve the transition from acute hospital care to home

from the perspectives of patients with traumatic brain injury, families, and providers. Clin Rehabil 2021;35(7):1056–72.

38. Bergquist-Beringer S, Daley CM. Adapting pressure ulcer prevention for use in home health care. Journal of Wound, Ostomy, and Continence Nursing/Journal of WOCN 2011;38(2):145–54.

39. Value-Based Care Spotlight | CMS, Available at: https://www.cms.gov/priorities/innovation-center/value-based-care-spotlight. (Accessed July 1, 2024).

# Ethnicity, Skin Tones, and Cultural Considerations in Wound Care: Challenges and Solutions

Melania Howell, DNP, RN, AGCNS-BC, CWOCN, DAPWCA[a],*,
Tuba Sengul, PhD, CWON[b], Holly Kirkland-Kyhn, PhD, FNP-c, GNP-c, CWCN, FAANP[c]

## KEYWORDS

- Ethnic disparities • Social determinants of health • Skin tone • Wound assessment
- Cultural competence

## KEY POINTS

- Assessing early signs of DTPI, PI, MASD, and DF in patients with darker skin tones can be challenging, leading to delayed treatment and misinterpretation.
- Social determinants of health, such as socioeconomic status and access to health care, significantly affect wound care outcomes and contribute to disparities in chronic wound complications.
- Cultural competence in health care is essential for improving patient outcomes, as understanding ethnic and cultural differences can enhance the accuracy of wound assessments and the effectiveness of treatment plans.
- Training health care providers to recognize skin tone variations and implement culturally sensitive care practices can reduce health disparities and improve wound care for vulnerable populations.

## BACKGROUND

Ethnicity and culture can influence healthcare delivery type, quality, and timeliness.[1] These concepts can also impact a patient's trust in the healthcare provider and system, thus impacting decisions such as when or if an individual will seek care. Alternatively, a provider's perception of a patient's ethnicity and culture can give rise to implicit biases delaying the recognition and treatment of disease processes, leading to suboptimal outcomes.[1] This two-way interplay plays a significant role in wound care outcomes for persons of color (POC).[1] Understanding the vulnerability of specific

[a] Winona State University WOCNEP, Winona, MN, USA; [b] Department of Nursing, Koç University School of Nursing, Davutpaşa Street No: 4, 34010 Topkapı, Istanbul, Turkey; [c] Betty Irene Moore School of Nursing, UC Davis Health, University of California, Davis, Davis, CA, USA
* Corresponding author. Winona State University WOCNEP, 175 West Mark Street, Winona, MN 55987.
*E-mail address:* Melania.Howell@winona.edu

Nurs Clin N Am 60 (2025) 165–174
https://doi.org/10.1016/j.cnur.2024.07.017
0029-6465/25/© 2024 Elsevier Inc. All rights reserved, including those for text and data mining, AI training, and similar technologies.
nursing.theclinics.com

populations starts with studying the gaps in societies and health care systems that contribute to these problems.[1]

Wealthier individuals and nations have reaped the benefits of reduced morbidity and mortality associated with particular diseases and increased life expectancy.[2] In recent years, the health care community, the public, and legislators have become acutely aware of disparities in health care.[2] Health inequities became a sharper focus during the Coronavirus disease (COVID-19) pandemic.[2] Before the global health emergency, however, investigators sought to understand why specific patient populations continued to experience poor health outcomes despite the standard of care.[2]

### Impact of Skin Tones on Wound Assessment and Healing

Wound and skin assessment is the basis for developing a plan for wound healing.[3] For patients with darker skin tones, assessing color changes may prove difficult (**Figs. 1** and **2**) when the early identification of color changes in red, blue, or maroon is necessary for early wound development.

Despite only a 10-day difference between the two images, the variation in skin tone can make detecting deep tissue pressure injuries (DTPI) challenging. Changes in skin coloration may lead to misinterpretation due to differences in the lighting of the photographs. This situation complicates accurate DTI assessment and may result in misunderstandings regarding the severity of the injury (see **Figs. 1** and **2**).

The wound healing process is complicated, requiring clinicians to consider the many attributes of the host that contribute to delayed healing.[3] These can include the patient's overall health, nutritional status, medications, lifestyle factors, and the specific characteristics and etiology of the wound.[3] Presented the demographics complete with skin tones (using the Fitzpatrick scale) and outcomes of 958 COVID-19-positive patients in a hospital who, while in the hospital, developed both COVID lesions and pressure injuries (PIs).[3] Findings from this study suggested that certain ethnicities and those with darker skin tones exhibited a higher disease burden, increased hospitalizations, longer lengths of stay, and adverse outcomes such as cerebrovascular accidents (CVAs), myocardial infarctions (MIs), chronic kidney disease (CKD), end-stage renal disease (ESRD), chronic wound, and amputations.[3] Health

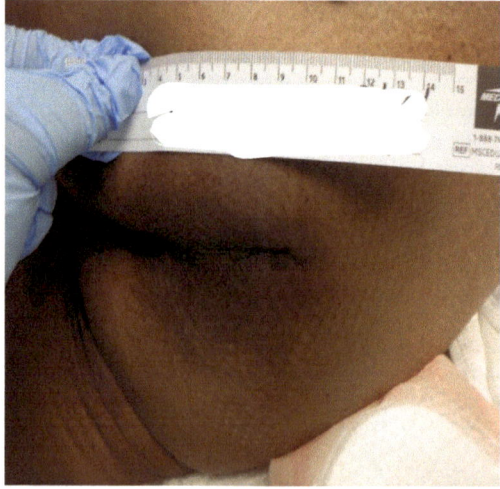

**Fig. 1.** DTPI 1 day.

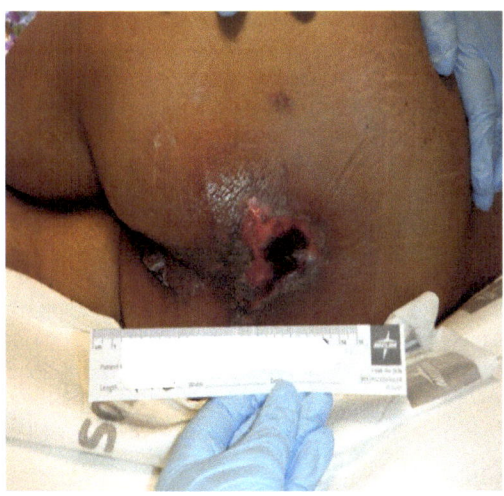

**Fig. 2.** Evolution of DTPI 10 days later.

disparities occur for multiple reasons and may be limited because of the type, amount, and quality of primary and specialized care available to vulnerable populations.[3] A significant portion of the existing evidence on skin tones pertains to PIs, while sufficient evidence on other types of wounds, such as incontinence-associated dermatitis (IAD) and diabetic foot (DF), is lacking.[4] Patients with darker skin tones tend to be diagnosed late with DTPI evolving into stage 3 and 4 PI,[5] whereas the initial "redness, maroon, or purple color seen in lighter skin tones may not be observed in darker skin tones.[6]

Skin problems such as incontinence-associated dermatitis (IAD) can also present differently due to ethnic-related skin tone differences. In individuals with darker skin tones, IAD may appear as dark spots or gray tones on the skin rather than redness.[7] Therefore, health care professionals must recognize IAD symptoms and the evolution distribution in different skin tones for accurate assessment, diagnosis, and treatment. Various challenges exist in diagnosing and treating moisture-associated skin damage (MASD), which differs from IAD as it can occur in areas that are not associated with incontinence but moisture alone in patients with darker skin tones.[8,9] MASD often presents as erythema or redness in a linear fashion or surrounding tubes and appliances. Additionally, health care providers may need to become more familiar with the visual appearance of MASD in patients with darker skin tones, leading to underdiagnosis and undertreatment.[8,9] For example, the Ghent Global IAD Classification Tool (GLOBIAD) relies on redness as the leading damage indicator. In contrast, patients with darker skin tones may present as paler, darker, or more purplish skin rather than red.[9] In addition to awareness-raising training, health care institutions should incorporate cultural competence principles into their policies and procedures. This will increase the continuity and prevalence of culturally sensitive care.[10]

### Social Determinants of Health

Health disparities and their outcomes result from a complex interplay of numerous issues. An individual's socioeconomic situation is influenced substantially by place of birth and race, skin tones, or ethnicity.[2] These uncontrollable factors make an individual more vulnerable to succumbing to the detriments of social determinants of health (SDOH), such as access to quality education, employment, housing, and food.[3]

Whereby individuals live can place them at risk for unreliable transportation, unsafe outdoor recreational spaces, limited community support systems, and insufficiently funded health care resources.[2] In some communities, lack of transportation, especially for low-income clients with mobility challenges, will impact the individual's ability to attend medical appointments.[2,11] As a result, patients, through no fault of their own, miss clinic appointments and are labeled noncompliant.[2,11]

SDOH impacts people in developed and developing economies.[2] Cardiovascular disease (CVD), a disorder significantly impacted by SDOH, is responsible for 80% of unexpected deaths not attributable to communicable diseases.[12] Several metabolic derangements increase a person's risk of developing CVD.[12] Type 2 diabetes mellitus (T2DM), increased body mass index (BMI), hypertension, and high cholesterol, each or in combination, can also increase the severity of CVD.[13,14] T2DM is the second leading metabolic factor impacting the development of CVD.[15] Globally, hyperglycemia and associated complications are rising, with developing economies disproportionately impacted.[16]

### Diabetes and Wounds

Interestingly, T2DM incidence is growing in developed countries despite more robust health care systems providing patient education and medication access.[6] Internationally, China, India, and the United States are the nations at the top of the T2DM prevalence list.[15–17] The U.S. populations with the most significant number of individuals diagnosed with the condition are native Alaskans and indigenous Americans, followed by nonHispanic blacks and Hispanics.[17] Despite a higher prevalence of the disorder in these populations, these patients do not receive timely evidence-based treatments.[18] As a result, these ethnicities exhibit a higher proportion of T2DM-related complications such as cerebrovascular accidents (CVAs), retinopathies, CVD, including peripheral vascular disease (PVD), end-stage renal disease (ESRD), and lower extremity amputations.[18] Patients with nonHispanic black T2DM experience lower limb loss at rates higher as compared with their white peers.[18] Major contributing factors identified for the disparity fall under the SDOH umbrella, with the significant influences of lack of education, income inequality, lack of or suboptimal insurance, and lack of access to transport or health care.[18–20]

Nontraumatic lower limb loss caused by T2DM-related complications is expensive.[21] The costs start with treating the diabetic foot ulcer (DFU), which can include surgical interventions, antibiotic therapies, dressing supplies, and professional medical care.[12,21] Patient recovery often requires hospitalizations, rehabilitation, and durable medical equipment (DME). Despite the standard of care and advanced therapies, most DFUs will recur within 1 year of healing.[13] Recalcitrant infections of the DFU result in amputation, often causing the patient's mortality within 5 years of the procedure, making the mortality much like a person with lung cancer.[12,20,21]

Reducing the morbidity and mortality associated with DFUs requires greater attention to individuals from vulnerable populations, especially those with darker skin tones.[21] Diabetic individuals are already at higher risk of DFU-related limb loss due to neuropathy, a common comorbidity that delays the detection of foot ulcers.[21] Additionally, coexisting PAD often blunts signs of infections, such as color changes such as erythema around the wound. Infection-related skin color difference is further confounded when the patient has a darker skin tone.[21] Furthermore, during initial assessments, clinicians could overlook more subtle clues, such as skin thickening in patients with darker skin tones.[21,22] More evidence is needed to understand how skin tone affects the appearance of chronic wounds and associated complications, delaying treatment and resulting in disparate patient outcomes.[4,23]

## IMPROVING OUTCOMES OF VULNERABLE POPULATIONS

Clinicians must commit to understanding how ethnicity, skin tones, and culture impact the evaluation/assessment, timely intervention, and quality of care they provide.[24] This can be accomplished by increasing the impact of ethnicity, skin tones, and cultural awareness, promoting competence, including learning about the cultural practices and beliefs of different patient populations and applying this knowledge in the care of individual patients.[25] Cultural competence in wound care is not just a desirable attribute but a critical element that directly influences the quality and outcome of patients' health care experiences.[25] Health care providers must understand and integrate patients' cultural backgrounds, beliefs, and values into the care processes. By promoting cultural competence, clinicians can significantly improve patient outcomes and satisfaction.[25]

### Importance of Nutrition

Optimizing nutritional intake to promote healing is essential to any wound care plan.[26] This becomes more critical through the lens of reducing the morbidity and mortality associated with chronic conditions such as T2DM.[26] Glycemic control is instrumental to the organized progression of the healing cascade.[26] The process, which also requires increased energy expenditure, should be met by improving quality calorie intake through the appropriate balance of micro and macronutrients.[27] Establishing a nutritional plan to promote wound healing should be done collaboratively with the client.[27] An individual's ethnicity, culture, and race impact food preferences and established eating habits.[27,28] Food choices and preparation methods are essential ways communities hold on to and pass down cultural and ethnic identity, especially in multicultural societies.[28] SDOH can complicate the type, amount, quality, preference, and availability of foods in some communities.[28]

### Community Health Needs Assessment

The Patient Protection and Affordable Care Act of 2010 (ACA) mandates that all health care tax-exempt hospitals collaborate with public health and community organizations to gather data on their communities every 3 years by conducting community health needs assessments (CHNA).[29] The type of data collected is not prescriptive.[29,30] The information is used to generate a health summary of those living in their region and identify opportunities to improve the health outcomes of those vulnerable communities.[29,30] Data from CHNA reports have highlighted food deserts and areas whereby suboptimal food choices exist widely. Classic characteristics of food desserts include a predominance of fast food and mini-marts embedded in economically distressed settings whereby ethnic minorities reside.[29] These businesses offer cheap, overly processed food options with long shelf life and scarce or no high-quality foods such as fresh fruits and vegetables.[29] Vendors often select these items for sale due to their reasonable rate of return, allowing them to remain in business.[29] In other instances, especially in rural areas, delivering fresh food is too risky and cost-prohibitive.[30] Due to these factors, residents in these food deserts exhibit a higher incidence and prevalence of diet-related chronic diseases and complications, including chronic wounds.[31] Partnering with registered dieticians to develop medically suggested and acceptable foods that respect cultural considerations and availability can increase the likelihood of a patient's adherence to the nutritional care plan.[29–31]

## TRADITIONAL MEDICINE, ETHNICITY, AND DRESSING SELECTIONS

Varying cultures use traditional healers to address their mental and physical health.[32] Communities using traditional healers hold them in high esteem and use them as medical practitioners to treat psychological and physical disorders and, sometimes, forgoing health care in primary care clinics and hospitals.[32] Traditional Chinese Medicine (TCM) and herbal remedies from other cultures, which have existed for over a millennia, have a proven track record of improving numerous ailments.[33] Today, the ingredients used in TCM and other traditional practices exist primarily in larger cities.[32,33] POCs living in rural regions or places unfamiliar with their traditions and already at increased risk of lack of access to health care are further disenfranchised when they cannot access their traditional therapies.[32,33] Recently, research has borne out what has been observed by traditional practitioners for years: TCM is used as adjunctive therapy and improves blood glucose and lipid levels.[32] Additionally, some traditional Chinese medical regimens confer cardioprotective benefits by reducing vascular inflammation.[32] In Ethiopia, healers use plants medicinally for topical wound care.[30] Some herbs are used to treat lymphedema, and additional studies are needed to determine if these compounds have a role in limb salvage.[30–34] Research has yielded valuable information on how naturally occurring drugs influence the different phases of wound healing. Several of these natural remedies influence the various stages of the wound healing cascade, resulting in good healing outcomes, including minimal scar formation.[31–34]

Wound care practitioners, increasingly challenged with finding innovative solutions to healing complex chronic wounds, are looking into the past. Commercially available "drawing agents" or hyperviscosity dressings rely on ancient technologies. to draw out the liquid and break down slough and eschar.[30–34] Products with irradiated honey, highly salinated dressings, and naturally occurring bacteriostatic properties used in yesteryear when dealing with open wounds are now commercially available.[10,30–34]

## STRATEGIES TO OVERCOME CHALLENGES CARING FOR MULTI-ETHNIC POPULATIONS
### Education for Health Care Professionals

Comprehensive education and awareness programs are needed to enhance health care professionals ' cultural competence. These trainings help health care professionals understand the health and care needs of various cultural and ethnic groups.[35] Cultural competence training enables health care professionals to communicate effectively and provide appropriate care in diverse cultural contexts. For example, providers should have information on traditional treatment methods used in wound care by some cultural groups. More importantly, teams should consider strategies for integrating these methodologies into modern medical practices.[36]

### Regulations Considering Ethnic and Cultural Diversity

Publications regarding regulations considering ethnic and cultural diversity in health care services are precious.[25,37] These regulations are crucial for addressing inequalities in health care, ensuring access to quality care, and developing inclusive policies.[25,37] Ensuring that all health care workers possess cultural competence is fundamental in today's diverse societies.[25,37] These regulations promote the provision of equitable and effective health care by recognizing the unique needs of various ethnic and cultural groups.[25,37] In many countries, health care regulations consider ethnic and cultural diversity. For example, in the United States, the Affordable Care Act (ACA) mandates the collection of data on race, ethnicity, and language to identify and address disparities in health outcomes.[29] Moreover, organizations such as the Joint Commission require hospitals to implement strategies to enhance cultural competence as part of their accreditation process.[38] Globally, various countries implement regulations that account for cultural diversity in health care services. Australia's National Safety and Quality Health Service (NSQHS) Standards require providing culturally safe and respectful health care services.[39] Despite these regulations, challenges such as insufficient training for health care workers in cultural competence and limited resources to support the implementation of these regulations persist.[25] Involving community leaders in designing and implementing health care services ensures that the services meet the needs of diverse populations.[25,40] Strengthening existing rules and developing new policies in areas whereby gaps exist is necessary.[25]

### *Needs and Recommendations*

Regulations that consider ethnic and cultural diversity in health care are critical for enhancing the quality and equity of health care services.[25] In this context, specific needs arise:

*Cultural Competence Training:* Health care workers need comprehensive training programs to understand the needs of different ethnic and cultural groups and provide appropriate care.[35] These trainings enhance health care workers' cultural sensitivity, enabling more effective and empathetic communication with patients.[36]

*Data Collection and Analysis:* Collecting demographic data such as race, ethnicity, and language is essential for identifying disparities in health care services and developing strategies to address these disparities.[41] Data collection objectively assesses the current situation and helps policymakers make informed decisions.[41]

*Community Involvement:* In the design and implementation phases of health care services, teams need to ensure the involvement of community leaders and members.[25] This participation allows the customization of health care services based on the community's real needs and increases their acceptability.[40]

*Language Services:* Overcoming language barriers in health care requires effective translation and interpretation services.[38] Language barriers can prevent patients from receiving accurate information and benefiting from health care services during assessments.[37] Teams should consider leveraging technology through translation applications and digital health services to facilitate providing services in different languages.[41,42]

*Policy Development and Implementation:* New policies should consider ethnic and cultural diversity.[25] Effective implementation and continuous evaluation of existing policies are necessary.[35] These policies should promote justice and equity in health care services.[40]

*Increasing the diversity of the healthcare workforce:* Diversity, equity, and inclusion in health care improves patient outcomes.[25,35] A diverse and inclusive health care workforce can foster a sense of trust between the clinician, health system, and patient, resulting in greater uptake of health information and disease avoidance behavior.[37]

### SUMMARY

Regulations considering ethnic and cultural diversity in health care are crucial for delivering fair and effective wound care services. Cultural competence training and community-based approaches are critical for improving the quality and equity of patient care. These classes need to include implicit and explicit bias concepts with real-world examples. Education can be enhanced by inviting patients impacted by micro and macroaggressions that they have encountered in health care. Case examples from different ethnic groups and multidisciplinary approaches provide a comprehensive understanding of every aspect of wound care. Moreover, technological innovations are making significant advancements in wound care, but considering the effects of these innovations on different skin tones is essential for providing equitable and effective care. Health care professionals' ability to use these technologies effectively and their sensitivity to the needs of patients with different skin tones will lead to more successful outcomes in wound care. In this regard, developing and implementing regulations considering ethnic and cultural diversity in health care will support continuous improvement in patient care.

## CLINICS CARE POINTS

> Ethnicity, skin tones, and patient culture significantly impact healthcare delivery, quality, and timeliness.
> - Social determinants of health (SDOH) further impact and complicate the health disparities experienced by POCs.
> - Additional regulations and implicit and explicit bias training for all healthcare personnel are needed to address the challenges of caring for multi-ethnic populations.

## DISCLOSURE

The authors have nothing to disclose.

## REFERENCES

1. Vela MB, Erondu AI, Smith NA, et al. Eliminating explicit and implicit biases in health care: evidence and research needs. Annu Rev Public Health 2022;43: 477–501.
2. Gostin LO, Friedman EA. Health inequalities. Hastings Cent Rep 2020;50(4):6–8.
3. Kirkland-Kyhn H, Teleten O, Wilson M, et al. Comparing demographics, treatments, and outcomes of patients with COVID-19 lesions versus hospital-acquired pressure ulcers/injuries during the first year of COVID-19. Wound Manag Prev 2024;70(1). https://doi.org/10.25270/wmp.23018.
4. Mukwende M, Tamony P, Turner M. Mind the gap: a handbook of clinical signs on Black and Brown skin. 1st edition. London, UK: St. George's University; 2020.
5. Dhoonmoon L, Nair HKR, Abbas Z, et al. International consensus document: wound care and skin tone signs, symptoms and terminology for all skin tones. Wounds International 2023. Available at: www.woundsinternational.com.
6. Smith EM. Addressing skin color in dermatological education. J Am Acad Dermatol 2019;80(4):1164–5.
7. Baich L, Wilson D, Cummings GG. Care considerations in patients with dark skin tones. Adv Skin Wound Care 2018;31(2):62–8.
8. Cole N, Waller S. Challenges in skin tone assessment in moisture-associated skin damage. medicareplus International; Addenbrookes Hospital. In: Voegeli N, editor. Moisture-associated skin damage (MASD). UK: The Wound Care People Limited; 2023. p. 45–9.
9. Beeckman D, Campbell J, Campbell K, et al. The ghent global IAD categorisation tool (GLOBIAD): development and evaluation. J Wound Care 2018;27(3):150–61.
10. Brocke T, Barr J. The history of wound healing. Surg Clin North Am 2020;100(4): 787–806.
11. Artiga S, Orgera K, Pham O. Disparities in health and health care: five key questions and answers. 2020. Available at: https://deancare.com/getmedia/

e00c9856-28d0-4c63-b2c0-9bf68cadcebb/Disparities-in-Health-and-Health-Care-Five-Key-Questions-and-Answers.pdf. Accessed July 22, 2024.

12. Rippe JM. Lifestyle strategies for risk factor reduction, prevention, and treatment of cardiovascular disease. Am J Lifestyle Med 2018;13(2):204–12.

13. Community Relations Services Toolkit for Policing, understanding bias: a resource guide bias policing overview and resource guide, Available at: https://www.justice.gov/d9/fieldable-panel-panes/basic-panes/attachments/2021/09/29/understanding_bias_content.pdf. (Accessed 12 July 2024).

14. An introduction to community health needs assessment (CHNA). Available at: www.communitycommons.orghttps://www.communitycommons.org/collections/An-Introduction-to-Community-Health-Needs-Assessment-CHNA. (Accessed 18 June 2024).

15. Khan MAB, Hashim MJ, King JK, et al. Epidemiology of type 2 diabetes - global burden of disease and forecasted trends. J Epidemiol Glob Health 2020;10(1):107–11.

16. Centers for Disease Control and Prevention, National diabetes statistics report, Available at: https://www.cdc.gov/diabetes/php/data-research/index.html. (Accessed 25 June 2024).

17. Haw JS, Shah M, Turbow S, et al. Diabetes complications in racial and ethnic minority populations in the USA. Curr Diab Rep 2021;21(1):2.

18. Saelee R, Hora IA, Pavkov ME, et al. Diabetes prevalence and incidence inequality trends among U.S. adults, 2008-2021. Am J Prev Med 2023;65(6):973–82.

19. McDermott K, Fang M, Boulton AJM, et al. Etiology, epidemiology, and disparities in the burden of diabetic foot ulcers. Diabetes Care 2023;46(1):209–21.

20. Lin C, Liu J, Sun H. Risk factors for lower extremity amputation in patients with diabetic foot ulcers: a meta-analysis. PLoS One 2020;15(9):e0239236.

21. Armstrong DG, Swerdlow MA, Armstrong AA, et al. Five year mortality and direct costs of care for people with diabetic foot complications are comparable to cancer. J Foot Ankle Res 2020;13(1):16.

22. Schaper NC, van Netten JJ, Apelqvist J, et al. Practical Guidelines on the prevention and management of diabetic foot disease (IWGDF 2019 update). Diabetes Metab Res Rev 2020;36(Suppl 1):e3266.

23. Bps W. Best practice statement addressing skin tone bias in wound care: assessing signs and symptoms in people with dark skin tones assessment and diagnosis common wound types and issues to consider product selection education and the future, Available at: https://wounds-uk.com/wp-content/uploads/sites/2/2023/02/191ac9b79f47de2896cf1a30f39037f5.pdf, (Accessed 18 July 2024). 2021.

24. Rotenstein LS, Reede JY, Jena AB. Addressing workforce diversity - a quality-improvement framework. N Engl J Med 2021;384(12):1083–6.

25. Betancourt JR, Green AR, Carrillo JE, et al. Defining cultural competence: a practical framework for addressing racial/ethnic disparities in health and health care. Public Health Rep 2016;131(4):293–302.

26. Seth I, Lim B, Cevik J, et al. Impact of nutrition on skin wound healing and aesthetic outcomes: a comprehensive narrative review. JPRAS Open 2024;39:291–302.

27. Reddy G, van Dam RM. Food, culture, and identity in multicultural societies: insights from Singapore. Appetite 2020;149:104633.

28. Stoto MA, Davis MV, Atkins A. Making better use of population health data for community health needs assessments. EGEMS (Wash DC) 2019;7(1):44.

29. An introduction to community health needs assessment (CHNA). Available at: www.communitycommons.org https://www.communitycommons.org/collections/An-Introduction-to-Community-Health-Needs-Assessment-CHNA.

30. Nigussie D, Makonnen E, Tufa TB, et al. Systematic review of Ethiopian medicinal plants used for their anti-inflammatory and wound healing activities. J Ethnopharmacol 2021;276:114179.

31. Fazil M, Nikhat S. Topical medicines for wound healing: a systematic review of Unani literature with recent advances. J Ethnopharmacol 2020;257:112878.

32. Xu Z, Dong M, Yin S, et al. Why traditional herbal medicine promotes wound healing: research from immune response, wound microbiome to controlled delivery. Adv Drug Deliv Rev 2023;195:114764.

33. Wei Y, Ding QY, Yeung C, et al. Evidence and potential mechanisms of traditional chinese medicine for the adjuvant treatment of coronary heart disease in patients with diabetes mellitus: a systematic review and meta-analysis with trial sequential analysis. J Diabetes Res 2022;2022:2545476.

34. Barrow BE, Alur AA, Kasdan ML, et al. Wine, honey, and boiling oil: a modern understanding of ancient wound care practices. Am Surg 2023;89(5):2150–3.

35. Saha S, Beach MC, Cooper LA. Patient centeredness, cultural competence and healthcare quality. J Natl Med Assoc 2008;100(11):1275–85.

36. Purnell L. The purnell model for cultural competence. J Transcult Nurs 2002; 13(3):193–201.

37. Nair L, Adetayo OA. Cultural competence and ethnic diversity in healthcare. Plast Reconstr Surg Glob Open 2019;7(5):e2219.

38. The Joint Commission. A roadmap for hospitals. 2021. Available at: https://www.jointcommission.org/-/media/tjc/documents/resources/patient-safety-topics/health-equity/aroadmapforhospitalsfinalversion727pdf.pdf?db=web&hash=AC3AC4BED1D973713C2CA6B2E5ACD01B. Accessed July 16, 2024.

39. Australian Commission on Safety and Quality in Health Care. National safety and quality health service standards. Sydney, NSW: Australian Commission on Safety and Quality in Health Care; 2017.

40. Haldane V, Chuah FLH, Srivastava A, et al. Community participation in health services development, implementation, and evaluation: A systematic review of empowerment, health, community, and process outcomes. PLoS One 2019; 14(5):e0216112.

41. James CV, Haley JM, Allen EH, et al. Using race and ethnicity data to advance health equity: examples, promising practices, remaining challenges, and next steps. Grantmakers in health. Washington, DC: The Urban Institute; 2023.

42. Kirkland-Kyhn H, Howell-Taylor M, Senestraro J, et al. Leveraging EMR to improve wound care delivery and transitions of care. Nurs Manage 2021; 52(11):24–8.

# The Multidisciplinary and Interdisciplinary Teamwork Across Care Settings and Transitions of Care

Diane Rita Maydick Youngberg, EdD, ACNS-BC, CWOCN[1,*],
Irene Jankowski, RN, MSN, ANP, CWOCN/Ret/Emeritus[2]

## KEYWORDS

- Interdisciplinary • Health care • Neuropathic/diabetic foot ulcers • Pressure injury
- Care transition

## KEY POINTS

- Interprofessional teamwork and communication are crucial in today's increasingly complex health care environment, where people live longer with multiple diagnoses and specialized providers.
- Interdisciplinary teams have inherent advantages such as enhancing care, improving outcomes, reducing error rates, expediting and improving efficiency, as well as satisfaction.
- The role of interdisciplinary teams in health care will continue to strengthen, providing more effective responses to the evolving needs of individuals and health care systems.

## INTRODUCTION

The increasing complexity of health care and the growing demand for safe, high-quality health care have underscored the crucial need for interdisciplinary teams in health care.[1–3] As people live longer, many complex health care needs arise, necessitating specialized care from various health care professionals.[4] Interdisciplinary teams include a group of health care professionals with various areas of expertise who work together to achieve mutual goals on behalf of a patient and their other significant individuals. The team is pivotal in bringing clarity, consistency, and continuity to patient care across different settings and preventing service duplication among diverse providers.[5] Specifically, there are ongoing areas for improvement in teamwork across care settings and transitions for individuals coping with life-changing health conditions, including wounds and ostomies.[6–12]

---

Care Improvement Strategies, LLC, East Elmhurst, NY, USA
[1] Present address: 54 Valencia Avenue, Staten Island, New York, NY 10301.
[2] Present address: 71-06 30th Avenue, East Elmhurst, NY 11370.
* Corresponding author.
*E-mail address:* dianemaydick@careimprovementstrategies.com

Nurs Clin N Am 60 (2025) 175–183
https://doi.org/10.1016/j.cnur.2024.07.010
0029-6465/25/© 2024 Elsevier Inc. All rights reserved, including those for text and data mining, AI training, and similar technologies.
nursing.theclinics.com

The advantages inherent in an interdisciplinary approach encompass enhanced care and outcomes, reduced error rates, expedited treatment processes, improved operational efficiency, and heightened staff morale.[13,14] Consequently, the role of interdisciplinary teams in health care continues to strengthen, providing more effective responses to the evolving needs of individuals and health care systems.

## BACKGROUND

Health professionals include patient-centeredness as a core value; however, each profession has its values, beliefs, norms, and practices that may create conflict and communication failure when delivering patient care. Interdisciplinary teamwork, collaboration, and communication are needed to minimize patient harm.[15] Failure to communicate has been cited as a leading cause of sentinel events and a primary contributing factor to near misses and adverse events.[16] In this context, it is understood that communication problems in health care have severe effects on the safety of patients.[17] Health care is shifting toward interdisciplinary teamwork and collaboration in education and practice, which addresses the mandate that health care workers must be more than professional. They must be interprofessional.[18] This change demonstrates that when we consider that health care is delivered in various settings, interdisciplinary teamwork and communication are critical in preventing impending dangers, reducing adverse events, and improving outcomes.[1]

## WHAT IS INTERDISCIPLINARY COLLABORATION?

An interdisciplinary team is a group of health care professionals with various areas of expertise who work together toward a mutual goal for the patient and their other significant individuals. Interprofessional collaboration has been described as a process by which these different health and social care professionals work together to impact care positively.[2] Thus, interdisciplinary teamwork is when professionals from various disciplines collaborate to manage complex health care for a patient with physical and psychological needs. Teams may consist of assorted medical and social professionals, the patient, and their significant other(s).

As the population and health care systems evolve, there has been a gradual shift toward interdisciplinary teamwork, where multiple providers collaborate with their patients to deliver care to improve health care delivery.

### Improved Care and Outcomes

Specialized health care professionals have unique knowledge and skills and will likely focus on their specialty areas. However, when working as a member of an interdisciplinary team with other specialty providers, a comprehensive treatment plan can address multiple symptoms and likely result in better outcomes. Experts in their respective fields stand out in health care with specialized knowledge and skills. For example, an endocrinologist may focus on health issues related to diabetes, while a wound care specialist may specialize in diabetic foot ulcers. However, the true strength lies in the collaborative efforts of these specialists within an interdisciplinary team.

Consider a patient with diabetes, particularly one grappling with the challenge of a diabetic foot ulcer. In a nontraditional, collaborative environment, each expert may work independently in their specific domain but could overlook interconnected aspects of the patient's health. For example, Maydick and Acee[11] highlighted the challenges of managing diabetes and diabetic foot ulcers (DFUs). Diabetes, comorbid depression, and DFU place a substantial burden on the US health care system.

Thus, the authors recommended managing comorbid depression and DFU using an interdisciplinary team approach including the patient, other significant individuals, primary nurses, psychiatric nurse practitioners, wound care nurses, diabetes educators, physicians, endocrinologists, psychologists, psychiatrists, social workers, infectious disease specialists, podiatrists, rehabilitation team, vascular surgeons, neurologists, and dieticians.

When experts collaborate seamlessly within an interdisciplinary team, the possibility of formulating a comprehensive care plan emerges. Interdisciplinary collaboration for a patient dealing with a DFU enables the endocrinologist and wound care specialist, along with other relevant health care professionals, to gain a more profound understanding of the patient's condition.[11] This collaborative approach is tailored to address the specific needs of DFU treatment, encompassing psychological, endocrinological, and wound care aspects. Consequently, the treatment plan offers a comprehensive strategy to expedite the healing process of the ulcer and prevent future complications.

This comprehensive strategy does not merely address the immediate wound issues but also considers the long-term effects of diabetes. The patient can undergo a more effective and tailored treatment with a more integrated approach and interdisciplinary support. The synergy among specialists in an interdisciplinary team creates a robust framework for delivering effective and personalized health care for a patient with a DFU.

## WHAT MAKES FOR A SUCCESSFUL INTERDISCIPLINARY TEAM?

While team members may vary by specialty, some basic concepts will contribute to the success of an interdisciplinary team. There are fundamental concepts that team members should embrace regardless of their area of expertise. Team members must understand their and their colleagues' professional cultures, values, and ethics. This understanding allows for precise comprehension of the roles and responsibilities among different health professions, fostering a harmonious collaboration. Emphasis is placed on collaborative decision-making, advanced communication, and effective teamwork within the team. Ideally, these elements lead to increased trust among team members, successful collaboration, and more efficient delivery of health care services.

Additionally, gathering information about the patient and other significant individuals is essential, ensuring that care is patient centered, considering their needs and preferences. A critical factor is including the patient and their other significant individuals in the care planning process. This involves active participation in discussions, decisions, and care planning by the patient and their significant others. Such an approach contributes to the patient feeling heard and valued. The team should collaboratively establish a mutually agreed upon goal, which may encompass enhancing overall operational efficiency, improving quality of life, or saving a life or limb.

Following the identification of the goal, intervention strategies should be continuously shaped through an ongoing assessment. In this process, team members play a vital role by engaging in effective communication through sharing knowledge and expertise and evaluating the effectiveness of the care plan. Continuous consideration of the perspectives and feedback from the patient and other significant individuals is paramount. This interactive and participatory approach is the foundation of successful interdisciplinary care within the team.

### Importance of Interdisciplinary Teamwork

Health care professionals deliver care within their scope of practice and have different areas of expertise. Improving the health of populations worldwide by providing efficient, effective, and equitable care (preventive, curative, rehabilitative, and palliative) is a commitment of the World Health Professions Alliance.[19]

Patients accessing health care may experience duplication, gaps, and discontinuity of care as they transition from one provider to another and from one setting to another. The World Health Organization (WHO) has described interprofessional collaboration as occurring "when multiple health workers from different professional backgrounds work together with patients, families, carers, and communities to deliver the highest quality of care across settings."[20] This is important and is designed to improve access to and coordination of health care interventions for patients and families. Additional benefits of working together with health care professionals include comprehensive, coordinated, safe care, efficient use of resources, reduced incidence and prevalence of disability, and reduced stress and burnout of health professionals.[19] Interdisciplinary teams should have members with the appropriate and complementary skills depending on the purpose of the team, patient needs, and the practice setting. Ideally, the patient can access the right professional at the right time. Multidisciplinary and interdisciplinary teams function most effectively when there is adequate and clear communication among the professionals to meet the needs of the patient and their significant others.

## INTERDISCIPLINARY COMMUNICATION
### Electronic Health Records

In 2005, the WHO suggested there was a potential impact that technologies might have on health care delivery,[21] and this was affirmed in 2016[22] when the advantages of the Electronic Health Record (EHR) were highlighted in the third global survey on eHealth. The WHO purports that EHRs (1) improve the quality, accuracy, and timeliness of patient information at the point of care; (2) provide insights into health care costs, utilization, and outcomes; (3) promote quality of care, reduce costs, support patient mobility, increase the reliability of information, and provide access to patient information to multiple health care providers; and (4) data from the EHR can highlight areas of concern and health services delivery.[22]

The use and adoption of EHRs fostered meaningful use of health care technology for all citizens in the United States and have essentially replaced paper health care records. Implementing electronic medical records has been posited to improve the quality and efficiency of health care documentation. Uslu and Stausberg[23] conducted a literature review and summarized their findings about the value of EHRs for hospital care. The researchers reviewed 18 studies that examined the effect of an EHR on the quality and efficiency of health care and found a positive effect on health care, an increase in health care quality, and a reduction of costs; not one failed to demonstrate a positive effect on health care.[23]

Kirkland-Kyhn and colleagues[24] conducted a quality improvement intervention and described the value of expanding the use of the EMR by including handheld EMR devices to upload wound photographs, improve wound care documentation and care, and improve communication for transitioning of care to alternate settings. The investigators created a database to identify patients with complex needs, frequent readmissions, and social determinants of health that must be addressed. Information about multiple admissions, social determinants of health, wound presence on admission or discharge, stage of pressure injury, photographic image of the wound(s), and the latest note for wound management was captured. This was designed for use by a multidisciplinary team comprised case managers, medical social workers, physicians, nurses, and psychologists. It has the potential to link to patient education and community resources to reduce readmissions. Results monitored overtime revealed less time completing incident reports, increased documentation of pressure injury stage and photographs, and identification of multiple admissions.[24]

One primary value of the EHR is the ability "to provide the correct information at the right time and place."[5] There may be reduced time spent on documentation, improved adherence to guidelines, and fewer medication errors and adverse drug events.[25] Zlabek and colleagues[26] examined the early cost and safety benefits of using the EMR. They reported decreased costs of care and improved patient safety in the following categories: decreased laboratory tests, radiology examinations, transcription and paper costs, and medication errors. An additional means for communication among team members is the availability of secure messaging systems within the EMR. This allows for timely communication among selected multidisciplinary and interdisciplinary team members.

### Health Information Exchange

Beyond the use of the EMR, there has been progress with the ability to share health information, such as "the electronic transfer of patient data and health information between health care providers," also known as health information exchange or HIE.[27] The use of this feature by the interdisciplinary team may reduce errors by establishing a thorough and accurate record of diagnoses, medications, test results, and treatments ordered by other providers. Capabilities within the EMR also exist to provide rapid notification of test results, thus reducing waiting time and allowing for faster treatment and improved efficiency. The record is accessible to all disciplines and provides a comprehensive overview of the history, physical, medications, treatments, laboratory results and other tests, and notes written by caregivers, including but not limited to providers, nursing, social work, and discharge planning, to name but a few. The EMR allows for communication across care settings and among providers.

An additional benefit of the EMR is the ability to conduct telehealth visits: During a recent pandemic, we saw a surge in telehealth. The ability to consult a provider using a smartphone or computer provides another level of access.

### Warm handoff or bedside handover

Ideally, when sharing patient information, it is best to do it in person and include the patient. A warm handoff or bedside handover is described as a handoff conducted in person, between 2 health care team members, in front of the patient (and family if present).[28]

### Care Transition Examples

Care transition occurs when patients with acute or chronic conditions receive health care from multiple providers in various settings.[29] Improving care transition is pivotal to improving patient satisfaction and quality outcomes for patients with complex health care needs. Prevention and treatment of pressure injury, neuropathic/DFUs, venous or arterial ulcers, or complications related to an ostomy provide some examples of interdisciplinary care transition.

### Care Transition for Individuals with Spinal Cord Injury

Soegaard and colleagues[30] conducted an evidence-based review of the literature. They looked at initiatives, organizational measures, and stakeholder perspectives for the prevention of skin injury for individuals with spinal cord injuries. They sought to determine whether adding an interdisciplinary communication written tool and verbal communication would improve the patient, their family, and the receiving facility's clinical outcomes and satisfaction (of the transfer).

While international pressure injury prevention guidelines for SCI were cited in studies, they reviewed that there was not always a close collaboration between providers after transitioning to an alternate setting. The authors concluded that communication is essential for successfully transitioning multiple details across an extensive health care system.

### Care Transitions for Individuals with Pressure Injury

Kirkland-Kyhn and colleagues[24] performed a quality improvement by examining existing pressure injury documentation in an extensive health care system. The researchers first examined workflows, including incident reports and the validity and reliability of wound documentation. Baseline data revealed an opportunity to streamline EHR documentation. To improve documentation capabilities, the EHR was expanded. Handheld mobile devices were implemented for wound photography to be uploaded directly into the EHR and made accessible to all interdisciplinary team members, patients, and other significant individuals. The clinician is prompted to document the etiology, anatomic location, and stage if the wound is a pressure injury. Leveraging technology for documentation and communication with the interdisciplinary team has improved efficiency and increased staff satisfaction.[24]

### Care Transitions for Neuropathic/Diabetic Foot Ulcers

Diabetes has become a worldwide epidemic.[11] An interdisciplinary approach to treating this severe and chronic disease is recommended.[11,31] Maydick and Acee[11] highlighted the prevalence of comorbid depression and diabetes and recommended screening for depression and the risk of DFUs followed by interdisciplinary care planning and communication.

Using a case study approach, Xu and colleagues[31] discussed a strategy for a patient with diabetes and foot ulceration, which included vascular surgery, wound care center specialists, trauma orthopedics, endocrinology, plastic surgery, and pharmacology. Patient–provider interaction and health education, in combination with topical wound care, contributed to preparing the wound for full closure with skin grafting after 3 months.[31]

### Care Transitions for Individuals with a Permanent Ostomy

Approximately 1 million people in the United States have an ostomy.[8] An ostomy is a passage created during surgery to eliminate stool or urine after removing diseased organs.[8] Physiologic and psychological needs accompany this life-altering change, and professionals widely support individuals with an ostomy.[32,33] Improving care transitions after life-altering surgery could improve the quality of life for patients living with an ostomy. Facilitating the transition from hospital care to home health care and self-care requires providing education and resources throughout all transition phases, including the patient's life span. The transition of care from one professional to another should include information about the patient, other significant individuals, the diagnosis leading to ostomy creation, the ostomy type (ileostomy, urostomy, colostomy), whether the ostomy is temporary or permanent, and the recommended plan of care (skincare, pouching supplies, physical and psychological support). Individuals with a permanent ostomy require life-long support and access to health professionals to achieve optimal quality of life.

## SUMMARY

Interprofessional teamwork and communication are crucial in today's increasingly complex health care environment, where people live longer with multiple diagnoses and specialized providers. Interdisciplinary teams have inherent advantages such as enhancing care, improving outcomes, reducing error rates, expediting and improving efficiency, as well as satisfaction. The role of interdisciplinary teams in health care will continue to strengthen, providing more effective responses to the evolving needs of individuals and health care systems.

## CLINICS CARE POINTS

- Interdisciplinary healthcare is crucial to meet the need for safe, high-quality care for complex healthcare.
- A "warm handoff" is preferred when sharing patient information.Interdisciplinary care has ainherant advantages to impove patient care and outcomes, reduce error rates, improve efficiency, and patient satisfaction with healthcare.
- Interdisciplinary care has ainherant advantages to impove patient care and outcomes, reduce error rates, improve efficiency, and patient satisfaction with healthcare.

## REFERENCES

1. American College of Healthcare Executives and National Patient Safety Forum Lucian Leape Institute. Leading a culture of safety: a blueprint for success. Chicago, IL: American College of Healthcare Executives; 2017. Available at: http://www.npsf.org/custom_form.asp?id=F1845654-1D95-4869-8924-738D4CC8E06D.
2. Reeves S, Pelone F, Harrison R, et al. Interprofessional collaboration to improve professional practice and healthcare outcomes. Cochrane Database Syst Rev 2017;6(6):CD000072.
3. Schmutz JB, Meier LL, Manser T. How effective is teamwork really? The relationship between teamwork and performance in healthcare teams: A systematic review and meta-analysis. BMJ Open 2019;9(9).
4. Starfield B. Threads and yarns: weaving the tapestry of comorbidity. Ann Fam Med 2006;4(2).
5. Tobias J, Stewart-Weeks M, editors. Could 9: connecting clinicians for better health care. Sydney: Cisco Systems/Intel Corporation; 2007.
6. Berti-Hearn L, Elliott B. A resource guide to improve nursing care and transition to self-care for patients with ostomies. Home Healthc Now 2018;36(1):43–9.
7. Jackson PD, Biggins MS, Cowan L, et al. Evidence summary and recommendations for improved communication during care transitions. Rehabil Nurs 2016; 41(3):135–48.
8. Maydick D. Individuals with a permanent ostomy: Quality of life and out-of-pocket financial costs for ostomy management. J Nurs Economic$ 2014;32(4): 204–18.
9. Maydick D. A descriptive study assessing quality of life for adults with a permanent ostomy and the influence of preoperative stoma site marking. OstomyWound Manage 2016;62(5):14–24.
10. Maydick D. A descriptive study assessing quality of life for adults with a permanent ostomy and the frequency of peristomal complications. OstomyWound Manage 2017;63(5):10–23.

11. Maydick DR, Acee AM. Comorbid depression and diabetic foot ulcers. Home Healthc Now 2016;34(2):62–7.
12. Maydick-Youngberg D, Acee A. The challenge of self-managing comorbid depression and diabetes. Medsurg Nurs 2017;26(6):371–3.
13. Bendowska A, Baum E. The Significance of Cooperation in Interdisciplinary Health Care Teams as Perceived by Polish Medical Students. Int J Environ Res Publ Health 2023;20(2):954.
14. Taberna M, Gil Moncayo F, Jané-Salas E, et al. The Multidisciplinary Team (MDT) Approach and Quality of Care. Front Oncol 2020;10:85.
15. Maydick-Youngberg D, Liao J, Francis K, et al. An evidence-based interprofessional collaborative practice approach to decrease tracheostomy related pressure injury. Medsurg Nurs 2020;29(3):189–91.
16. The Joint Commission. Sentinel event alert 58: Inadequate hand-off communication. 2017. Available at: https://www.jointcommission.org/resources/patient-safety-topics/sentinel-event/sentinel-event-alert-newsletters/sentinel-event-alert-58-inadequate hand-off communication/.
17. Institute of Medicine. To err is human: building a safer health system. Washington, DC: National Academy Press; 2000.
18. Institute of Medicine. The future of nursing: leading change, advancing health. Washington, DC: National Academies Press; 2010.
19. World Health Professions Alliance. Statement on Interprofessional Collaborative Practice. 2019. Available at: https://www.whpa.org/news-resources/statements/whpa-statement-interprofessional-collaborative-practice. [Accessed 10 March 2024].
20. World Health Organization. Framework for action on interprofessional education and collaborative practice. Geneva, Switzerland: World Health Organization; 2010. Available at: https://www.who.int/hrh/resources/framework_action/en/.
21. World Health Organization. Resolutions and Decisions. WHA58.28 eHealth. 2020. Available at: https://www.who.int/healtacademy/media/WHA58-28-en.pdf.
22. World Health Organization. Report of the third global survey on eHealth. Geneva, Switzerland: World Health Organization; 2016. Global Observatory for eHealth. Global diffusion of eHealth: Making universal health coverage achievable.
23. Uslu A, Stausberg J. Value of the electronic medical record for hospital care: update from the literature. J Med Internet Res 2021;23(12):e26323.
24. Kirkland-Kyhn H, Howell M, Senestraro J, et al. Leveraging technology to improve wound care delivery and care transitions. Nurs Manag 2021;52(11):24–8.
25. Campanella P, Lovato E, Marone C, et al. The impact of electronic health records on healthcare quality: A systematic review and meta-analysis. Eur J Publ Health 2016;26(1):60–4.
26. Zlabek JA, Wickus JW, Mathiason MA. Early cost and safety benefits of an inpatient electronic medical record. J Am Med Inf Assoc 2011;18(2):169–72.
27. Esmaeilzadeh P, Sambasivan M. Health Information Exchange (HIE): A literature review, assimilation pattern and a proposed classification for a new policy approach. J Biomed Inf 2016;64:74–86.
28. Agency for Healthcare Policy and Research. Guide to Patient and family Engagement in Primary Care. Available at: https://www.ahrq.gov/sites/default/files/wysiwyg/professionals/quality-patient-safety/patient-family-engagement/pfeprimarycare/warm-handoff-guide-for-clinicians.pdf.
29. Rojas Smith L, Ashok M, Morse Dy S, et al. Contextual Frameworks for research on the implementation of complex system interventions. Rockville (MD): Agency for Healthcare Research and Quality (US); 2014.

30. Soegaard K, Sollie M, Beeckman D, et al. Interventions, stakeholders, and orga-nisation related to pressure ulcer prevention for individuals with spinal cord in-juries in transition from hospital to home - A scoping review. J Tissue Viability 2023;32(2):194–205.
31. Xu B, Song X, Weng Y. A multidisciplinary team approach for diabetic foot ulcer: a case study. Adv Skin Wound Care 2023 Apr;36(4):1–4. PMID: 36940382.
32. American Society of Colon and Rectal Surgeons Committee Members, Wound, Ostomy, Continence Nurses Society Committee Members. ASCRS and WOCN joint position statement on the value of preoperative stoma marking for patients undergoing fecal ostomy surgery. J Wound, Ostomy Cont Nurs 2007;34(6):627–8.
33. American Urological Association Committee Members, Wound, Ostomy, Conti-nence Nurses Society Committee Members. Society joint position statement on the value of preoperative stoma marking for patients undergoing creation of an incontinent urostomy. J Wound, Ostomy Cont Nurs 2009;36(3):267–8.

# The Role of the Wound, Ostomy, and Continence Nurse in an Earthquake

Ayise Karadag, PhD, ET/WOC[a],*, Tuba Sengul, PhD, CWON[a],
Holly Kirkland-Kyhn, PhD, FNP-c, GNP-c, CWCN, FAANP[b]

## KEYWORDS

• Disaster • Earthquake • Wound care • Nurse • Wound care nurse

## KEY POINTS

- The Wound, Ostomy, and Continence (WOC) nurses play a critical role in the immediate aftermath of earthquakes by triaging and providing initial treatment to individuals with injuries.
- The most important contributions of WOC nurses in earthquake injuries are reducing the risk of infection and preventing amputations.
- WOC nurses provide compassionate support and reassurance to patients experiencing distress or trauma related to their injuries.
- Despite the critical roles of WOC nurses in earthquake situations, the literature suggests that they may not be adequately prepared for this context.

## INTRODUCTION

Every year, more than a million earthquakes occur worldwide, roughly about 2 per minute.[1] Historically, some major earthquakes occurring worldwide have led to the deaths of tens of thousands of people and billions of dollars in material losses.[2] The effects of earthquakes have been felt over wide areas, as seen in events such as the Roman Empire's collapse, the city's destruction by the 1906 San Francisco earthquake, or the upheaval caused by the 2010 Haiti earthquake.[3,4] Many wound specialty professionals were recruited to work in Haiti after the 2010 earthquake due to the number of traumatic amputations and post-trauma infections.[3,4] Earthquakes in the twentieth century resulted in approximately 1.87 million deaths, with an average of 2052 deaths per earthquake event between 1990 and 2010.[5] The 9.5 magnitude earthquake in Chile in 1960 and the 9.2 magnitude earthquakes in the United States in 1964 are among the most destructive earthquakes known worldwide.[6] Additionally, it is

[a] Koç University School of Nursing, Istanbul, Turkey; [b] Betty Irene Moore School of Nursing, UC Davis Health, CA, USA
* Corresponding author.
*E-mail address:* akaradag@ku.edu.tr

Nurs Clin N Am 60 (2025) 185–195
https://doi.org/10.1016/j.cnur.2024.07.009
0029-6465/25/© 2024 Elsevier Inc. All rights reserved, including those for text and data mining, AI training, and similar technologies.
nursing.theclinics.com

estimated that the number of casualties from the 7.1 magnitude earthquake in China in 1976 exceeded 650,000.[7]

Turkey is in a seismically active region known as the Mediterranean–Asian seismic belt, which has been prone to earthquakes throughout its history. In Turkey, earthquakes are the most common natural disasters, resulting in the most injuries and fatalities.[8] In 1939 Erzincan earthquake, which measured 7.8 magnitude, 33 thousand people perished, while in the 1999 Gölcük and Düzce earthquakes, over 18 thousand people lost their lives, leaving 500 thousand people homeless.[9,10] The 2 earthquakes measuring 7.7 and 7.6 magnitude that occurred in Kahramanmaraş on February 6, 2024, have been among the largest earthquakes of this century regarding their intensity and the damage and losses they caused. In these earthquakes, more than 50 thousand people lost their lives, and over 100 thousand people were injured.[11] As a result, earthquakes have historically left deep scars on humanity and have influenced civilizations. Increasing efforts to mitigate the effects of earthquakes in the future will significantly strengthen our ability to combat natural disasters.

Earthquakes and natural disasters have always brought about immense challenges to health care systems. Nurses play a vital role in any major disaster relief, which has led to the development of disaster nursing as a particular field within the nursing discipline. However, disaster nursing has different challenges and obstacles in developed and developing countries.[12] Although nurses have good intentions and put considerable effort into saving lives, disaster relief practices go beyond normal daily nursing practices. Turkey is a country prone to both natural and man-made disasters, which requires a high level of preparedness for those involved in disasters, including the Wound, Ostomy, and Continence (WOC) Nursing. Existing literature, in combination with the 7.8 Mw earthquake that affected the southern and central parts of Turkey on February 6, 2023, at 04:17 TRT (01:17 UTC), heightened our awareness of the WOC nurse's experience in earthquake conditions. There is a need to improve nurses' competencies in managing injured people in earthquakes. WOC nurses are expected to assume crucial responsibilities in mass casualty situations like earthquakes. However, unlike disaster nurses, they do not receive training to help injured people in these urgent, critical, and complex situations. The role of nurses in disasters has been defined internationally[13]; there is a need to define the roles and functions of nurses involved in these processes, including WOC nurses.

Studies conducted on disaster nursing in Turkey have revealed a need for knowledge among nurses and nursing students. There is a lack of legal regulations regarding the role of the WOC nurse in disasters. Studies have also shown that disaster-related training, especially simulation exercises, effectively enhances nurses' knowledge[14] and competency. It is noteworthy that even in the latest revision of the Nursing National Core Curriculum, dated March 1, 2022, there is no specific topic addressing the roles of nurses in disasters.[15] This is a matter that requires consideration.[16]

In this article, we present the significance and roles of WOC nurses in the earthquake and the roles and functions performed by 4 WOC nurses who actively participated in the February 2023 Turkey earthquake, the challenges they encountered, and their suggestions for the future. It is anticipated that this article will contribute to developing the roles and responsibilities of WOC nurses during earthquakes and the content of training programs.

Nurses are the largest human resource group in disaster response within the health care sector.[17] Despite often being earthquake victims, nurses endeavor to carry out their services with an extraordinary sense of professional responsibility and a desire to assist. Nurses fulfilled different roles in the period after the disaster (eg, as a clinician, a communicator, a leader, and a provider of psychosocial support).[13] In earthquakes, the role of WOC nurses is crucial because they play a critical role in saving lives and improving the health conditions of the injured. When examining the limited literature on this subject,[16,18] the roles and functions performed by WOC nurses in earthquakes are summarized in **Fig. 1**.

The data obtained from interviews with 4 WOC nurses working in a university hospital with a capacity of 1598 beds in the recent earthquake zone provided valuable insights into the challenges nurses faced regarding wound management during earthquakes. They offered significant contributions to the proposed solutions (**Table 1**). In addition, the statements of these nurses closely parallel the difficulties and expectations stated in the literature.[17]

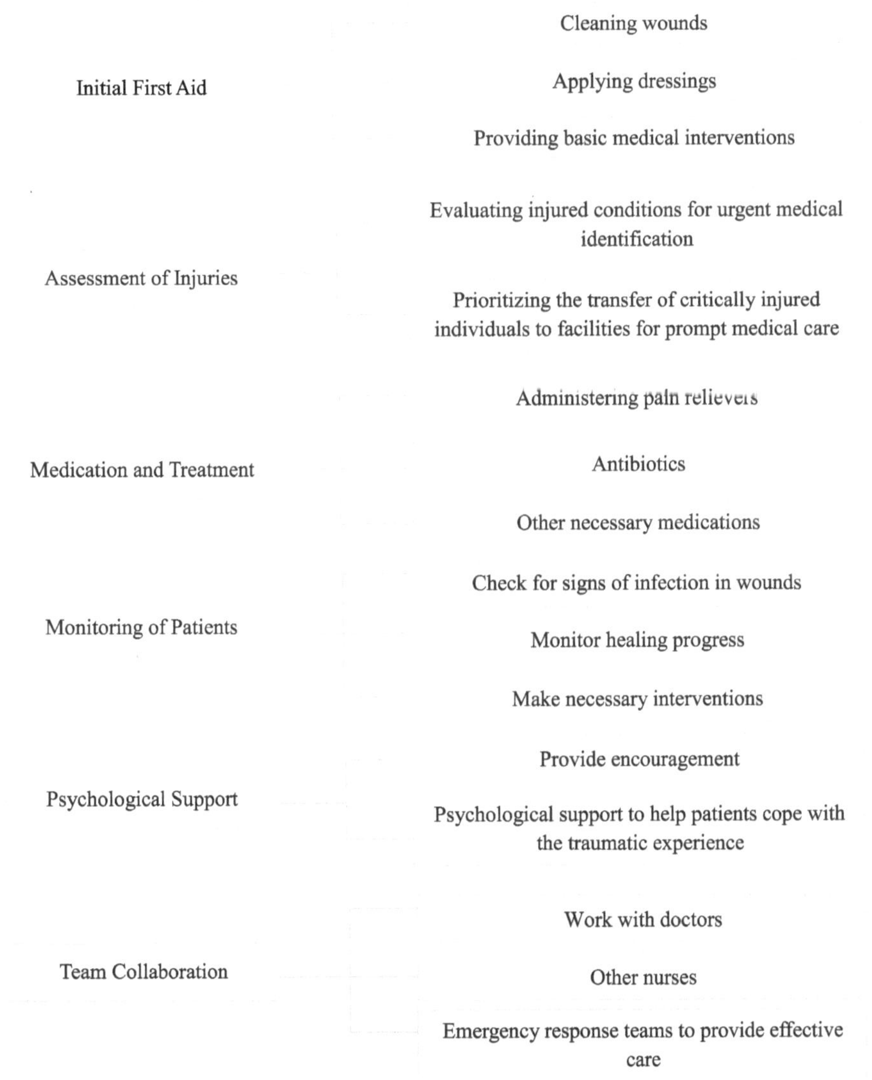

| | |
|---|---|
| **Initial First Aid** | Cleaning wounds |
| | Applying dressings |
| | Providing basic medical interventions |
| **Assessment of Injuries** | Evaluating injured conditions for urgent medical identification |
| | Prioritizing the transfer of critically injured individuals to facilities for prompt medical care |
| **Medication and Treatment** | Administering pain relievers |
| | Antibiotics |
| | Other necessary medications |
| **Monitoring of Patients** | Check for signs of infection in wounds |
| | Monitor healing progress |
| | Make necessary interventions |
| **Psychological Support** | Provide encouragement |
| | Psychological support to help patients cope with the traumatic experience |
| **Team Collaboration** | Work with doctors |
| | Other nurses |
| | Emergency response teams to provide effective care |

**Fig. 1.** The roles and functions of nurses in earthquakes.

**Table 1**
Characteristics of the nurses (n = 4)

| Nurse Code | Work Experience/ Wound, Ostomy, and Continence Nurse Experience (Year) | Level of Education | Certification | Status of Receiving Disaster Training | Mean Number of Patients/per d | Previous Earthquake Experience |
|---|---|---|---|---|---|---|
| N1 | 26/21 | MsN | WOC nurse certification | In-service training | At least 15 for each team member. | No |
| N2 | 22/14 | PhD in Nursing | | | | No |
| N3 | 34/34 | RN | | | 250–300 patients/ per d | Yes |
| N4 | 31/22 | RN | | | | No |

On October 27, 2023, almost 9 months after the earthquake on February 6, 2024, a meeting was held using the Zoom platform with 4 nurses working as WOC nurses in a large state university hospital located in the earthquake zone. These nurses also comprise the Turkish Wound Ostomy Incontinence Nursing Society (TWOINS). The identifying characteristics of the nurses interviewed are presented in **Table 1**, while the interview questions are provided in **Box 1**. Before starting the interview, an explanation was provided to the nurses, and their consent was obtained for recording audio and video and using the interview contents in scientific articles. Each question was directed to each nurse, who was asked to share their experiences. The answers provided by the nurses to the questions were grouped under the following headings.

## BACHELOR'S AND WOUND, OSTOMY, AND CONTINENCE-CERTIFIED TRAINING PROGRAMS

Nurses expressed that anatomy, pharmacology, wound physiology and classification, and crisis management topics in their bachelor's education significantly contributed to their knowledge, particularly benefiting from their experiences in wound management. They expressed that having more theoretic knowledge and practical skills in wound management during their bachelor's education would help them provide more effective service during emergencies like earthquakes. Another suggestion regarding a bachelor's education was to enhance teamwork and communication skills. Nurses

---

**Box 1**
**Interview questions**

1. How did your undergraduate education contribute to your management of wound care during the earthquake?

2. What would be your suggestions for undergraduate education programs?

3. How did you use your education in the certificate program in this process?

4. What did you need most when managing wounds?

5. What were the areas where you had difficulty managing wounds? How did you manage it? What knowledge, skills, and abilities did you need?

6. How prepared did you feel yourself?

7. What were your perceived challenges and coping strategies?

8. What would you do if you lived again?

9. What would be your suggestions regarding the role of the wound care nurse in an earthquake?
   - Basic training
   - Certified training programs
   - Professional organizations

10. Have you had challenges with legal regulations?

11. How has your wound management process differed from your normal practice?

12. How did your emotions during that period differ from regular?

13. How ready do you think WOC nurses are to respond to an earthquake?

14. What ethical dilemmas have you experienced?

15. What was the case/situation that affected you the most?

stated that by developing these skills during their bachelor's education, they could act more coordinated and effectively during emergencies, such as earthquakes. These suggestions highlight the significance of acquiring competencies, such as "strong theoretic knowledge, practical skills, communication skills, and teamwork," as the end-of-program student learning outcomes, enabling nurses to deliver wound care services more effectively during emergencies like earthquakes.[19]

However, nurses have suggested that WOC-certified training programs should incorporate topics such as the roles of WOC nurses in disasters and interventions for earthquake injuries. They also proposed conducting simulations using scenarios related to earthquake injuries in these training programs. Relevant literature indicates that nurses have knowledge and experiential needs during disasters, and simulation training contributes to increasing their knowledge and experience levels.[20–23] WOC nursing was initiated in Türkiye in the early 2000s, and the standards for certified training programs were established in 2014.[24] However, upon reviewing these standards, it is evident that the course content does not include topics related to wound management in disasters.[25]

*Nurse informants' statement regarding simulation training*: "...Simulation training should be included. I would prepare a simulation scenario on how wound care is performed. Additionally, during the earthquake period, within the first 24 to 72 hours, I would create a simulation scenario on how a wound care nurse should organize themselves before patients arrive. I would want students to learn how to manage the process through this scenario."

## MAINTAINING PROFESSIONAL VALUES

Nurses have expressed a significant need for regulations in the domain of law and ethics,[26] one of the domains identified by the International Council of Nurses for competency in disaster nursing. WOC nurses have faced challenges in making ethical decisions while providing wound care services to individuals injured in earthquakes in line with professional values and with rapid adaption to changing situations.

## THE ETHICAL ISSUES EXPRESSED BY WOUND, OSTOMY, AND CONTINENCE NURSES

*Working conditions and planning*: (1) intensive working conditions, (2) extended working hours, (3) lack of materials and equipment, (4) inconsistencies and conflicts in the work plans, and (5) coordination with different departments.

*Decision-making related to patient care*: (1) rapid decision-making due to emergencies, (2) lack of clarity in legal regulations leading to indecision and uncertainty, (3) emotional difficulties and anxieties experienced by nurses and families, and (4) providing care for pediatric patients.

*Issues related to teamwork and communication*: (1) lack of coordination and collaboration between different departments, (2) discrepancies between management's expectations and the realistic capabilities of WOC nurses, and (3) poor communication channels for making rapid decisions.

Nurses indicated that the cases that most significantly impacted them professionally and emotionally were severe injuries and limb losses in pediatric patients. Nurses expressed emotional difficulties while caring for pediatric patients, often reflecting on their children.

The nurse informants' statement regarding access to supplies was "We experienced material shortages. However, being affiliated with the association (referring to TWOINS) was very important; they contacted us and quickly organized to deliver materials to us. The value of being a member of the association was significant; in being able to rely on our associates. The value of wound care congresses and relationships with wound care corporations who contacted us with donations of supplies."

Thus, nurses highlighted the importance of belonging to their respective specialty associations, attending scientific congresses, and the presence of corporations providing products during earthquakes, emphasizing the significance of material supply.

## DIFFERENCES IN WOUND MANAGEMENT DURING EARTHQUAKES

During earthquakes, the wound management process significantly deviates from normal working conditions. Nurses interviewed faced a much higher patient load and higher acuity, with greater shortages of supplies. The workload raised from 25 patients per Wound Ostomy Continence Nurse (WOCN) to 250 to 300 patients daily, with more emergency cases. Nurses needed to determine wound care priorities and rapidly conduct emergency interventions. Nurses stressed that they constantly had to change their plans to provide services effectively with limited resources.[1] Nurses expressed challenges with intense workloads, stressful situations, and emotional difficulties requiring more energy and resilience than usual. For example, to perform fasciotomy in post-earthquake providing a suitable environment for sedation and nerve block application is necessary.[27] In crush syndrome, the role of nurses is crucial. During both emergency intervention and hospital care stages, nurses' accurate and prompt interventions can save the patient's life and prevent limb loss. Playing a supportive role in the patient's acute care and rehabilitation process. In the face of earthquake disasters, nurses having up-to-date literature knowledge and providing care to their patients accordingly will play a key role in public health.[28]

A statement from N3, a highly experienced WOC nurse, regarding wound care organization, "I was the first to initiate communication with other departments. I reached out initially. We created WhatsApp groups and provided written updates here. We tried to gather evidence and took photographs. There was no time to wait for permission for amputations. When we consulted with other departments, they would often say 'wait, hold on,' but the time passing was working against the patient's favor…".

## LEGAL REGULATIONS

WOC nurses expressed issues regarding permissions and authority, legal gaps and uncertainties, and patient rights. Particularly in emergency interventions like amputations, the limited time to obtain permissions made it difficult for them to perform their duties. They experienced uncertainties regarding the extent of their authority in interventions like surgical debridement. Dealing with unidentified patients or those without family members posed challenges regarding patient rights and family relationships. The lack of legal regulations concerning patients without relatives or identification documents, especially in the care of pediatric patients, created difficulties.

A quote from Nurse 2 (N2's) statements regarding legal regulations: "At first, due to intense emotions, laws didn't come to our minds. I felt anxious, especially when thinking about caring for children. Although there was a responsible physician and we had communication using WhatsApp, initially, I wasn't anxious because it was a crisis. However, later, I became worried. There were unidentified patients, both children and adults, but they had no relatives. Medical and nursing students stayed with the patients as attendants. For example, a student had to feed a 6-month-old baby with a bottle. Initially, it seemed like this might be the case during a crisis period, but there are some legal gaps. I don't know what will happen in the future; we need to take precautions and make regulations for the future."

Similar challenges are found in the relevant literature, and general guidelines regarding the duties, authority, and responsibilities of WOC nurses in disasters should be established when making legal regulations.[29] These regulations should also be included in the content of training programs.

## COPING STRATEGIES

Nurses highlighted professional competence and experience, collaboration and solidarity, and personal and professional support as coping strategies. These nurses, all with over 20 years of professional experience, have emphasized the importance of their professional competence and experience in coping with earthquakes. They mention that the knowledge and skills they acquired through their undergraduate education and certification programs helped them provide more effective services in emergencies like earthquakes. They stated that effective communication and collaboration with teams of different health disciplines played a crucial role in coping with challenging situations. Nurses emphasized the significance of receiving personal and professional support during the earthquake process. They pointed out the need for more effective implementation of psychosocial support programs and meeting the emotional needs of employees.

The expressions regarding whether nurses experienced acute stress or post-traumatic stress syndrome indicated that they also needed much more support.

Nurse 3 (N3) "...We experienced all of them. Most of the time, my friend held me. You're angry at the situation. We started experiencing this stress after the earthquake was over. We couldn't overcome it. We're still under that earthquake ... still there. Also, I realized something: when you think of an earthquake, you always think of death. I never thought about it; now, I'm thinking about which organ I might lose."

Nurse 4 (N4) "We are experiencing the definition of post-traumatic stress. For example, I noticed that I didn't talk to my coworker all day when we normally chat. I have two children, and when the earthquake happened, I started to fear not death but where I would end up under the rubble. Because I have seen many cases involving children, I think if there is an earthquake, should I protect my children's heads, legs, or arms? Unfortunately, it still continues."

## SUMMARY

In conclusion, WOC nurses strive to carry out their services with extraordinary professional responsibility and altruism in earthquake situations. In this extraordinary circumstance, they must cope with various issues ranging from physical conditions to managerial processes, ethical dilemmas, and material supply while caring for complex acute wounds in patients with polytrauma. To ensure effective wound management, competencies in disaster management and organization should be added to the training programs of WOC nurses. It is crucial to establish clear boundaries regarding nurses' duties, authorities, and responsibilities in such conditions through legal regulations. WOC nurses, especially in countries located in earthquake-prone zones, should be prepared for these conditions, and organization should be preplanned. Additionally, encouraging interested nurses to undergo educational training regarding disaster assistance is essential. Professional organizations, such as the Turkish Wound Ostomy Incontinence Nurses Society,[30] should provide their members with continuous professional education programs and support.

## CLINICS CARE POINTS

- *Psychological support*: WOC nurses play a critical role in providing psychological support to help patients cope with the traumatic experience of an earthquake. This includes offering encouragement and making necessary interventions to address emotional and mental health needs.

- *Emergency response*: Effective care during earthquakes requires immediate action from emergency response teams. WOC nurses must be prepared to administer pain relievers, prioritize the transfer of critically injured individuals to medical facilities, and provide primary medical interventions promptly.

- *Collaboration and communication*: Team collaboration is essential for efficient disaster response. WOC nurses must work closely with doctors and other health care professionals to monitor healing progress, apply dressings, clean wounds, and check for signs of infection.

- *Material and resource management*: Nurses often face material shortages during disasters. Establishing strong affiliations with associations and companies that can provide necessary supplies quickly is crucial. Nurses highlighted the importance of being part of professional associations like TWOINS to support obtaining materials.

- *Legal and ethical challenges*: Disaster situations often create legal and ethical dilemmas. WOC nurses need to be aware of their legal responsibilities and have clear guidelines on their authority to make rapid decisions, especially in emergency interventions like amputations. Legal regulations should provide clarity and support for nurses in such critical situations.

## DISCLOSURE

The authors have nothing to disclose.

## REFERENCES

1. Naghii M. Public health impact and medical consequences of earthquakes. Rev Panam Salud Públic 2005;18:216–21.
2. Oluwafemi J, Ofuyatan O, Sadiq O, et al. Review of world earthquakes. Int J Civ Eng Technol 2018;9(9):440–64.
3. Bonilla MG. The Marina District, San Francisco, California: Geology, history, and earthquake effects. Bull Seismol Soc Am 1991;81(5):1958–79.
4. Bilham R. Lessons from the Haiti earthquake. Nature 2010;463(7283):878–9.
5. Doocy S, Daniels A, Packer C, et al. The human impact of earthquakes: a historical review of events 1980-2009 and systematic literature review. PLoS currents 2013;5. https://doi.org/10.1371/currents.dis.67bd14fe457f1db0b5433a8ee20fb833.
6. Coffman JL, Von Hake CA, Stover CW. Earthquake history of the United States, 55. US Department of Commerce, National Oceanic and Atmospheric Administration; 1982.
7. Zheng-Xiang F, Gui-Ping L, Hui-Cheng S, et al. An overview on shallow strong earthquake activity and earthquake live losses of Chinese mainland in the centenary from 1901 to 2001. Acta Seismol Sin (Chin Ed) 2005;18: 392–401.
8. Ünal Y, Işık E, Şahin S, et al. Assessment of individual earthquake preparedness levels of health disaster workers: UMKE (National Medical Rescue Teams) association as an example. DEU J Fac Med 2017;31(2):71–80.

9. Haçin İ. 1939 Erzincan Büyük Depremi. Atatürk Araştırma Merkezi Dergisi 2014; 30(88):37–70.
10. Bahadır H, Uçku R. Uluslararası acil durum veri tabanına göre Türkiye Cumhuriyeti tarihindeki afetler. Dog Afet Cev Derg 2018;4(1):28–33.
11. Türkiye earthquake, External situation report no. 9: 1 May–4 June 2023, World Health Organization (WHO). Document number: WHO/EURO:2023-7145-46911-70035. Available at: https://iris.who.int/bitstream/handle/10665/370621/WHO-EURO-2023-7145-46911-70035-eng.pdf?sequence=1. [Accessed 2 March 2024].
12. Yang YN, Xiao L, Cheng HY, et al. Chinese nurses' experience in the Wenchuan earthquake relief. Int Nurs Rev 2010;57(2):217–23.
13. Kako M, Ranse J, Yamamoto A, et al. What was the role of nurses during the 2011 Great East Earthquake of Japan? An integrative review of the Japanese literature. Prehospital Disaster Med 2014;29(3):275–9.
14. Şimşek P, Gündüz A. Türkiye'de afet hemşireliği. Uludağ Üniversitesi Tıp Fakültesi Dergisi 2021;47(3):469–76.
15. Hemsirelik Ulusal Cekirdek Egitim Programı (HUCEP). 2022. Available at: https://www.yok.gov.tr/Documents/Kurumsal/egitim_ogretim_dairesi/Ulusal-cekirdek-egitimi-programlari/hemsirelik_cekirdek_egitim_programi.pdf. [Accessed 2 March 2024].
16. Cullen B. Roles for the WOC nurse in a disaster. JWOCN 2008;35(3):282–6.
17. Çopur EÖ, ÖÜF Karasu. Depremde Hemşire Olmak: Deprem Günlükleri. Yaşam Boyu Hemşirelik Dergisi 2023;4(2):224–35.
18. Miura S, Kondo A, Takamura Y. Practices and challenges of disaster nursing for Japanese nurses sent to Nepal following the 2015 earthquake. Health Emerg Dis Nurs 2020;7(1):46–54.
19. Aims of the Program and the End of Program Student Learning Outcomes, Koç University Faculty of Nursing. Available at: https://nursing.ku.edu.tr/en/education/undergraduate/aims-of-the-program-and-the-end-of-program-student-learning-outcomes/. [Accessed 2 March 2024].
20. Noh J, Oh EG, Kim SS, et al. Development and evaluation of a multimodality simulation disaster education and training program for hospital nurses. Int J Nurs Pract 2020;26(3):e12810.
21. Hasan MK, Younos TB, Farid ZI. Nurses' knowledge, skills and preparedness for disaster management of a Megapolis: Implications for nursing disaster education. Nurse Educ Today 2021;107:105122.
22. Mirzaei S, Eftekhari A, reza Sadeghian M, et al. The effect of disaster management training program on knowledge, attitude, and practice of hospital staffs in natural disasters. J Disaster Res 2019;2(1):9–16.
23. Said NB, Chiang VC. The knowledge, skill competencies, and psychological preparedness of nurses for disasters: a systematic review. Int Emerg Nurs 2020;48:100806.
24. Öztürk D, Karadağ A. Historical development of ostomy and wound care nursing: Turkey sample. J Educ Res Nurs 2019;16(1):73–8.
25. Sağlık Bakanlığı Sertifikalı Eğitim Yönetmeliği, Resmî Gazete. Available at: https://www.resmigazete.gov.tr/eskiler/2014/02/20140204-2.htm. Accessed March 2, 2024.
26. International Council of Nurses (ICN). Fact sheet: disaster response. International Council of Nurses. 2009. Available at: http://www.icn.ch/matters_disaster_response.htm. [Accessed 26 February 2024].
27. Walters T, Crush Syndrome-Prolonged Field Care (CPG ID: 58). Joint trauma system clinical practice guideline (JTS CPG). Publication Date; 2016.

28. Karahan F, Ünal S, Tezol Ö, et al. Thromboprophylaxis in pediatric patients with earthquake-related crush syndrome: a single centre experience. Pediatr Surg Int 2023;39(1):248.
29. Hemşirelik Yönetmeliğinde Değişiklik Yapılmasına Dair Yönetmelik, T.C Sağlık Bakanlığı. 2011. Available at: https://www.saglik.gov.tr/TR-10413/yonetmelikler.html?Sayfa=3. [Accessed 2 March 2024].
30. Wound Ostomy Incontinence Nurses' Society YOIHD, Available at: https://www.yoihd.org.tr/en (Accessed March 2 2024).

# Wound Care Education in Undergraduate and Graduate Nursing Settings

Tuba Sengul, PhD, CWON[a],*, Ayise Karadag, PhD, ET/WOC[a],
Holly Kirkland-Kyhn, PhD, FNP-c, GNP-c, CWCN[b]

## KEYWORDS

- Chronic wound care • Nursing education • Nursing students education
- Competency • Nursing curriculum • Educational programs

## KEY POINTS

- Wound care education is crucial in nursing due to the high incidence and complex treatment of chronic wounds, impacting over 6 million people in the United States.
- Comprehensive wound care education should start at the undergraduate level, emphasizing evidence-based practices and practical skills.
- Integrating wound care education into nursing curricula can improve patient outcomes and reduce health care costs.
- Nurses require continuous education and training in wound care to maintain competence and provide high-quality care.
- Wound care certification programs and postgraduate education opportunities enhance nurses' skills and professional development.

## THE IMPORTANCE OF WOUND CARE EDUCATION IN NURSING

Chronic wounds are defined as wounds whose anatomic and functional integrity cannot heal promptly and regularly, and the healing process takes longer than expected.[1,2] The incidence of chronic wounds affects more than 6 million people in the United States, and annual expenses are estimated to be over $10 billion.[1] The most common types of chronic wounds include lower extremity ulcers (diabetic foot, venous, and arterial ulcers) and pressure injuries (PIs). The treatment and care process for such wounds are quite complex.[1,3] The literature emphasizes the severe burden that the prevalence of chronic wounds imposes on hospitals and the misreporting of chronic wounds, and this burden is directly related to the increased use of

[a] Koç University School of Nursing, Istanbul, Turkey; Koç University Adress: Davutpaşa st No:4, 34010 Topkapı, Istanbul, Turkey; [b] Betty Irene Moore School of Nursing, UC Davis Health, 2570 48th Street, Sacramento, CA 95817, USA
* Corresponding author.
E-mail address: tsengul@ku.edu.tr

Nurs Clin N Am 60 (2025) 197–206
https://doi.org/10.1016/j.cnur.2024.07.002  **nursing.theclinics.com**
0029-6465/25/© 2024 Elsevier Inc. All rights reserved, including those for text and data mining, AI training, and similar technologies.

personnel, materials, and other resources.[4] On the other hand, chronic wounds pose a significant additional burden for health care systems because they require correct and appropriate care practices.[4,5] Additionally, the shortage of health care professionals globally harms the delivery of health care services and the quality of care.[6] According to the current data from the World Health Organization (WHO), in more than 45% of countries, there are more than 1 thousand patients for one nurse and one doctor (WHO 2024). Furthermore, inaccurate reporting can hinder the effective management of chronic wounds and negatively impact the overall performance of health care services.[4] Therefore, accurately identifying and reporting chronic wounds are essential to reduce costs and improve patient care.[6–8] For these reasons, health care professionals must have the necessary competencies to provide adequate level and quality of care. At the same time, developing practical, cost-effective, and comprehensive education approaches is essential.[9]

Competence acquisition in health care is fundamental to nurses' education and clinical practice.[10] Competence acquisition consists of many dimensions, including the appropriateness of health professionals' knowledge, skills, and attitudes.[10] At the same time, wound care is a critical factor that affects patients' health and determines the healing process[11,12] and stands out as a significant field in nursing practice.[13] Chronic wound care is thought to be more complex than acute wound care, especially by postgraduate nurses.[13] Therefore, pre-graduate nurses must receive comprehensive education on chronic wound care in the nursing curriculum, evaluate their wound care competencies, and learn the most up-to-date practices in this field.[10,13] This may allow for an accurate assessment of the effectiveness of wound care education and current competency requirements.[10] Because the level of competence of health care professionals in wound care is vital to ensure patient safety and quality of care.[11,12] It is emphasized in the literature that in cases where adequate wound care is not achieved, patient outcomes may be negatively affected, and the quality of patient care and patient satisfaction may decrease.[11,12] Assessing wound care competencies is an important step to ensure quality and safety in health care.[10]

Systematic analysis and the results of many studies on the subject show that, in general, wound care competence needs to be improved among nursing professionals and students.[14–19] Specifically, most studies attempt to determine levels of knowledge, prevention, or attitudes toward certain types of wounds, such as PI, or focus on specific types of wounds, such as lower extremity ulcers.[20–27] Additionally, studies evaluating the competencies of nurses and nursing students in all chronic wound care and management are limited.[21] A systematic review highlights that the evidence on wound care needs to be stronger, the link between this evidence and practice is inadequate, ritualistic practices are standard, and there needs to be more structured education at the pre-graduate and postgraduate levels.[14] Simultaneously, another critical point is creating more structured wound care education programs at pre-graduate/graduate and professional development levels.[14]

### An Educational Perspective on Chronic Wound Care

#### Wound care education status of nursing students

Although wound care is a crucial requirement in nursing practice, nurses' competence in wound care is established during undergraduate education.[17] However, courses on chronic wound management are not included in the curricula of many nursing schools during undergraduate education.[28] Therefore, to standardize wound care education in health care practices, nursing curricula must begin in undergraduate programs and develop content with consistent learning objectives.[17] Because in the expected results of many research findings in the literature, nursing students' chronic wound care knowledge levels were unfortunately insufficient.[13,18,22,23,29] One of the reasons for the lack of students' knowledge about chronic wound care is not only the lack of wound care education in the curriculum, but the difficulties experienced by students in transferring theoretic knowledge to clinical care environments and putting evidence-based knowledge into practice are also essential factors.[29] A significant obstacle in fully implementing evidence-based practice stems from nursing students' limited knowledge and attitude levels.[30] When students need more knowledge about preventing and treating chronic wounds, they cannot adopt and implement proper care interventions.[30]

On the other hand, a recent systematic analysis found that almost all nursing students' studies on chronic wound care and chronic wound types were related to PI. Their level of knowledge about other chronic wound etiologies, such as diabetic foot and venous/arterial leg ulcers, emphasizes a gap in the literature.[2] According to the information in the literature, it needs to be fully understood why many studies are primarily conducted on PIs. However, there is an intense interest in studies on PI because the prevalence of such injuries, response to treatment, and potential complications are essential indicators that determine the quality of nursing care in a health care facility.[2,31] The National Pressure Ulcer Advisory Panel revised its registered nurse competency-based curriculum for PI prevention in 2013.[32] It was stated that this revision aims to integrate the education module on PI into the education curriculum of nursing students.[32] In the same revision, it is emphasized that successful nursing education should include evidence-based practices, which can be achieved with an interactive and comprehensive curriculum.[32] The nursing curriculum should be structured to incorporate quality indicators and best practices for preventing and managing PIs while emphasizing and integrating it with interprofessional education.[32] This approach may contribute to the modern challenge of establishing the most effective education to improve the incidence of PIs and overall wound care outcomes.[02]

### Wound care education status of nurses

While chronic wounds are a significant concern for health care practices and patients, they also play an essential role in determining the costs of care for health care systems and the quality of life for society.[14,16] Chronic wound care is a specific clinical area where nurses play an essential role and require multidisciplinary teamwork.[14,16] Effective management of chronic wounds is complex, and nurses involved in the care and treatment process must have the correct knowledge and skills to optimize best practices and improve patient care outcomes.[14] Therefore, academic education and education in wound care, both in basic nursing and postgraduate knowledge, are essential in developing adequate and satisfactory competence and the specific skills that are directly relevant.[10,15-19] Chronic wound care education provided to nurses directly contributes to establishing professional standards, improving patient safety, and, more generally, the quality of care in the clinical field.[10,15-19] There are few studies on nurses' knowledge, skills, and competence levels in wound care education.[14,33] It is also emphasized that nursing research on chronic wound management is generally less produced, and nurses show less participation in research and a reluctance to engage in academic activities as compared to other health care colleagues.[14] According to the results of many descriptive and systematic analysis studies examining the knowledge level of nurses on chronic wound care, the knowledge level of nurses was generally found to be low.[14,21] Additionally, interesting results of these studies can be summarized as follows[14,21]: (1) insufficient knowledge on staging the correct classification of PI (which is the most chronic wound type); (2) awareness of clinical guidelines/protocols; and (3) selection of the proper and appropriate wound dressings.

Although wound care knowledge is generally sufficient, nurses need help adequately transferring this knowledge into practice in the clinical setting.[14,21] At the same time, a study by Gillespie and colleagues[34] found that although nurses working in acute care in Australia had an excellent theoretic knowledge of wound assessment, there needed to be a better relationship between knowledge and practice and negative outcomes related to poor application of clinical guidelines. According to the literature, nurses should receive education on chronic wounds to improve their evidence-based practice and research. It is acknowledged that there are shortcomings in wound care instruction, particularly in the context of undergraduate nursing. It is advised that programs for wound care education be put in place.[35–37] These education programs are significant in the clinical and primary health care sectors, providing public health services.[35–37] In addition, another interesting study on the subject, the lack of chronic wound care education, stands out as a problem that can even affect the cost of care for patients. On the other hand, it is emphasized that chronic wound education given to nurses is crucial in reducing patients' outpatient treatment costs.[38,39] It is anticipated that developing strategies for nurses who work and specialize in home health care to receive chronic wound education can significantly reduce the overall cost of ambulatory wound care management (https://www.facs.org/education/Patient-education/skills-programs/wound-care).

In conclusion, the results of many current systematic and meta-analysis studies emphasize the need for sufficient evidence on the effectiveness of educational interventions for nurses, especially in the hospital setting, and that nurses need more knowledge in chronic wound care.[14,19,21,40–44] The importance of focusing on the competency areas of nurses in chronic wound care, standardizing education on wound care, and integrating it into evidence-based practices is emphasized.[14,19,40] The development of more systematic and comprehensive wound care education programs for both associate degree students and nurses at professional development levels is effective in promoting innovation and best practices through ongoing monitoring and supervision by nurse leaders and managers.[14,19,40] This indicates the presence of various educational strategies that could be effective in chronic wound management within hospital settings.[14,19,40]

## THE STATUS OF WOUND CARE EDUCATION IN EUROPE, TURKEY, AND AMERICA

Wound care is a specialized field with a long history within the nursing discipline, and the leadership and contributions of nurses have shaped the development of knowledge and practices in this field.[45] In this historical process dating back to Florence Nightingale, nurses have pioneered by providing direct care to nonhealing wounds.[45] With advances in dressing techniques and moist wound healing, professionals such as the Wound, Ostomy, and Continence Nursing (WOCN) can access guidelines to promote leadership, research, and primary care for patients with wounds.[45] The increase in alternative treatment methods for diabetic foot ulcers, with growth factor treatments, biologic skin equivalents, and negative pressure wound therapy, has partially led physicians to this field.[45] Although wound care is traditionally carried out by nursing, wound care education is not included in the basic nursing curricula of many countries.[46] For instance, tissue viability nurses in the United Kingdom receive a specialized education program that includes multifaceted roles and skills (ie, communication and technical skills) to manage chronic wounds.[47] In the United States, nurses' scope of practice varies by state and hospital policy, which may limit nurses with advanced knowledge of wound care certification from performing even the most basic procedures.[46] In the literature, the nursing curriculum must adequately

> **Box 1**
> **Examples of different wound care educational opportunities and degrees in Europe**
>
> Wound consultant education at the Erasmus Medical Centre, the Netherlands
>
> Akademie für zertifiziertes Wundmanagement (ZWM), Germany
>
> Bachelor of Science module in the Principles of Wound Care Management, University of Glamorgan, the United Kingdom
>
> Master of Science in Wound Healing and Tissue Repair, Cardiff University, the United Kingdom
>
> Master of Science in Wound and Tissue Viability, Catholic University, Portugal
>
> World Council of Enterostomal Therapists (www.wcetn.org)
>
> Wound Care Education Institute (www.wcei.net),
>
> Tissue Viability Nurses Association (www.tvns.org),
>
> One years masters' program, England
>
> Wound Care Education (ewma.org/what-we-do/education/ewma-e-learning)

include primary wound care education.[46] Similarly, it is stated that insufficient time is allocated to wound care-related subjects in many medical schools in the United States, Germany, and the United Kingdom.[46] The wound care course is offered as an elective in the medical school curriculum and is not among the minimum or standard qualifications.[46]

For those who want to focus more on the nursing profession in wound care, the various postgraduate education opportunities offered in Europe offer an essential step toward specialization in health care.[40] In Europe, various educational opportunities are available at the postgraduate level to specialize in wound care nursing.[48] These opportunities include wound care course programs at different levels (**Box 1**). However, nurses still need clarification about their expectations from wound care course programs and the scope of practice.[48] The use of different titles such as "advanced wound care nurse," "tissue vitality nurse," "wound consultant," and "wound specialist" to describe nurses who will specialize in this field increases uncertainty.[48] Major decisions about nursing curricula are often based on informal consensus or local initiatives and may vary depending on the context of the health care organization.[48] On the other hand, determining the content and level of the wound care curriculum is an educational challenge.[48] The European Wound Management Association (EWMA) approves nurses' wound care certification after evaluating and accepting each education program.[49] In Europe and many countries, wound management education is available in

> **Box 2**
> **Examples of different educational opportunities and degrees in Turkey**
>
> Stoma and Wound Care Nursing Program, SANERC, Koç University, İstanbul
>
> Wound Care Course, SANERC, Koç University, İstanbul
>
> Health Facilities Authorized to Perform Stoma and Wound Care Nursing Certified Education, Certificate programs approved by the Ministry of Health, Turkey
>
> German ICW Association (initiative chronishe wunde [ICW]) Wound Care Specialist Education, Acıbadem University
>
> *Abbreviation:* SANERC, Semahat Arsel Nursing Education, Practice and Research Center.

---

**Box 3**
**Examples of different educational opportunities and degrees in USA**

R. B. Turnbull, Jr. School of ET/WOC Nursing, Cleveland, Ohio

Emory University School of Medicine WOCN, Education Center, Atlanta

Wicks Educational Associates-Harrisburg Area WOC Nursing Education Program, Mechanicsburg

VA Eastern Kansas Wound Management Academy, Leavenworth

University of Virginia Graduate Program in WOC Nursing, Charlottesville

University of Washington School of Nursing, Seattle

WebWOC Nursing Education Program Winona State University, WOCNEP's program

---

the form of 46 hour courses (lasting 3 years) or the EWMA e-learning courses (for wound management for health care professionals) approved by the EWMA.[49]

In Turkey, with the decision taken by the Ministry of Health on August 21, 2010, procedures and principles were determined for acquiring professional qualifications based on special knowledge and skills in certified education to be implemented after graduation in the health field.[50] The first program was started in 2001 as the 56-Hour Stoma and Wound Care Nursing Education Program.[50] Since 2015, the standards of wound and stoma care-certified education programs have been determined, and courses have been conducted accordingly[50] (**Box 2**). In this context, 3 day (16 hour) primary chronic wound care courses and a 240 hour course have been offered for the first time in 2018 by the Semahat Arsel Nursing Education and Research Center (SANERC) affiliated with the Koç University Faculty of Nursing since 2015. Certificate programs are organized.[51] Additionally, the Wound Care and Tissue Repair Association organizes 3 day courses for all health care professionals.[52] Courses covering basic and advanced wound care, including topics such as chronic wound management, wound and stoma case management, and advanced chronic wounds, have been integrated into the Koç University Faculty of Nursing course curriculum within the scope of the Ostomy and Wound Care Nursing Track Program (OWCNTP).[53]

Many wound care certification courses are available in America, both online and in person.[46] These certification courses offer the rigorous and comprehensive education necessary to treat complex patients.[46] The WOCN certification is offered at basic and advanced practice levels. This program includes highly respected and rigorous education with a comprehensive recertification process.[46] However, only wound-certified advanced practice nurses (wound ostomy care-advanced practice registered nurses [WOC-APRNs]) are authorized to prescribe and bill for their services independently[46] (**Box 3**).

## SUMMARY

In conclusion, despite the significant role of nurses in chronic wound management, more wound care education is needed, and competency checks should be included in the nursing curriculum. It is vital to make changes in the education curriculum of nursing students regarding chronic wound education for all continents. The authors recommend that more time should be devoted to wound management education in nursing schools. Wound care education can be supported not only through traditional workshops, conferences, home health nursing rotations, and internships but also by leveraging modern technologies such as Web-based interactive programs, digital educational materials, simulation applications, online live classes, and interactive mobile apps that are compatible with today's educational environment. Providing wound care education to students in the preclinical years can lead to using this knowledge in clinical practice and contribute to better care outcomes for millions of patients. This approach supports graduating nurses to tackle the complexities of chronic wound care and improve patient outcomes. Continuing chronic wound care education from student life to graduation improves nurses' competencies and provides them with up-to-date information. This plays a critical role in preventive and protective maintenance practices. Therefore, it is essential to prioritize education focusing on chronic wound care in the nursing curriculum and increase resources in this field.

The resources presented in this article show that the knowledge level of graduate or experienced nurses working in a clinical environment on chronic wound care is generally not at the desired level. Many of these studies were conducted in various regions, highlighting the need to consider and plan multiple strategies to improve nurses' knowledge of chronic wound care globally. In this context, steps need to be taken, such as developing more effective methods in chronic wound care education, investing in continuous education and updating opportunities for nurses, and encouraging information sharing at the international level. By increasing their knowledge and skills, these strategies can enable nurses to be more effective and efficient in patient care.

## CLINICS CARE POINTS

- *Evidence-based Practice*: Incorporate evidence-based wound care practices in clinical settings to ensure effective and up-to-date patient care.
- *Skill development*: Focus on practical skill development during nursing education to enhance student's ability to manage chronic wounds effectively.
- *Interprofessional collaboration*: Encourage collaboration between nurses and other health care professionals to improve wound care outcomes and patient management.
- *Ongoing training*: Provide continuous education and professional development opportunities to update nurses on the latest wound care techniques and guidelines.
- *Resource management*: Emphasize the importance of proper resource management, including appropriate wound dressings and materials, to optimize care and reduce costs.

## DISCLOSURE

The authors have nothing to disclose.

## REFERENCES

1. Jiang T, Li Q, Qiu J, et al. Nanobiotechnology: Applications in Chronic Wound Healing. Int J Nanomed 2022;17:3125–45. Published 2022 Jul 20.
2. Martinengo L, Yeo NJY, Tang ZQ, et al. Digital Education for the Management of Chronic Wounds in Health Care Professionals: Protocol for a Systematic Review by the Digital Health Education Collaboration. JMIR Res Protoc 2019;8(3). https://doi.org/10.2196/12488. PMID: 30907743; PMCID: PMC6452282.
3. Sen CK, Gordillo GM, Roy S, et al. Human skin wounds: a major and snowballing threat to public health and the economy. Wound Repair Regen 2009;17(6):763–71.
4. Posnett J, Franks PJ. The burden of chronic wounds in the UK. Nurs Times 2008;104(3):44–5.

5. Campbell J, Buchan J, Cometto G, et al. Human resources for health and universal health coverage: fostering equity and effective coverage. Bull World Health Organ 2013;91(11):853–63.
6. Olsson M, Järbrink K, Divakar U, et al. The humanistic and economic burden of chronic wounds: A systematic review. Wound Repair Regen 2019;27(1):114–25.
7. González-Consuegra RV, Verdú J. Quality of life in people with venous leg ulcers: an integrative review. J Adv Nurs 2011;67(5):926–44.
8. Green H, Barkham M, Kellett S, et al. Therapist effects and IAPT Psychological Wellbeing Practitioners (PWPs): a multilevel modeling and mixed methods analysis. Behav Res Ther 2014;63:43–54.
9. Mosadeghrad AM. Factors influencing healthcare service quality. Int J Health Pol Manag 2014;3(2):77–89.
10. Kielo-Viljamaa E, Suhonen R, Ahtiala M, et al. The development and testing of the C/WoundComp instrument for assessing chronic wound-care competence in student nurses and podiatrists. Int Wound J 2021;18(1):62–78.
11. Kajander-Unkuri S, Metetoja R, Katajisto J, et al. Self-assessed level of competence of graduating nursing students and factors related to it. Nurse Educ Today 2014;34(5):795–801.
12. Numminen O, Laine T, Isoaho H, et al. Do educational outcomes correspond with the requirements of nursing practice: educators' and managers' assessments of novice nurses' professional competence. Scand J Caring Sci 2014;28(4):812–21.
13. Sengül T, Shoqirat N, Singh C, et al. A qualitative evaluation of online active learning modalities in the chronic wound management lecture of nursing students' experiences in Turkey. J Tissue Viability 2022;31(4):746–50.
14. Welsh L. Wound care evidence, knowledge and education amongst nurses: a semi-systematic literature review. Int Wound J 2018;15(1):53–61.
15. Kielo E, Suhonen R, Salminen L, et al. Competence areas for registered nurses and podiatrists in chronic wound care, and their role in wound care practice. J Clin Nurs 2019 Nov;28(21–22):4021–34. Epub 2019 Jul 31. PMID: 31294490.
16. Kielo-Viljamaa E, Suhonen R, Jalonen L, et al. Nursing competence areas in acute wound care: A focus group study. Collegian 2022;29(1):44–53.
17. Kielo-Viljamaa E, Viljamaa J, Suhonen R, et al. Learning objectives and content of wound care education in nursing education in Finland: A Delphi study. Nurse Educ Today 2022;110:105278.
18. Kielo E, Salminen L, Stolt M. Graduating student nurses' and student podiatrists' wound care competence – An integrative literature review. Nurse Educ Pract 2018;29:1–7.
19. Kielo E, Salminen L, Suhonen R, et al. Theoretical competence in wound care among graduated student nurses and foot care specialists: A cross-sectional study. J Wound Care 2019;28(3):136–45.
20. De Meyer D, Verhaeghe S, Van Hecke A, et al. Knowledge of nurses and nursing assistants about pressure ulcer prevention: A survey in 16 Belgian hospitals using the PUKAT 2.0 tool. J Tissue Viability 2019;28(2):59–69.
21. Sengül T, Karadag A. Determination of nurses' level of knowledge on the prevention of pressure ulcers: The case of Turkey. J Tissue Viability 2020;29(4):337–41.
22. Sengül T, Kaya N, Kirkland-Kyhn H, et al. Investigation of nursing students' knowledge levels and attitudes in incontinence-associated dermatitis management through game-based learning: a mixed methods study. Wound Manag Prev 2024 Jun;70(2). https://doi.org/10.25270/wmp.23077. PMID: 38959349.
23. Dag Sucu G, Firat Kilic H. Knowledge and attitudes of Turkish nursing students towards pressure injury prevention. J Tissue Viability 2022;31(1):16–23.

24. Fulbrook P, Lawrence P, Miles S. Australian Nurses' Knowledge of Pressure Injury Prevention and Management: A Cross-sectional Survey. J Wound, Ostomy Cont Nurs 2019;46(2):106–12.

25. Ylönen M, Viljamaa J, Isoaho H, et al. Internet-based learning program to increase nurses' knowledge level about venous leg ulcer care in home health care. J Clin Nurs 2017;26(21–22):3646–57.

26. Kumarasinghe SA, Hettiarachchi P, Wasalathanthri S. Nurses' knowledge on diabetic foot ulcer disease and their attitudes towards patients affected: a cross-sectional institution-based study. J Clin Nurs 2018;27(1–2). https://doi.org/10.1111/jocn.13917.

27. Kaya Z, Karaca A. Evaluation of Nurses' Knowledge Levels of Diabetic Foot Care Management. Nurs Res Pract 2018;2018:8549567.

28. Shipton NH, Luctkar-Flude M, Tyerman J, et al. The use of clinical simulation in wound care education for nurses: a scoping review protocol. Br J Nurs 2023;32(15). https://doi.org/10.12968/bjon.2023.32.15.S26.

29. Simonetti V, Comparcini D, Flacco ME, et al. Nursing students' knowledge and attitude on pressure ulcer prevention evidence-based guidelines: A multicenter cross-sectional study. Nurse Educ Today 2015;35(4):573–9.

30. Usher K, Woods C, Brown J, et al. Australian nursing students' knowledge and attitudes towards pressure injury prevention: a cross-sectional study. Int J Nurs Stud 2018;81:14–20.

31. Öner B, Karadağ A. Determination of Nursing-Sensitive Indicators for Intensive Care Units in Turkey: A Qualitative Study. J Innov Healthc Pract 2023;4(1):9–21.

32. Ayello EA, Zulkowski K, Capezuti E, et al. Educating Nurses in the United States about Pressure Injuries. Adv Skin Wound Care 2017;30(2):83–94.

33. Porter-Armstrong AP, Moore ZE, Bradbury I, et al. Education of healthcare professionals for preventing pressure ulcers. Cochrane Database Syst Rev 2018 May 25;5(5). https://doi.org/10.1002/14651858.CD011620.pub2. PMID: 29800486; PMCID: PMC6494581.

34. Gillespie BM, Chaboyer W, Allen P, et al. Wound care practices: a survey of acute care nurses. J Clin Nurs 2013;23:2618–27.

35. Dugdall H, Watson R. What is the relationship between nurses' attitude to evidence based practice and the selection of wound care procedures? J Clin Nurs 2009;18(10):1442–50.

36. Ferreira A, Rigotti M, Barcelos L, et al. Knowledge and practice of nurses about care for patients with wounds. Rev Pesq Cuidado Fundam Online 2014;6:1178–90.

37. McCluskey P, McCarthy G. Nurses' knowledge and competence in wound management. Wounds U K 2012;8:37–47.

38. Sen CK. Human wounds and its burden: an updated compendium of estimates. Adv Wound Care (New Rochelle) 2019;8(2):39–48.

39. Corbett LQ, Ennis WJ. What do patients want? patient preference in wound care. Adv Wound Care (New Rochelle) 2014;3(8):537–43.

40. Kitamura JC, Nicolosi JT, Paggiaro AO, et al. Educational interventions on preventing pressure injuries targeted at nurses: systematic review and meta-analysis. Br J Nurs 2023 Nov 1;32(Sup20). https://doi.org/10.12968/bjon.2023.32.Sup20.S40. PMID: 37949494.

41. Gocmen Baykara Z, Karadag A, Senol Celik S, et al. Impact of tailored education about pressure injuries on nurses' knowledge levels and pressure injury point prevalence: The case of Turkey. J Tissue Viability 2021;30(4):552–8.

42. Karadag A, Hanönü SC, Eyikara E. A Prospective, Descriptive Study to Assess Nursing Staff Perceptions of and Interventions to Prevent Medical Device-related Pressure Injury. Ostomy/Wound Manag 2017;63(10):34–41.
43. Aydın AK, Karadağ A, Gül Ş, et al. Nurses' Knowledge and Practices Related to Pressure Injury: A Cross-sectional Study. J Wound, Ostomy Cont Nurs 2019; 46(2):117–23.
44. Aydin AK, Karadağ A. Assessment of nurses' knowledge and practice in prevention and management of deep tissue injury and stage I pressure ulcer. J Wound, Ostomy Cont Nurs 2010;37(5):487–94.
45. Ennis WJ. Wound Care Specialization: The Current Status and Future Plans to Move Wound Care into the Medical Community. Adv Wound Care (New Rochelle) 2012 Oct;1(5):184–8.
46. Mahmoudi M, Gould LJ. Opportunities and Challenges of the Management of Chronic Wounds: A Multidisciplinary Viewpoint. Chron Wound Care Manag Res 2020;7:27–36.
47. Ousey K, Milne J, Atkin L, et al. Exploring the role of the tissue viability nurse. Wounds UK 2015;11(5):36–45.
48. Eskes AM, Maaskant JM, Holloway S, et al. Competencies of specialized wound care nurses: a European Delphi study. Int Wound J 2014 Dec;11(6):665–74.
49. Lindahl E, Holloway S, Bobbink P, et al. Wound curriculum for student nurses: European Qualification Framework Level 4. J Wound Manage 2021;22(3 Suppl 1).
50. Karadağ A. Stoma and Wound Care Nursing: Historical Development Process, Roles and Functions. Turk Klin J Pediatr Nurs-Special Topics 2015;1(1):1–8.
51. Koç University. SANERC: Center for Nursing Education and Research. Koç University. Available at: https://sanerc.ku.edu.tr/. [Accessed 8 July 2024].
52. Turkish Wound Care Association. Available at: https://yarabakimidernegi.org.tr/. [Accessed 8 July 2024].
53. Sengül T, Karadag A, Kilic H. Exploring Nursing Students' First Experiences Providing Wound and Ostomy Care to Patients: A Qualitative Study. Adv Skin Wound Care 2024 Jun 1;37(6):304–10. PMID: 38767422.

# Future Direction of Wound Care

Sanaz Martin, MS, FNP-c

## KEYWORDS

- Artificial intelligence • Machine learning • Digital photography • Telemedicine
- Mobile phone camera • Tissue analytics app • Deep learning techniques
- Predictability

## KEY POINTS

- Artificial intelligence (AI) in wound assessment and imaging.
- Predictive capabilities of AI for wound occurrence.
- Documentation and data integration of AI in wound care.
- Challenges and considerations for using AI in wound care specialty.
- Future direction of wound care with AI.

## INTRODUCTION

Artificial intelligence (AI) comprises a range of complex computational techniques, including machine learning (ML) algorithms and natural language processes, endorsed for improving clinical decision-making, patient care, and health care delivery.[1,2] AI may increase efficiency and accuracy in a few areas in the wound care specialty.[3,4] Assessment and evaluation of wounds with digital imaging offer more accurate measurement and assessment of tissue, volume, and surrounding skin.[5,6] The documentation using applications transferrable to electronic medical records (EMR) is more efficient and accurate.[7–9] Prediction of certain wound conditions, such as pressure injuries (PIs), using algorithms may offer more accurate intervention and harm prevention implementation for at-risk patients.[10–12] Natural language processing (NLP) allows clinicians to pull out notes to uncover valuable data from narrative clinical notes that can support machine-learning algorithms and pull out words and expressions from clinicians' notes. In one study, NLP helped recognize infection cases that would otherwise not be accurately captured for diagnosis and treatment. Utilizing this method (NLP) is particularly practical in wound care for home health settings since up to 50% of crucial wound information is kept in clinical notes.[1,2]

UC Davis Health System, 4860 Y Street, Sacramento, CA 95817, USA
*E-mail address:* snzmartin@ucdavis.edu

Nurs Clin N Am 60 (2025) 207–215
https://doi.org/10.1016/j.cnur.2024.07.011
0029-6465/25/© 2024 Elsevier Inc. All rights are reserved, including those for text and data mining, AI training, and similar technologies.
nursing.theclinics.com

As the wound care specialty evolves, data are essential in this journey. Consistent and effective valuable data capture is imperative in creating valuable data pulls to standardize the practice. Technology may be the best way to bridge the current gap and influence data capturing and sharing to provide transparency in approach and lead to necessary changes. AI will be a link for more informed wound care practice.[1,3,6,9] For example, by using "apps," practitioners may capture a significant volume of data, and through artificial and ML techniques, standardizing the practice may be accomplished more easily.[13] Combining AI and human intellect will lead to more robust standardization and specialization in wound care. It will also allow for the application of technology for patient and family engagement in the setting of limited clinician resources in remote locations. ML models can be trained to process large volumes of data and images kept in electronic medical records, with billions of data points, to help with the assessment analysis and the development of treatment plans. This is nearly impossible for humans to experience and process throughout their careers.[3] Although the growing use of AI in health care has the potential and many benefits of improving efficiency and patient outcomes, it may pose some risks. One of the risks is an algorithmic bias that might impact specific ethnic or religious backgrounds, those with differing sexual or gender preference backgrounds, and those with differing sexual or gender preferences when accessing health care.[1,4]

## CURRENT USE IN WOUND CARE

Technology advancements in improving the assessment and monitoring of wound sizes are transforming clinical practices in wound care. Innovations include integrating innovative imaging techniques like digital photography and 3 dimensional (3D) scanning and advanced modalities like thermal and infrared imaging. These technologies promise enhanced precision in measuring wound dimensions and tracking healing progress, which is crucial for timely medical interventions and treatment adjustments. The evolution of wound imaging technologies addresses longstanding challenges in wound assessment by providing clinicians with detailed, objective data. Early developments focused on commercial digital cameras capable of creating 3D maps of wounds with tissue labeling, significantly improving accuracy and usability in clinical settings. Subsequent advancements introduced handheld devices like the Silhouette Mobile and InSight systems, offering geometric measurements of wound area and volume, though initial iterations lacked tissue classification capabilities.[4]

Recent innovations have expanded to include sophisticated features such as 3D modeling and tissue labeling directly from handheld platforms like WoundZoom and InSight, demonstrating superior accuracy over manual methods. Emerging modalities like thermal and infrared imaging, multispectral and hyperspectral imaging, and fluorescence-based techniques like the MolecuLight and Kent Imaging Snapshot NIR devices provide insights into tissue health and wound healing potential by detecting oxygen saturation levels and bacterial presence. Integration of AI further enhances wound assessment capabilities through ML and deep learning (DL) algorithms. AI-driven technologies automate image analysis tasks, enabling precise tissue segmentation and classification essential for treatment planning. DL techniques like convolutional neural networks have shown promise in medical image analysis, achieving high accuracies in tissue classification tasks related to wound assessment.[4]

The future of wound imaging technology lies in standardizing imaging protocols, developing large, labeled datasets, and validating algorithms to ensure clinical applicability and reliability. Challenges such as data standardization, algorithm validation, and clinical integration remain critical for widespread adoption in routine clinical practice. Nevertheless, these advancements promise to revolutionize wound care by providing clinicians with accurate, real-time data essential for optimizing therapeutic decisions and improving patient outcomes.[4]

A study conducted at Valley Wound Healing Center in Modesto, California, compared Swift's digital AI-powered wound assessment tool's efficiency with that of traditional manual methods. Swift, equipped with AI capabilities, significantly outperformed manual methods in several key metrics. It reduced the time required for capturing and accessing wound images to 62 seconds compared to a standard digital camera. Importantly, Swift achieved a 77% reduction in the time needed to accurately measure and calculate wound surface area, taking only 45.05 seconds on average. Swift demonstrated a higher success rate (92.2%) in capturing high-quality wound images on the first attempt, compared to 75.7% with manual techniques, in various wound types, including venous, diabetic, and surgical wounds. Overall, Swift reduced the time spent on complete wound assessments by 79%, completing all necessary steps in approximately half the time required by traditional methods.[5]

The efficiency gains with Swift translate into potential annual savings of 21.8 to 51.7 clinician days per year, based on an average daily workload of 130 wound assessments. This improved efficiency times, enhanced clinical throughput reduced patient wait times, and potentially improved access to specialized wound care. Future integration of Swift with electronic health records (EHR) could further streamline workflows and enhance overall efficiency in wound management. It promises to optimize clinician time and improve patient care outcomes in wound care settings.[5,6]

### *Wound Healing Predictability*

Accurate wound assessment is crucial for effective treatment, yet current methods like manual ruler-based measurements and digital planimetry have limitations in accuracy and efficiency. Manual methods often lead to variability and overestimating wound area, while subjective visual estimation of granulation tissue hampers consistency among clinicians. AI offers a promising solution for automated wound assessment, potentially enhancing accuracy and clinical decision-making. However, the lack of standardized evaluation methods for AI-based tools compared to traditional measurements presents a challenge.

A retrospective study across 2 hospital wound care centers used photographs from routine clinical care involving manual tracings by wound care specialists and AI-based tracings using specific software. Key metrics such as false-positive area (FPA) and relative error (RE) were employed to evaluate differences between AI and human assessments. FPA identifies discrepancies where AI detects additional areas not identified by humans, while RE quantifies relative differences in area measurements. These metrics, alongside qualitative assessments by masked reviewers, provided insights into agreement and perception of accuracy between AI and human tracings. Findings from the qualitative evaluation revealed variability in agreement among reviewers on whether tracings met standardized definitions of wound area. Overall, this study underscores the potential of AI to improve consistency and accuracy in wound assessment despite existing challenges in perception and agreement among expert reviewers. Standardizing AI evaluation methods could further enhance its integration into clinical practice, offering significant benefits for health care delivery and patient outcomes in managing chronic wounds.[7]

Diabetic foot ulcers (DFUs) are prevalent complications of diabetes mellitus (DM), affecting approximately 6.3% of individuals globally, with a quarter of patients with DM developing a DFU during their lifetime. These ulcers are associated with significant morbidity, including heightened risks of lower extremity amputations (LEAs) and mortality. About half of DFUs are complicated by infections, and severe cases may lead to minor or major amputations in up to 20% of instances. The 10 year survival rate following DFU-related LEAs is notably low, underscoring the severity of these complications compared to several cancers. Adequate care of DFUs involves rigorous monitoring, frequent dressing changes, antibiotic therapy for infections, optimal diabetes management, and offloading to prevent further tissue damage from pressure. Despite the critical need for comprehensive care, challenges such as manpower shortages and logistical issues in multidisciplinary foot clinics often lead to delays in patient review, impacting treatment outcomes.

The coronavirus disease of 2019 (COVID-19) pandemic highlighted these challenges and prompted the exploration of telemedicine solutions, including telephone and video clinics, to facilitate remote patient monitoring during lockdowns. This period also accelerated interest in AI algorithms to enhance virtual clinic capabilities for DFU management. Photographic monitoring of DFU progression has become integral to clinical practice, aiding in continuity of care and prognostication across different health care providers. However, challenges persist, such as variations in photograph quality due to lighting and camera focus. Digital archiving of DFU photographs has replaced traditional printouts, offering advantages in accessibility and image preservation.

Mobile phone cameras have emerged as practical tools for patients and health care professionals to capture DFU images, facilitating early evaluation and management decisions. Despite initial skepticism, studies have demonstrated promising results in using mobile technology for DFU monitoring. Advancements in digital technology, including AI and smartphone applications, show promise in enhancing DFU care. However, further research and integration into clinical practice are necessary to optimize outcomes and address ongoing challenges in diabetic foot care services worldwide.[8]

### Current Use of Artificial Intelligence in Documentation

Despite being treated within specific medical silos, wound care is recognized as a co-morbid condition, leading to varied approaches across specialties and a lack of unified patient-centered care. Effective wound management necessitates accurate documentation covering variables such as wound size, location, surrounding skin condition, exudate levels, and patient-reported symptoms. However, there is a noted deficiency in comprehensive wound documentation across health care settings globally, as evidenced by studies from Australia, Norway, the United States, and beyond. These studies reveal significant gaps in wound assessment and management documentation within electronic medical records (EMRs) compared to written records, highlighting discrepancies in adherence to evidence-based guidelines. Challenges such as subjective wound assessment due to clinician variability, differences in camera quality for wound photography, and privacy concerns related to image upload and sharing further complicate wound care documentation.

Recent advancements in digital wound photography, facilitated by smartphone applications and AI-driven technologies like the Tissue Analytics app, promise to improve wound care documentation and management accuracy and efficiency. These applications enable real-time wound analysis, tracking of healing progress, and integration with EMRs, offering decision-support tools for clinicians. Despite some existing studies on specific wound types like DFUs, broader applications across various wound types are still underexplored in the literature. A study by Barakat-Johnson colleagues evaluated the usability and effectiveness of the Tissue Analytics app in enhancing wound assessment and management within a primary metropolitan health service in New South Wales, Australia. Utilizing TA showed a significant reduction in wound size among patients using the TA app, with a mean reduction of 54.0% over approximately 36 days across various wound types. The app also improved the completeness of wound documentation compared to standard care, achieving complete documentation of wound size (from 8.3% to 100%) and exudate levels (from 31.9% to 87.2%).

Patients using the TA app experienced cost savings related to reduced travel expenses, averaging $4.54 per visit for metropolitan patients and $72.90 per visit for rural patients. Both clinicians and patients expressed satisfaction with the app, noting its ease of use for wound assessment, monitoring, and remote communication. It was valuable during the COVID-19 pandemic for maintaining continuity of care while minimizing face-to-face visits. Overall, the TA app demonstrated feasibility and effectiveness in enhancing wound care through improved documentation, remote monitoring capabilities, and reduced patient travel burden, suggesting its potential for broader implementation across health care settings.[9]

### Wound Development Predictability

ML is pivotal in modernizing health care practices, emphasizing its potential to revolutionize patient care through data-driven insights and predictive analytics, particularly in preventing conditions like PIs. ML in health care has evolved from initial concerns about cost and depersonalization to improving health care delivery by facilitating easier data retrieval and uncovering insights that manual review might miss. ML augments or replaces traditional bedside risk assessments by analyzing extensive data points from EHRs and monitoring changes overtime. This holistic approach helps predict the risk of developing PIs risks, such as the risk of developing PIs earlier and, more accurately, potentially preventing injuries before they occur. DL techniques and hybrid models combining DL with other AI methodologies (such as traditional ML, transfer learning, metaheuristics, and fuzzy logic) are increasingly utilized. These models enhance predictive accuracy and address complexities in health care prediction tasks, including PI risk assessment. ML facilitates personalized care by combining objective assessment data with subjective insights gathered during patient interactions.

It supports health care providers in identifying care gaps, recognizing trends, and enhancing individualized treatment, thereby improving health care services' overall quality and efficiency. The future integration of ML into health care systems is expected to optimize patients further and streamline health care operations. Continued advancements in ML techniques and broader adoption and integration with clinical practice will improve patient outcomes and health care delivery.[10]

Medical errors are a global concern, contributing to fatalities and permanent disabilities among patients. Studies from various countries highlight the prevalence and consequences of avoidable medical errors, such as inappropriate treatments, misdiagnoses, surgical errors, and medication-related incidents. Medical errors incur substantial costs, estimated to be billions annually in the United States alone. These costs include additional medical treatments, prolonged hospital stays, legal expenses, and compensation for patients affected by errors. Hospital-acquired pressure injuries (HAPIs) are a significant subset of preventable medical errors. They occur due to prolonged pressure on the skin and underlying tissues, primarily in immobile patients, leading to pain, infections, prolonged hospitalizations, and increased health care costs. Wound, Ostomy, and Continence nurses are pivotal in preventing PIs. Their responsibilities include risk assessments, personalized care plans, patient education, and implementing preventive measures. Various tools like the Braden Scale aid in predicting PI risk based on factors such as mobility and skin condition, guiding preventive interventions. Despite the availability of assessment tools, consistent application and effectiveness in preventing HAPIs remain challenging. Integrating AI and decision support systems (DSSs) presents an opportunity to improve predictive capabilities and optimize interventions using electronic health records (EHR) data.[11]

HAPIs are a prevalent issue in the US health care system, leading to substantial annual costs and complications. Effective prevention strategies using standardized risk assessments, such as the Braden scale, are essential but costly due to labor and preventive materials. In recent years, ML has been used to predict HAPI development using electronic health records (EHR) to reduce incidence rates. However, existing literature lacks predictions on when HAPIs occur, complicating timely interventions. An integrated ML approach incorporating genetic algorithm, cost-sensitive learning, and grid search is promising for predicting both the likelihood and timing of HAPIs. This novel approach uses multiple data points overtime to optimize prevention strategies, improve resource allocation, and enhance overall care outcomes.[12]

ML algorithms have also emerged as powerful tools for predicting the risk of other conditions, such as wound infections, particularly in vulnerable populations such as home health care (HHC) patients. In HHC settings, infections can lead to severe outcomes like hospitalizations and mortality, increasing health care costs and burdening families. Timely diagnosis of wound infections is critical to initiating prompt treatments and preventing complications like sepsis. ML models capitalize on large datasets to detect patterns and identify infection risk factors, enhancing patient care quality. NLP techniques are highlighted for extracting pertinent information from unstructured clinical notes, enriching the accuracy and depth of data available for predictive modeling. Prior research has demonstrated NLP's efficacy in uncovering infection cases that traditional diagnosis codes might miss.

Developing predictive algorithms involves rigorous processes such as literature synthesis, expert validation, and iterative refinement to ensure precision in identifying infection-related categories from clinical notes. By integrating structured and unstructured data through advanced analytical techniques like NLP, health care providers can improve risk assessment and patient outcomes in HHC settings. This approach enables better identification and management of individuals at elevated risk of wound infections that may necessitate hospital care, optimizing resource allocation and enhancing overall health care delivery in home settings.[2]

### Artificial Intelligence Potential in Wound Care

The transformative potential of AI and ML in wound care is undeniable. AI, encompassing technologies like ML and NLP, allows machines to sense, comprehend, act, and learn without explicit programming. This capability is poised to revolutionize various industries, including health care, by enhancing productivity and innovation. Key parallels are drawn between the evolution of AI/ML and advancements in wound care, noting that both fields have seen significant developments since the early 1980s. AI plays a vital role in addressing challenges within wound care, such as the scarcity of real-world data and evidence, which have hindered progress in clinical specialties. AI and ML, facilitated by mobile apps, offer the potential to gather large volumes of real-world data efficiently. By applying AI/ML techniques to analyze these data, practitioners can gain deeper insights into wound care practices, leading to standardized protocols and improved patient outcomes. Moreover, AI can support the training and standardization of wound care across various levels of health care delivery, potentially empowering less-trained caregivers like family members or patients. AI will facilitate the specialization of wound care, enhancing both the efficiency and effectiveness of treatment. Health care providers are encouraged to embrace technological advancements and leverage AI to enhance caregiving and improve the quality of life for patients. Embracing AI and ML act as catalysts for advancing wound care practices, foreseeing a future where these technologies enable more informed, standardized, and specialized treatment approaches in health care.[13]

## Artificial Intelligence Challenges in Wound Care

While AI technologies like chatbots and AI-assisted search have gained popularity for tasks ranging from creative writing to data summarization, they pose significant challenges, such as potential misinformation and regulatory concerns.[14] AI, exemplified by models like ChatGPT and Google's Bard, can process vast amounts of data and generate human-like responses, revolutionizing information retrieval and content creation. This rapid adoption of AI, supported by significant investments from tech giants like Microsoft and Google, signifies a seismic shift in how AI integrates with daily life and professional activities. AI promises to enhance data management, assessment, and treatment approaches in wound care, which is inherently data rich due to its complex interactions with various health conditions. Generative AI can aid in summarizing complex research findings efficiently, transforming how researchers review and synthesize literature for clinical applications.

## Wound Care with Artificial Intelligence in the Future

The future lies where AI-driven communities of practice facilitate personalized data repositories and automate laborious research tasks, freeing researchers to focus on more substantive aspects of their work. Advancements in AI are drawing parallels to the initial resistance and eventual reliance on technologies like social media, suggesting that AI in wound care could similarly revolutionize the field with improved efficiency and outcomes.[15]

There is a paradigm shift in health care from reactive treatment to predictive, preventive, and personalized medicine (PPPM), particularly crucial for chronic conditions like wounds. The barriers are the significant economic burden and complexity associated with chronic wounds, influenced by modifiable and non-modifiable risk factors. Complex system thinking, exemplified by frameworks such as the "Wound Bed Paradigm" and "Triangle of Wound Assessment," has laid the groundwork but requires further innovation. AI is a transformative health care tool that leverages advanced algorithms and image processing to revolutionize diagnostics, treatment decisions, and patient management. DSSs based on ML promise to enhance diagnostic accuracy, workflow efficiency, and treatment outcomes, especially in wound care, where predicting healing is challenging due to multifactorial factors.

The evolution of AI in clinical care ranges from wound measurement and treatment decision support apps to advanced imaging devices. It stresses the need for AI-driven predictive models that move beyond isolated risk factors to recognize complex patterns in wound healing. However, challenges such as data privacy, biases in data selection, and interpretation issues that must be addressed for widespread clinical adoption remain.[16]

## SUMMARY

Technology in standardizing wound care practices across various health care settings plays a significant role and may reduce systemic burdens. The evolving relationship between clinicians and technology notes that while clinicians primarily think clinically, designing AI technologies with a clinical perspective enhances their acceptance and effectiveness in practice. Integrating existing electronic medical record (EMR) systems enhances transparency and facilitates better care delivery, ultimately benefiting patients, providers, and health care systems by improving care quality and reducing costs. AI and ML in wound care will improve patient outcomes and health care delivery. AI's role in wound care extends beyond diagnostics to prognosis, treatment optimization, and patient engagement. Embracing technological advancements will be crucial in overcoming current barriers and transforming wound care delivery into a more efficient and effective model for the benefit of patients and providers alike.[13]

## CLINICS CARE POINTS

- *Digital imaging*: AI enhances wound assessment accuracy through technologies like digital photography, 3D scanning, and advanced imaging modalities (thermal, infrared, multispectral, hyperspectral). These technologies provide detailed, objective data crucial for precise measurement and tracking healing progress.

- *ML models*: AI and ML models predict wound development and outcomes such as DFUs and PIs. They analyze large datasets from electronic health records (EHRs) to identify risk factors, optimize treatment plans, and potentially prevent complications like HAPIs.

- *Tissue analytics*: AI-driven applications like Tissue Analytics (TA) improve wound care documentation by enabling real-time analysis and integration with EHRs. They enhance completeness and accuracy of wound documentation, supporting remote monitoring and reducing patient travel burden.

- *NLP*: NLP techniques extract valuable data from clinical notes, improving AI's ability to assist in wound care management by uncovering insights that may not be captured through structured data alone.

- *Algorithmic bias*: Concerns about algorithmic bias in AI applications highlight potential disparities in health care outcomes for certain demographic groups.

- *Integration and adoption*: Challenges remain in standardizing AI evaluation methods, validating algorithms, and integrating AI technologies into routine clinical practice despite promising advancements.

- *Personalized medicine*: AI supports the shift toward PPPM in wound care, offering tailored treatment approaches based on individual patient data.

- *Clinical integration*: Continued research and development are essential to address challenges and maximize the clinical impact of AI in wound care, ensuring improvements in patient outcomes and health care delivery efficiency.

## REFERENCES

1. O'Connor S, Booth RG. Algorithmic bias in health care: Opportunities for nurses to improve equality in the age of artificial intelligence. Nurs Outlook 2022;70(6): 780–2.
2. Song Jiyoun, Woo K, Shang J, et al. Predictive risk models for wound infection-related hospitalization or ED visits in home health care using machine-learning algorithms. Adv Skin Wound Care 2021;34(8):1–12.
3. Queen D, Harding K. Data-driven specialisation of wound care through artificial intelligence. Int Wound J 2019;16(4):879–80.
4. Lucas Y, Niri R, Treuillet S, et al. Wound size imaging: ready for smart assessment and monitoring. Adv Wound Care 2021;10(11):641–61.

5. Mohammed HT, Bartlett RL, Babb D, et al. A time motion study of manual versus artificial intelligence methods for wound assessment. PLoS One 2022;17(7): e0271742.
6. Reifs David, Casanova-Lozano L, Reig-Bolaño R, et al. Clinical validation of computer vision and artificial intelligence algorithms for wound measurement and tissue classification in wound care. Inform Med Unlocked 2023;37:101185.
7. Howell RS, Liu HH, Khan AA, et al. Development of a method for clinical evaluation of artificial intelligence-based digital wound assessment tools. JAMA Netw Open 2021;4(5):e217234.
8. Pappachan JM, Cassidy B, Fernandez CJ, et al. The role of artificial intelligence technology in the care of diabetic foot ulcers: the past, the present, and the future. World J Diabetes 2022;13(12):1131–9.
9. Barakat-Johnson M, Jones A, Burger M, et al. Reshaping wound care: Evaluation of an artificial intelligence app to improve wound assessment and management amid the COVID-19 pandemic. Int Wound J 2022;19(6):1561–77.
10. Dweekat OY, Lam SS, McGrath L. An integrated system of multifaceted machine learning models to predict if and when hospital-acquired pressure injuries (Bedsores) occur. Int J Environ Res Publ Health 2023;20(1):828.
11. Toffaha KM, Simsekler MCE, Omar MA. Leveraging artificial intelligence and decision support systems in hospital-acquired pressure injuries prediction: A comprehensive review. Artif Intell Med 2023;141:102560.
12. Dweekat OY, Lam SS, McGrath L. Machine learning techniques, applications, and potential future opportunities in pressure injuries (Bedsores) management: a systematic review. Int J Environ Res Publ Health 2023;20(1):796.
13. Queen D. Artificial intelligence and machine learning in wound care-The wounded machine. Int Wound J 2019;16(2):311.
14. Gupta S, Gupta SS, McMath K, et al. Enhancing complex wound care by leveraging artificial intelligence: an artificial intelligence chatbot software study. Wounds 2023;35(8):E265–7.
15. Queen D. Could wound care benefit from the artificial intelligence storm taking place worldwide. Int Wound J 2023;20(5):1337–8.
16. Cross K, Harding K. Risk profiling in the prevention and treatment of chronic wounds using artificial intelligence. Int Wound J 2022;19(6):1283–5.

# Moving?

## Make sure your subscription moves with you!

To notify us of your new address, find your **Clinics Account Number** (located on your mailing label above your name), and contact customer service at:

**Email: journalscustomerservice-usa@elsevier.com**

**800-654-2452** (subscribers in the U.S. & Canada)
**314-447-8871** (subscribers outside of the U.S. & Canada)

**Fax number: 314-447-8029**

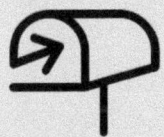

**Elsevier Health Sciences Division**
**Subscription Customer Service**
**3251 Riverport Lane**
**Maryland Heights, MO 63043**

*To ensure uninterrupted delivery of your subscription, please notify us at least 4 weeks in advance of move.

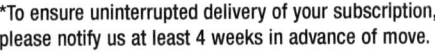
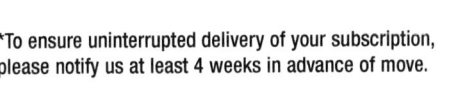